ALLE ZEIT WACH 1842

TREATMENT OF BURNS

Editors:
Yang Chih-chun, MD
Hsu Wei-shia, MD
Shih Tsi-siang, MD

Translation Supervisor:
Nyi Pao-chun, BS, MD

With 213 Figures, Some in Color

Shanghai Scientific and Technical Publishers
Springer-Verlag Berlin Heidelberg NewYork 1982

Prof. YANG CHIH-CHUN, MD

Lect. HSU WEI-SHIA, MD

Prof. SHIH TSI-SIANG, MD

Burn Unit, Rui Jin Hospital
Shanghai Second Medical College
Shanghai 200025
The People's Republic of China

ISBN-13:978-3-642-68102-8 e-ISBN-13:978-3-642-68100-4
DOI: 10.1007/978-3-642-68100-4

Library of Congress Cataloging in Publication Data. Main entry under title: Treatment of burns. Bibliography: p. Includes index. 1. Burns and scalds. I. Yang, Chih-chun, 1930– [DNLM: 1. Burns-Therapy. WO704T784] RD96.4.T73 617'.1106 81-18463 AACR2

2124/3130-543210

List of Contributors

CHANG DE-ZHEN, Senior Technician, Burn Research Laboratory, Shanghai Second Medical College, Shanghai

CHEN ZHI-RANG, MD, Associate Professor of Pathology, Shanghai Second Medical College; Chief, Department of Clinical Pathology, Rui Jin Hospital, Shanghai

HSU WEI-SHIA, MD, Lecturer of Surgery, Shanghai Second Medical College; Deputy Chief, Burn Unit, Rui Jin Hospital, Shanghai

HUANG ZONG-MING, MD, Visiting Anesthetist, Department of Anesthesia, Rui Jin Hospital, Shanghai

LI YING-YU, MD, Visiting Surgeon, Burn Unit, Rui Jin Hospital, Shanghai

LIU GUO-YU, MD, Lecturer of Surgery, Shanghai Second Medical College; Visiting Surgeon, Department of Surgery, Rui Jin Hospital, Shanghai

LIU YUE-LIANG, MD, Visiting Surgeon, Burn Unit, Rui Jin Hospital, Shanghai

SHIH TSI-SIANG, MD, Professor of Surgery, Shanghai Second Medical College; Chief Surgeon (I), Burn Unit and Burn Research Laboratory, Rui Jin Hospital, Shanghai

TANG SHEAN-SHI, MD, Lecturer of Surgery, Shanghai Second Medical College; Visiting Surgeon, Burn Unit, Rui Jin Hospital, Shanghai

TAO XIANG-LING, Head Nurse, Burn Unit, Rui Jin Hospital, Shanghai

XIAO YU-RUI, MD, Visiting Surgeon, Burn Unit, Rui Jin Hospital, Shanghai

XU WEI-ZHEN, MD, Lecturer of Surgery, Shanghai Second Medical College; Visiting Surgeon, Burn Unit, Rui Jin Hospital, Shanghai

YANG CHIH-CHUN, MD, Professor of Surgery, Shanghai Second Medical College; Chief Surgeon (II), Burn Unit and Burn Research Laboratory, Rui Jin Hospital, Shanghai

YANG ZENG-NIA, MD, Lecturer of Surgery, Shanghai Second Medical College; Deputy Chief, Plastic Section, Burn Unit, Rui Jin Hospital, Shanghai

List of Translators *

CHANG TI-SHENG, MD, Professor of Surgery, Shanghai Second Medical College; Chief, Department of Plastic Surgery, Ninth People's Hospital, Director, Ninth People's Hospital, Shanghai

LING LI-LI, BS, MD, Associate Professor of Pathology, Deputy Chief, Department of Pathology, Shanghai Second Medical College, Shanghai

NYI PAO-CHUN, BS, MD, Professor of Surgery and Advisor, Shanghai Second Medical College, Shanghai

WANG PAO-MEI, MD, Lecturer of Pathology, Department of Pathology, Shanghai Second Medical College, Shanghai

WANG ZHI-ZENG, MD, Visiting Anesthetist, Department of Anesthesia, Rui Jin Hospital, Shanghai

* Excluding those authors who also translated parts of the text

Preface

The greater the poverty,
The stronger the will.
In the face of hardship,
Soar, soar, soar on still

WANG BO
(650–676 A.D.)

In the late spring of 1958 a patient was admitted to Rui Jin Hospital with extensive burns; just minutes before he had been dexterously operating one of Shanghai's "productive converters" used in the making of steel. He resembled a mass of charcoal but was mentally alert, asserting that he must survive, not only because of the great expectations he had of life but also to continue working in his beloved post as first-generation steelworker in this newly liberated country.

The case presented a stern challenge; faced with this man yearning both for his own life and for that of the society in which he lived, we had no way of escaping either "poverty" (in the form of our limited facilities) or hardships. However, by pooling all our efforts we were able to ensure that the patient ultimately survived the extremely tortuous course that followed, in addition to which quite good functional recovery was achieved. So began our burn unit.

It was on this patient that we performed for the first time artificial hibernation (in the treatment of burns), early eschar excision, repeated autoskin cropping, and allografting. Not only were these the decisive measures which helped our patient to achieve his professed intention, but they also gradually evolved to become the characteristics of our present-day treatment.

We realize that, owing to the events of the past hundred years, we have made a late start in this field. As a result we must constantly assess our experiences, conduct exchanges with and learn from the outside world, and continue discovering, inventing, creating, and advancing. These are the driving forces behind the preparation of this book, the publication of which has been made possible by Dr. HEINZ GÖTZE. The work was kindly supported by Professor LAN XI-CHUN and Mr. CHEN XIAN-JIA, the president and vice-president, respectively, of Shanghai Second Medical College, and by Mr. WANG GUO-ZHONG, the director of Science and Technology Publishers, Shanghai. Mr. RICHARD MILLS contributed much in improving the language of the original manuscript, while Mrs. TH. DEIGMÖLLER provided considerable help in the production of the book. Mr. XU JIA-HUA and Miss SHI FENG-DI took care of most of the secretarial work involved in preparing the manuscript. To all of them the editors wish to express their gratitude.

C.C. YANG, MD
W.S. HSU, MD
T.S. SHIH, MD

Contents

Introductory Remarks

YANG CHIH-CHUN

Translated by YANG CHIH-CHUN

The Burn Unit of Rui Jin Hospital, Shanghai Second Medical College, was established in 1958. At that time we had just successfully treated a steel worker with burns to 89% of the body surface area (BSA), including third degree burns to 23% of the BSA. More than 5,000 patients have since been admitted. The present book is a summation of our clinical and laboratory experiences and reflects one aspect of the present state of burn treatment in China.

See through the appearance to perceive the essence: The complicated pathophysiologic disturbances and their clinical manifestations following burns can be traced to and are initiated by the wounds created by burn insults. The course begins after formation of the wound and ends with either spontaneous healing or covering of the wound by surgical means. If shock, infection, and bleeding ulcers are regarded as a knife, then it is the "wound" that brandishes it and threatens the life of the patients. This is the principal problem which warrants our attention, and efforts have been made during the past few years to achieve its solution.

Second degree burns or even deep second degree burns, if handled properly, can be healed spontaneously by regeneration of the epidermis from the dermal adnexal elements. But in the case of third degree burns, only small wounds (less than, for example, 1 cm) can be healed by scar formation. In all other cases, grafts must be used. Allografts, xenografts, or any kind of artificial skin can only survive or adhere transiently as "biological dressings."

In extensive third degree burns, the amount of grafting material needed is large, but the donor site is comparatively limited; this is the principal contradiction in handling such burns. From where could the autografts be obtained when third degree wounds cover more than half of the body surface? Through repeated medical practice we have finally discovered the solution, namely staged excision of third degree eschar and covering of the wound with large sheets of allograft with insertion of small areas of thin split-thickness autografts harvested repeatedly from the scalp. In 1966 a patient with burns to 98% of the BSA, including third degree burns to 90% of the BSA, was cured by employing the above-mentioned method. The intermingled transplantation of auto- and allografts modifies the conventional process of rejection of the allograft.

Since 1966, better results have been achieved in the treatment of burns in our unit (Tables 1, 2). From 1958 through 1978, a total of 4,684 severely burned patients were admitted: 1,573 between 1958 and 1965 and 3,111 between 1966 and 1978. The general data are listed in Tables 1–8. Linear regression

Table 1. Deaths of patients according to the total BSA burned (1958–1978)

Total	BSA burned (%)	0–	5–	10–	15–	20–	25–	30–	35–	40–
1958–1965	No. of patients	190	262	215	190	142	105	115	68	58
	Deaths	0	2	3	2	9	8	10	8	9
	Death rate	0	0.76	1.39	1.05	6.33	7.61	8.69	11.76	15.51
1966–1978	No. of Patients	360	472	425	349	295	212	185	128	116
	Deaths	2	6	5	5	10	6	10	11	14
	Death rate	0.55	1.27	1.17	1.43	3.38	2.83	5.4	8.59	12.06
1958–1978	No. of patients	550	374	640	539	437	317	300	196	174
	Deaths	2	8	8	7	19	14	20	29	23
	Death rate	0.36	1.08	1.25	1.29	4.34	4.41	6.66	9.69	13.21

Table 2. Death rate of different third degree burn groups[a] (1958–1978)

III°	(%)[b]	0–	5–	10–	15–	20–	25–	30–	35–	40–
1958–1965	No. of patients	407	150	84	50	43	17	28	30	11
	Deaths	4	8	10	6	11	3	15	12	7
	Death rate	0.98	5.33	11.9	12	25.58	17.64	53.57	40	63.63
1966–1978	No. of patients	741	386	196	119	91	66	58	39	43
	Deaths	3	18	15	11	15	9	12	9	19
	Death rate	0.4	4.66	7.65	9.24	16.48	13.63	20.68	23.07	44.18
1958–1978	No. of patients	1,148	536	280	169	134	83	86	69	54
	Deaths	7	26	25	17	26	12	27	21	26
	Death rate	0.6	4.85	8.92	10.05	19.4	14.45	31.39	30.43	48.14

[a] The percentage of second degree burns is excluded, only the percentage of the third degree being counted (e.g., 80% BSA burned with 50% third degree burn is counted as 50%)
[b] III° (%) = Percentage of BSA affected by third degree burn

Table 3. Linear regression equation of total BSA burned and mortality probit

Period	Linear regression equation	LA_{50}
1958–1965	$y=0.0394x+2.1761$	71.69
1966–1978	$y=0.0301x+2.3939$	85.97
1958–1978	$y=0.0319x+2.3940$	81.66

Table 4. Linear regression equation of amount of BSA affected by third degree burns and mortality probit

Period	Linear regression equation	LA_{50}
1958–1965	$y=0.0718x+2.7552$	31.28
1966–1978	$y=0.0476x+2.6495$	49.28
1958–1978	$y=0.048x+2.7728$	46.4

Table 5. Age distribution of patients admitted (1958–1978)

Age (years)	No. of patients	%
< 2	503	10.74
2–12	1,534	32.75
12–50	2,259	48.23
50–60	208	4.40
>60	180	3.83

45–	50–	55–	60–	65–	70–	75–	80–	85–	90–	95–	Total
37	32	18	25	20	18	8	18	12	18	22	1,573
9	7	7	7	10	7	6	7	7	14	20	152
24.32	21.87	38.88	28	50	38.88	75	38.88	58.33	77.77	90.09	9.66
1	93	61	64	37	47	26	30	36	42	52	3,111
16	14	9	15	8	13	13	9	15	29	39	249
19.75	15.05	14.75	23.43	21.62	27.65	50	30	41.66	69.04	75	8
118	125	79	89	57	65	34	48	48	60	74	4,684
25	21	16	22	18	20	19	16	22	43	39	401
21.18	16.8	20.25	24.71	31.57	30.76	55.88	33.33	45.83	71.66	79.71	8.56

45–	50–	55–	60–	65–	70–	75–	80–	85–	90–	95–	Total
5	12	2	5	3	5	2	3	5	3	4	869
3	12	2	4	3	5	2	3	5	3	4	122
0	100	100	80	100	100	100	100	100	100	100	14.04
6	36	8	15	13	10	8	15	6	15	11	1,902
3	22	6	8	5	7	7	13	6	11	11	220
0	61.11	75	53.33	38.46	70	87.5	86.66	100	73.33	100	11.56
1	48	10	20	16	15	10	18	11	18	15	1,771
6	34	8	12	8	12	9	16	11	14	15	342
1.61	70.83	80	60	50	80	90	88.88	100	77.77	100	12.34

Table 6. Sex distribution of patients admitted (1958–1978)

Period	No. of patients	Male (%)	Female (%)
1958–1965	1,573	1,087 (69.1)	486 (30.9)
1966–1978	3,111	2,206 (70.9)	905 (29.1)
1958–1978	4,684	3,293 (70.3)	1,391 (29.7)

Table 7. Different causes of burns (1958–1978)

Cause	No. of cases	%
Electrical	214	4.57
Chemical	510	10.89
Thermal	3,960	84.54

Table 8. Causes of death (1958–1978)

Cause of death	1958–1965	%	1966–1978	%	1958–1978	%
Shock	26	17.1	48	19.28	74	18.45
Septicemia	101	66.44	50	20.08	151	37.65
Wound sepsis	–	–[a]	127	51.00	127	31.67
Acute renal failure	1	0.65	9	3.61	10	2.49
Stress ulcer	2	1.31	3	1.20	5	1.24
Pneumonia	1	0.65	4	1.61	5	1.24
Respiratory failure	10	6.57	8	3.21	18	4.48
Miscellaneous	11	7.15	0	0	11	2.74
Total	152	100	249	100	401	100

[a] Before 1966 "wound sepsis" was classified under "septicemia".

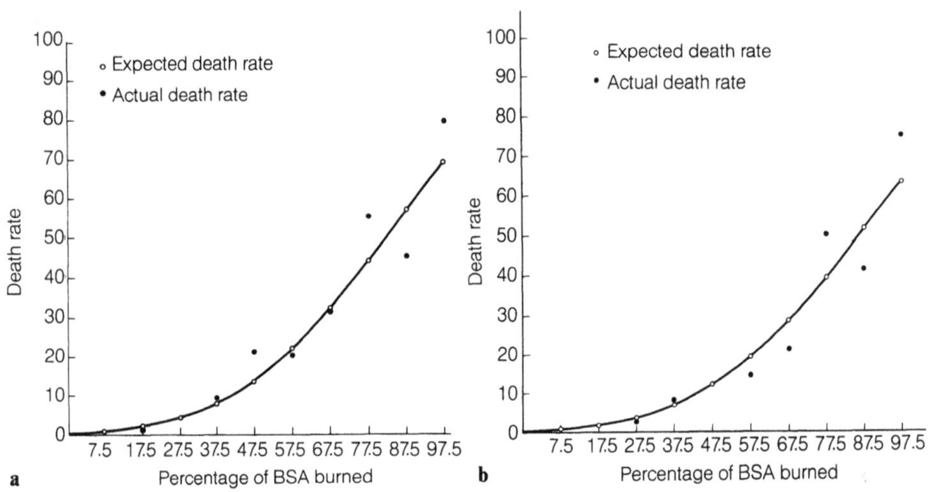

Fig. 1. a Expected and actual death rates in relation to the total BSA burned ($LA_{50}=81.66\%$) for the period 1958–1978. **b** Expected and actual death rates in relation to the total BSA burned ($LA_{50}=85.97\%$) for the period 1966–1978. **a** and **b** are the result of probit analyses on 4,684 and 3,111 cases respectively

equations with burn area x and probit y were produced through transformation of mortality percentage to probit according to the normal distribution law (Tables 3, 4). When the values of y in the equations shown in Tables 3 and 4 were substituted by mortality percentage, sigmoid curves as shown in Figs. 1 and 2 were produced. The regression coefficients of the equations were statistically significant ($P<0.01$). For the sake of comparison, linear graphs were produced on the basis of the equations (Figs. 3, 4). The LA_{50} s (i.e., the percentage of BSA burned which proved lethal for 50% of the patients) were calculated for the periods 1958–1965 and 1966–1978. The results showed that the improvement achieved in patients with third degree involvement (LA_{50} of third degree

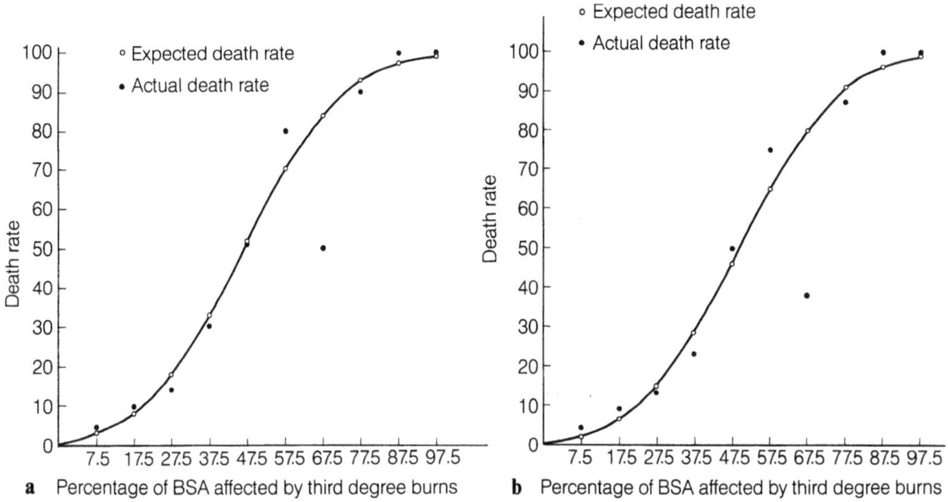

Fig. 2. a Expected and actual death rates in relation to the amount of the BSA affected by third degree burns ($LA_{50}=46.4\%$) for the period 1958–1978. **b** Expected and actual death rates in relation to the amount of the BSA affected by third degree burns ($LA_{50}=49.28\%$) for the period 1966–1978. **a** and **b** are the result of probit analyses on 2,771 and 1,902 cases respectively

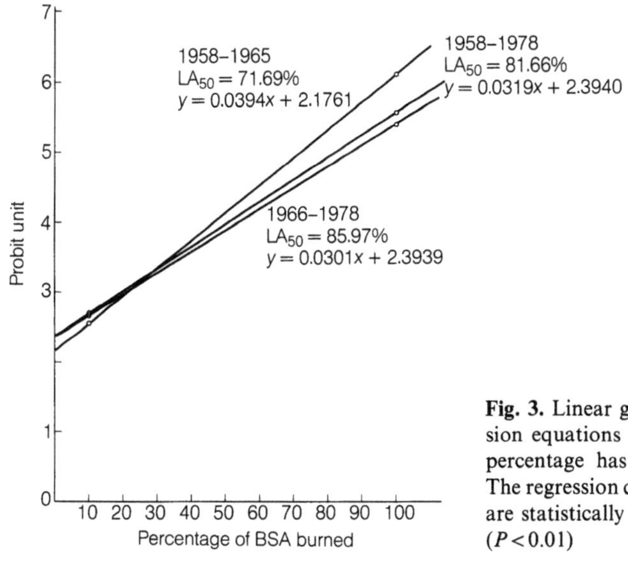

Fig. 3. Linear graph derived from linear regression equations of total BSA burned. Mortality percentage has been transformed into probit. The regression coefficients of the three equations are statistically significant ($P<0.01$)

burns rose from 31.28% to 49.28%) was greater than that achieved when the total BSA is considered (LA_{50} rose from 71.69% to 85.97%).

This book has been completed with the cooperation of the Departments of Anaesthesiology, Laboratory Diagnosis, and Pathology of this hospital. Photographs were taken and donated by the Section of Medical Photography of Shanghai Second Medical College. All the line drawings and some of the color illustrations were made by the Shanghai Scientific and Technical Publisher.

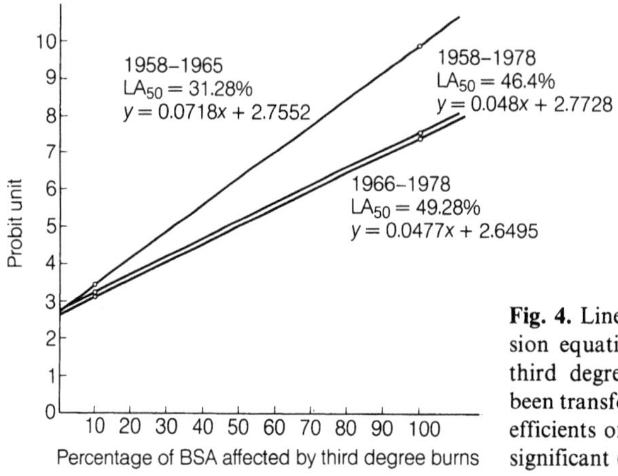

Fig. 4. Linear graph derived from linear regression equations of amount of BSA affected by third degree burns. Mortality percentage has been transformed into probit. The regression coefficients of the three equations are statistically significant ($P < 0.01$)

Movement is in progress: new things lie ahead and are emerging in an endless stream. So it is with our medical practice. There are still many problems in burn treatment, such as prolonged course, high costs, excessive hospital stay, and unacceptably high mortality, but we are convinced that by conscientious study and painstaking work we can further raise the survival rate, lower the disability rate, and continuously improve treatment.

Chapter I Early Management of Burn Patients

LIU GUO-YU

Translated by NYI PAO-CHUN

1 Emergency Care and Transportation

Priorities in the emergency care of burn patients are (a) rapid eradication of the cause of burn and (b) taking effective measures for initial care, giving necessary emergency treatment (cf. Chap. III), or preparing the patient for transportation. When emergency care needs to be given to mass casualties, resuscitation should be well organized.

1.1 Eradication of the Cause of Burn

When the clothing is on fire, the victim should immediately lie down and put out the fire by rolling slowly on the ground. Alternatively, the clothing should be taken off right away or sprayed with large quantities of water, or the fire should be smothered with heavy clothing, blankets, or other suitable means at hand. The patient should never be allowed to run around, since the fire may be fanned by the wind and burns to the head, face, and neck may be incurred. If the patient is burned by jellied gasoline, the body should be covered with many layers of wet cloth.

All clothing wetted by hot water or other hot fluids should be removed immediately. Limbs with small- or medium-sized burns may be immersed in cold water in order to decrease pain as well as to lessen injury.

Again, when the clothing is wetted by acids, alkali, or other caustic chemicals, it must be removed right away. The wound should then be irrigated with large quantities of tap water for a long time. When the burn is caused by dry lime, the particles should be removed first and the wound cleansed with water. It is important to note that a copious amount of water must be used, since if the lime is only moistened it will generate heat and thereby increase the severity of the burn. Particular attention should be paid to whether the eyes are burned or not. If they are, they should be irrigated first, using a suitable amount of tap water. There is a very close relationship between the severity of burning of the eyes and the time when irrigation is started, as well as with the efficiency with which it is carried out.

When the burn is caused by phosphorus, the wound should immediately be covered with well-wetted cloth or immersed in water in order to prevent the flare-up of the phosphorus by its contact with air. One patient was brought to our emergency room with phosphorus burns of both hands, which were immersed in a bucket of cold water – this is an excellent method. In the early care of this kind of burn, particles of phosphorus should be thoroughly removed and the wound bandaged with wet dressings. Oily dressings are contraindicated, because phosphorus may be dissolved in oil and large quantities of phosphorus may be absorbed, resulting in phosphorus poisoning.

In high tension electric injuries, the electric current must be cut off immediately; flames caused by electric sparks should be extinguished and necessary first aid given.

1.2 Resuscitation of Critically Ill Patients

If respiratory and cardiac arrest occur in critically ill patients, cardiopulmonary resuscitation should be carried out immediately. When the respiratory tract is severely burned and is accompanied by obstruction of the air passage, tracheotomy should be performed immediately. When the burn trauma is complicated by hemorrhage, hemostasis should be achieved at once. If fractures are a complication, immobilization with simple means should be implemented.

1.3 Relief of Pain

After burn injury, all patients are in pain, the degree of which varies, and are irritable and restless. Measures for the relief of pain should be taken. Dolantin or morphine may be chosen (they are contraindicated in patients with burns of the respiratory tract and brain injuries). In burn patients during the stage of shock, analgesics given by intramuscular injection may not be absorbed owing to poor peripheral perfusion; therefore they should be given intravenously. As shock does not necessarily take place in lightly burned patients, analgesics may be given by intramuscular injection or orally. Dolantin and morphine are contraindicated in infants under 1 year of age. The name, dosage, route, and time of administration of the drug should be recorded in detail. Irritability and restlessness may not necessarily be caused by pain. It is quite possible that they are a manifestation of inadequate blood volume. Therefore, before the cause of irritability is clarified, repeated injections of analgesics should be avoided (especially by intramuscular injection). Failure to do so may produce a danger of intoxication due to accumulation.

1.4 Protection of the Wound Surface

The wound surface should be covered with sheets or clothes, or by the application of Chinese herb medication when available, to avoid contamination and additional trauma.

1.5 Transportation

When condition permits, burn patients may be treated on the spot. When transportation of the patient is deemed necessary, it should be carried out as quickly as possible under the prerequisite of safety.

1. It is best to get the severely burned patient to the hospital within 2–3 h after injury; otherwise it is safer to wait until he has passed the shock stage. To transport the patient at the peak of the shock stage should never be allowed. If transportation requires more than 1 h, physiologic saline solution should be given by intravenous infusion before and during the journey in order to prevent shock. Injection of large amounts of glucose solution or intake of water orally should be prohibited, because it will not prevent shock and may have serious consequences, such as edema of the brain. If shock has already appeared, the blood volume should first be replenished, and the patient may be transported after the shock has become stable. During transportation, the patient should be kept warm and rocking should be avoided. For old people and infants with light or medium burns, or adults whose condition is complicated by other traumas, precautions against the occurrence of shock should be taken if the journey is long.

2. As obstruction of the air passage may occur in patients with burns of the respiratory tract during the course of transportation, measures for tracheotomy should be kept in readiness.

3. During transportation, the patient should be laid crosswise if possible, or in a position with the feet toward the direction of travel. When the patient is carried up or down stairs, the head should be kept lower than the feet. When an extensively burned patient is transported during the shock stage on an airplane, if he is laid with his head toward the front, then in the takeoff blackout will inevitably occur due to acute ischemia of the brain.

4. Artificial hibernation drugs are contraindicated before and during transportation.

2 Estimation of BSA Burned; Assessment and Classification of Depth of the Burn Wound

Although factors affecting the prognosis of burns are numerous, the extent of burn surface area and the depth of the burn wound are the principal factors by which the severity of burn is determined and plans for treatment are formed. Therefore, it is very important to assess the burn surface area and the depth of the burn wound accurately.

2.1 Estimation of BSA Burned

The "new rule of nines": The head and neck cover 9% of the BSA (the front and back of the neck occupying 1% each); the upper limbs cover 18% (the upper arms, 4% each; the forearms, 3% each; the hands, 2% each); the trunk covers 27% (the front and back, 13% each; the perineum, 1%); the buttocks cover 5%; and the lower limbs cover 41% (the front and back of the thigs, 5% each; the front and back of the legs, $3\frac{1}{2}$% each; the dorsal and plantar surfaces of the feet, $1\frac{3}{4}$% each) (Table I.1).

For small areas of burn, the palm method may be used (Fig. I.1), i.e., the palmar surface, with all five fingers close together, of the patient's own

Table I.1. The new rule of nines (applies to adults)

Site	Percentage of BSA	Site	Percentage of BSA
Head, neck	9 (1×9)	Torso, including perineum	27 (3×9)
Upper limbs	18 (2×9)	Lower limbs, Buttocks	46 (5×9+1)

hand is 1% of the BSA. By this method, the area of burn may be quickly estimated. When the burn is very extensive, this method may be also used to calculate the total burn area indirectly by estimating the area unburned. It may also be used to estimate small areas of third degree burn.

In clinical practice the aforementioned two methods may be used in conjunction with each other, e.g., when an upper extremity is not totally burned then we can estimate the burned area by subtracting the unburned surface as assessed by the palm method from nine, which is the percentage of BSA occupied by the upper extremity. If the burn areas are recorded on charts as exemplified by Fig. I.2, then their percentages and depths may be clearly recorded. As the depth of burn may undergo changes, it is not possible to assess it accurately in the early stage of burn, rather it is necessary to check it periodically. Consequently the charts may also serve as a valuable record for comparison.

When the burn surface area is estimated in children, the characteristics of their anatomy should be kept in mind. That is to say, the percentages of their BSA occupied by their head and lower limbs are not the same as those of adults; therefore the method of calculation is also different. The younger the child, the more of its BSA is accounted for by the head and the less

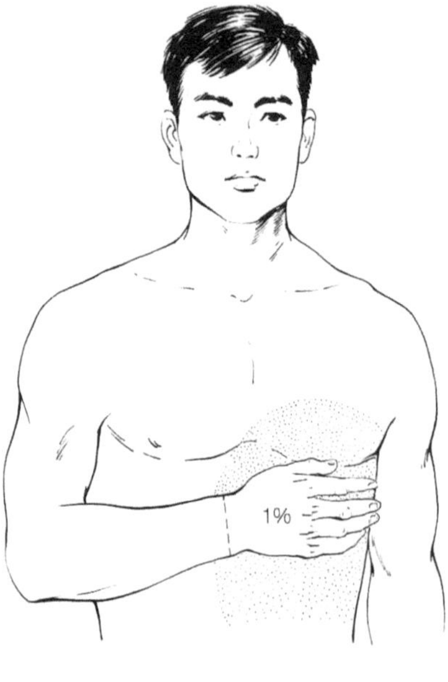

Fig. I.1. Palm method for calculating percentage of BSA burned

BURN CHART

Name Sex Age Bed number Hospital number

Cause of burn Date and time of burn

Coexisting traumas

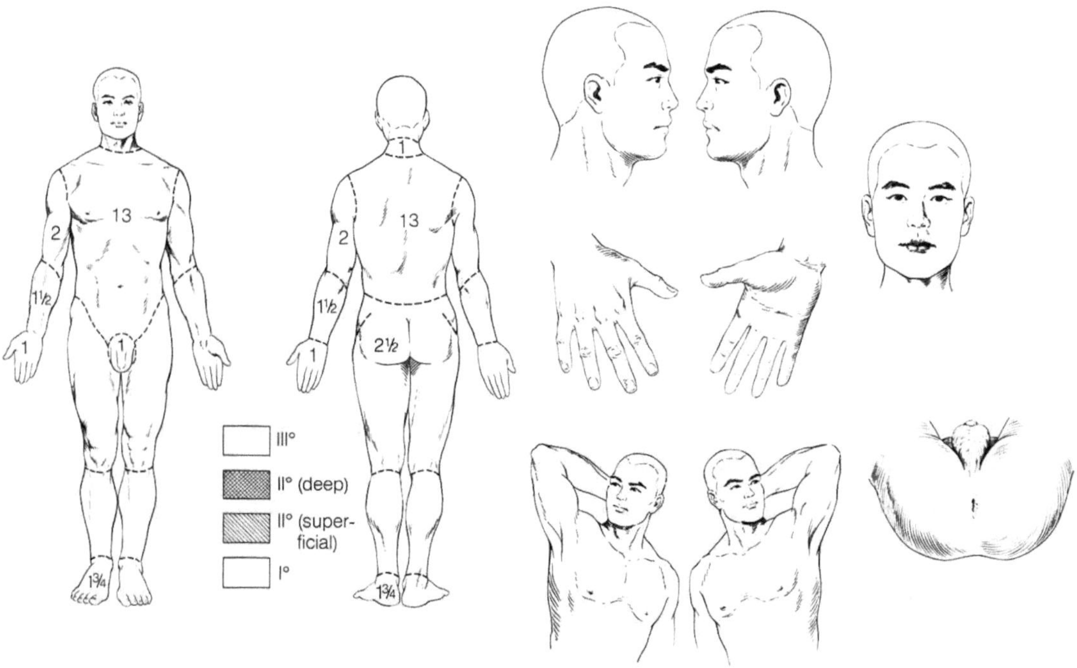

Sites	Age in years <1	1	5	10	15	Adult
1/2 of head	9.50%	8.50%	6,50%	5.50%	4.50%	3.50%
1/2 of thigh	2.75%	3.25%	4.00%	4.25%	4.50%	5.00%
1/2 of leg	2.50%	2.50%	2.75%	3.00%	3.25%	3.50%

BSA burned (%)

Possible I°, II° burn

Head	Neck
Trunk	Upper arms
Forearms	Hands
Perineum	
Buttocks	Thighs
Legs	Feet
Total	%

Possible III° burn

Head	Neck
Trunk	Upper arms
Forearms	Hands
Perineum	
Buttocks	Thighs
Legs	Feet
Total	%

Total BSA burned %

Fig. I.2. Burn chart for depicting the distribution of BSA burned

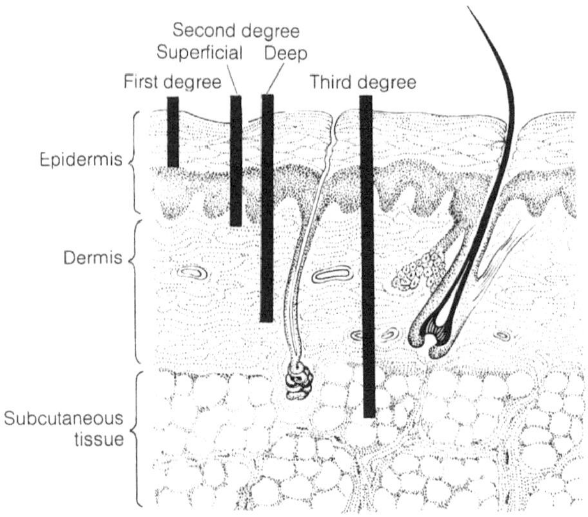

Fig. I.3. Grading of depth of burn

by the lower limbs. As age increases, the percentages occupied by their head and lower limbs gradually approach those of adults. The percentages may be calculated using the following formulaes:

Area of children's head and neck is $9+(12-\text{age})=\%$
Area of children's lower limbs is $41-(12-\text{age})=\%$

The results of calculation with the above formulas are the same as those which we have obtained from actual measurements of children in our country.

2.2 Assessment of Depth of the Burn Wound

The depth of the burn wound is generally classified into three degrees and four divisions (Fig. I.3), i.e., first degree burn (I°), superficial second degree burn (superficial II°), deep second degree burn (deep II°), and third degree burn (III°). The characteristics of their local pathologic changes and clinical manifestations are as follows.

First Degree Burn. The stratum corneum of the epidermis is injured. The injury may spread to the stratum lucidum and the stratum granulosum, and even to the stratum spinosum and the stratum basale. Clinically, it is manifested as erythema of the skin, also called erythematous burn. There is slight swelling and pain. As first degree burn involves only the cells of the superficial layer, and necrosis does not occur in some of the injured cells, they may recover their original function in due time. In general, redness, swelling, and pain disappear after 2–3 days. The necrotic cells of the epidermis will be replaced by hyperplasia of the cells of the deeper layers, and desquamation will appear clinically. No scars will be formed. Sometimes there may be slight local pigmentation. Since first degree burn has little effect on treatment and prognosis, when the burn surface area is calculated, that of the first degree burn is not included.

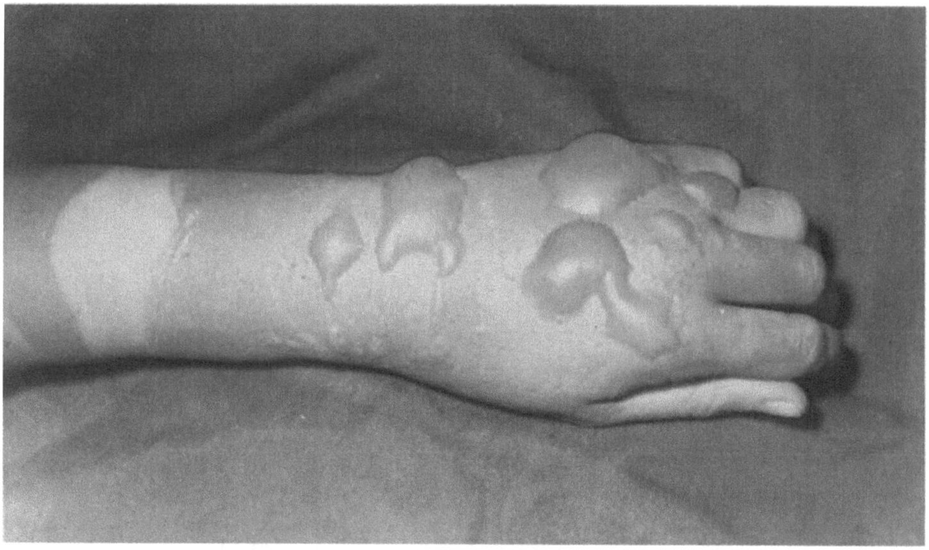

Fig. I.4. Typical superficial second degree burn showing blisters

Superficial Second Degree Burn. The entire epidermis and the superficial layer of the dermis are involved in superficial second degree burn. It is characterized by the separation of the epidermis from the dermis, with accumulation of exudates in between to form blisters under the epidermis, therefore it is also called blister-type burn. Generally speaking, the thinner the skin of the injured parts of the body (such as the skin of the abdominal wall or the medial aspect of the limbs), the bigger the blisters. Blisters may be formed immediately after the burn or within 24 h (Fig. I.4). The contents of the fluid inside the blisters are similar to those of plasma, but with slightly less protein. Therefore, after a comparatively long time, the fluid may coagulate to form a jelly-like substance. When the epidermis of the blisters is peeled off, a pinkish base may be seen, and on it bright red spots are evenly distributed. These are congested vascular plexuses of the dermal papillary layer. The patient feels a good deal of pain due to the stimulation of exposed nerve endings. There is constant exudation of body fluids, local swelling occurs very quickly, and in 3–4 days a thin layer of brownish crust is formed. If the wound is not infected, healing takes place in 10–14 days by regeneration and eversion of dermal appendages. After the wound is healed, there may be pigmentation or decrease of pigment of the skin, but there is no scarring.

Deep Second Degree Burn. This denotes that the burn injury has reached the deeper layer of the dermis, but remnants of cutaneous appendages may exist. Owing to the presence of a large amount of necrotic tissue, infection can easily occur. There may or may not be blister formation. If the already separated necrotic epidermis is peeled off, a pale base containing numerous scarlet red spots of various density may be seen. These spots are most conspicuous 12 h–24 h

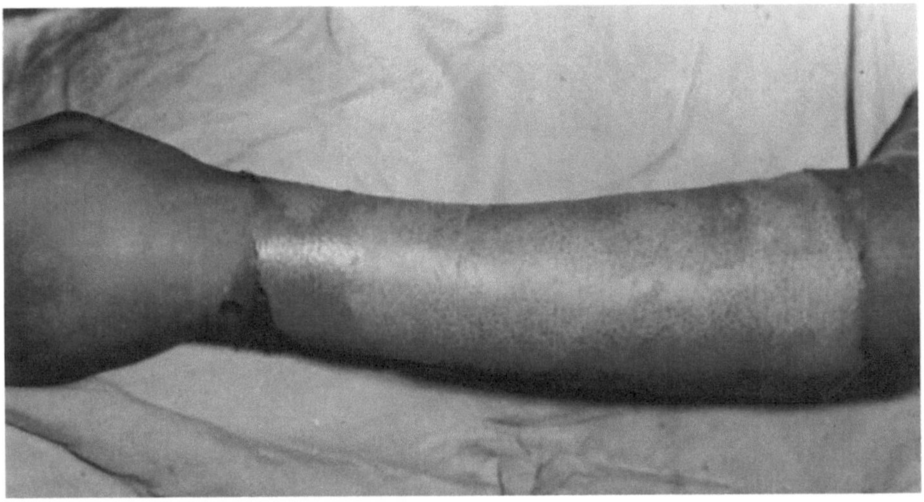

Fig. I.5. Deep second degree burn. The necrotic epithelium has been removed, revealing scarlet spots scattered on a pale-white base. These spots are most prominent 12–24 h postburn

after burn (Fig. I.5). The wound surface gradually becomes dry 1–2 days postburn, and sometimes fine and dense reticular vascular thrombi are seen. Healing of deep second degree burns takes place generally after the local necrotic tissues have been cast off or absorbed by phagocytosis, by the regeneration of epithelium from the adjacent deeper layers of the epidermis, or by hyperplasia of epidermal elements of the remnant hair follicles and sweat glands. Therefore, complete healing requires longer, usually ca. 3–4 weeks. When there is no infection, the rapidly extending hyperplastic epidermis may also cover the wound before the necrotic tissues are cast off. This is so-called subeschar healing, but the epithelium is rather flimsy and may easily be wiped off. Furthermore, the anti-infectious power of such epithelium is rather weak, and small pustules may easily form. Scar formation is inevitable. After a deep second degree burn is infected, all the remnant skin appendages may be destroyed, and the wound is converted into a third degree one.

Third Degree Burn. In a third degree burn, the whole layer of the skin is involved, while the muscles and even bone may also be affected. Depending upon the severity of the burn and whether there is vascular response and exudation, the wound may appear pale, brown, or burned black. The skin has lost its elasticity and is hard and dry, but in the interspaces of the subdermal tissue there is a large quantity of exudate. However, the patient does not feel much pain from that area, because the nerve endings have been destroyed by the burn. One or two days afterwards, if the necrotic tissue (eschar) becomes dry, branching thrombosed blood vessels will appear in the wound (Fig. I.6).

The time of eschar separation is influenced by the position and depth of the wound, the degree of infection, and the age of the patient. Separation occurs earlier on the face, the movable parts of the joints, and parts of the

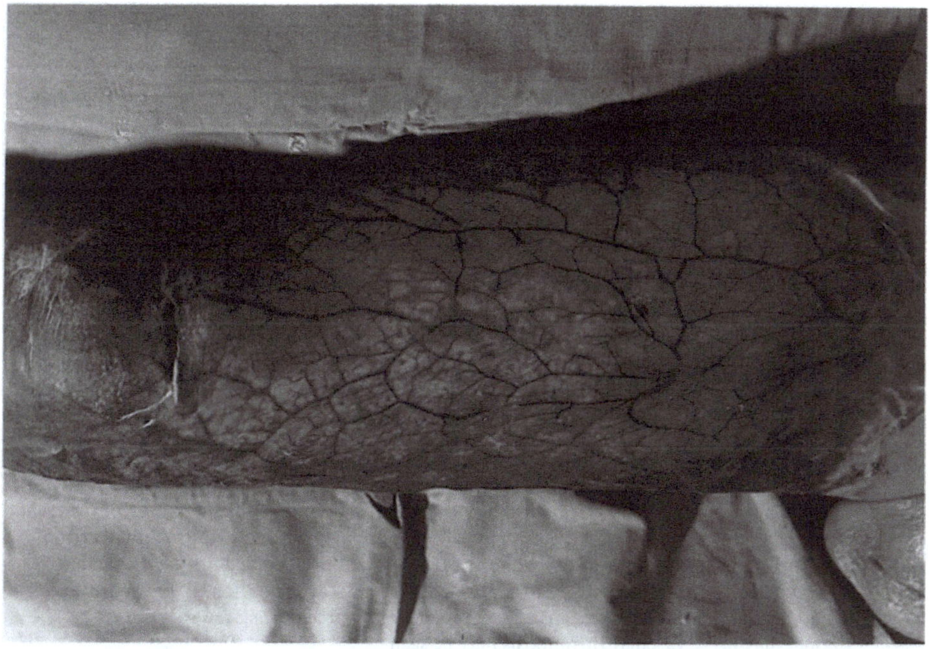

Fig. I.6. After desiccation of eschar in third degree burn, branching thrombosed vessels appear

body under pressure. The eschar separates earlier in children and later in the aged. The deeper the third degree burn, the later the separation of the eschar. The eschar separates earlier when infection is heavy. Generally the eschar separates 3–5 weeks postburn, and the granulation surface is thus exposed. Third degree burn with a small wound area can be healed by epithelium advancing from the rim of the wound as well by contraction of the wound itself, but severe scarring will be the result. For a large third degree burn wound surface, autologous skin must be transplanted. A summary regarding differentiation of the depth of the burn wound is provided in Table I.2.

Differentiation Between Second and Third Degree Burns

At first sight it is rather difficult to differentiate deep second degree burn from third degree burn (especially shallow third degree burn). The diagnosis and treatment of these two burns of different depths are closely related to their prognosis, so that accurate assessment is vital. The following points may be of help in judging the depth of the burn.

1. Position of the wound: The thickness of the skin varies in different parts of the body. The appendages of the skin lie at different depths; therefore the depths of the various degrees of burn will differ accordingly. For example, as the skin of the back and buttock region and the lateral aspect of the thighs is comparatively thick, a second degree burn may often be mistaken for third degree burn. On the other hand, as the skin of the abdomen and the medial

Table I.2. Differentiation of depth of burns

Degree	Depth	Clinical manifestations	Healing process
I°	Epidermis	Erythema, mild redness, swelling, and pain. Hyperesthesia. No blister formation	Symptoms will disappear in 2–3 days, followed by desquamation; no scar
II° (superficial)	Superficial layer of dermis	Severe pain, hyperesthesia, blister formation. Marked swelling	Heals ca. 2 weeks postburn; no scar formation, but pigmentations are possible
II° (deep)	Deep layer of dermis	With or without blisters with thick walls. Beneath necrotic epidermis, the base is wet and white with small petechial spots. Marked swelling, hypoesthesia. A few days later, reticular vascular thrombosis may be seen	Heals 3–4 weeks postburn by advancement of the adjacent epidermis or eversion growth of the epidermal elements of the dermal adnexa. Subeschar healing after the sloughing of the scabs. If badly infected the dermal adnexa may be destroyed, forming third degree wounds
III°	Whole layer of skin, the subcutaneous tissues, or even muscles and bones may be involved	The skin is leatherlike, with loss of elasticity and sensation. The wound may appear dry white or carbonized. No blister formation. Severe subeschar edema. Arborescent vascular thrombosis may be seen a few days afterward	Spontaneous separation of the eschar 3–5 weeks postburn. Small area of third degree burn can be healed by scar formation. Extensive third degree burns need skin grafting

side of the limbs is comparatively thin, a third degree burn may be mistaken for a second degree burn.

In the thick corneum of the palm and plantar surface, there are many more and deeper-seated sweat glands than elsewhere; the epidermal and dermal layers of the scalp are both comparatively thick and contain a large number of hair follicles which are distributed deep down in the tissues under the skin. Consequently, although the skin in the aforesaid positions may be burned quite deeply, the remnant epithelium of the sweat glands or hair follicles may still regenerate and cover the surface of the burn wound. Therefore, a deep second degree burn may sometimes be mistaken for a third degree burn.

2. Age of the patient: As the skin of children and old people is thin, a third degree burn can easily be mistaken for a second degree burn.

3. Sex of the patient: As the skin of women is thinner than that of men, a third degree burn in women can easily be mistaken for a second degree burn.

4. The cause of burn and the condition under which the burn is sustained: In certain acid burns or flash burns of high temperature and short duration, the quick occurrence of coagulation and necrosis of the superficial layer of the skin often leads to their being mistaken for third degree burns in the primary examination; in fact the deep layer has not been destroyed and they are discovered to be deep second degree burns in the course of illness. The caustic action of trichloroacetic acid and caustic soda is very strong; tissues burned

by these agents become white and soft, and most of these burns are of third degree. Burns caused by high tension electric current often go deep into the muscles and bones, whereas burns by electric spark are generally superficial.

5. The depth of burn wounds is not static and unchangeable, but, just like any other matter, is changed as the condition is changed. Generally speaking, the depth of burn can be more accurately judged about 48 h after injury. In the course of the illness, a deep second degree burn may be changed into a third degree burn due to pressure on the wound, thrombosis of the blood vessels, or severe infection. Therefore it is often necessary to confirm the diagnosis during the early phase of burn, after 48 h, at the time of eschar separation, and during the process of healing. It is only then that final assessment of the depth of the burn wound can be made.

2.3 Classification of Burn Wounds

The degree of severity of the burn wound is determined by the extent, depth, position, and cause of the burn, by the presence or absence of complications of trauma and poisoning, by the age of the patient, and by his physical condition before burn. Of these factors, extent and depth of the burn are the most important, especially the depth. At present, classification of burn wounds is based on these two factors. The criteria of classification set by the China National Burn Congress in 1970 are as follows:

1. Light burn: Second degree burns to less than 10% of the BSA
2. Medium burn: 11%–30% of the BSA, or third degree burns to less than 10% of the BSA
3. Severe burn: 31%–50% of the BSA, or third degree burns to 10%–20% of the BSA, or burns to less than 30% of the BSA, but with the following manifestations:
   a) General condition of the patient is poor or shock is already present.
   b) Severe trauma or chemical poisoning.
   c) Severe burn of the respiratory tract (with involvement below the larynx).
4. Very severe burn: Burns to more than 50% of the BSA, or third degree burn to more than 20% of the BSA.

In this book, we have used the terms small burn, medium burn, extensive burn and very extensive burn to express the degree of severity of the burn. Small burn is equal to light burn as established by the above criteria. Medium burn is equal to medium plus severe burn. Extensive burn is equal to very severe burn. The term "very extensive burn" in our classification denotes burns to more than 80% of the BSA and at the same time with third degree burns to more than 50% of the BSA.

3 Early Care of Burns

Early care of burns denotes the emergency diagnosis and treatment of the burn patient at the receiving unit or hospital after resuscitation of the patient at the spot where the burn was sustained and/or after transportation. The condition of the burn patient must be rapidly and concretely analyzed, with particular attention being paid to life-threatening factors. Emergency management should then proceed rapidly and orderly according to the degree of urgency.

3.1 Maintaining the Patency of the Respiratory Tract

If the patient has remained for a long time in a closed environment full of smoke and his oral mucous membrane appears pale and edematous with accompanying hoarseness and respiratory distress, or if there are deep burns of the head, face, and neck, especially around the mouth and nose, with signs of obstruction of the air passage, then tracheotomy should be performed as soon as possible.

3.2 Ascertaining Concomitant Traumas and Poisonings

Careful and meticulous examination should be made to ascertain whether there are concomitant intracranial injuries, thoracic and abdominal trauma, rupture and perforation of viscera, internal hemorrhage, fracture of the limbs and spinal column, and carbon monoxide poisoning. With the exception of fracture of the limbs and the spinal column, if there are severe traumatic complications such as rupture of the liver and the spleen, massive internal hemorrhage, tension pneumothorax and extradural hematoma, then emergency operation should be performed. It is imperative that attention should not be paid only to the management of the wound, while measures to treat traumas or poisonings threatening the life of the patient are neglected. Of course, if there are absorbable poisonous substances on the wound surface, they should be eradicated in the period of early care.

3.3 Establishment of Intravenous Lines

At the same time as the above-mentioned examinations are being conducted, lines for intravenous replacement of fluids should be established and crystalloid and colloid solutions should be given to those patients who are liable to shock. Generally venipuncture is employed. If the patient is already in shock and the peripheral veins are empty or if the patient is very irritable and restless, venipuncture and fixation of the needle are difficult. If the veins of the limbs are destroyed or if rapid replacement of fluids is necessary in severe burns, then fluids may be replaced by catheterization of the superior vena cava by way of (a) the cephalic vein or (b) the internal or external jugular vein. Assessment of the burn surface area and budgeting of the replacement fluid are done simultaneously with the above procedure.

3.4 Use of Analgesics

After the venous inlet has been established, diluted analgesics should be given intravenously. For this purpose Dolantin (pethidine) 1–2 mg/kg (contraindicated in infants under 1 year of age) and promethazine 0.5–1 mg/kg may be chosen; morphine 0.2 mg/kg may also be used (contraindicated in intracranial injuries, burns of the respiratory tract, and in infants under 1 year of age). Special attention is demanded if the patient is still irritable and restless after the analgesic has been given. This may not be due to pain: it may be a manifestation of blood volume inadequacy or hypoxemia. The respiratory passage should be examined again to see whether it is patent, and the rate of replacement of colloids should be increased, but injection of analgesics should not be repeated.

When primary debridement is performed in patients with extensive burns, artifical hibernation drugs may be used to alleviate pain. Yet it must be pointed out at the same time that among the artificial hibernation drugs, chlorpromazine and acetyl promazine possess vasodilation properties; therefore if they are used when the blood volume is inadequate, shock may be aggravated, even leading to sudden cardiac arrest. Consequently, once the intravenous route is established, crystalloids and colloids should be infused first, *not* artificial hibernation drugs. In other words, artificial hibernation drugs may be used only in the presence of adequate blood volume. Furthermore, when they are used, urine output, pulse, respiration, and blood pressure should be observed by a special attendant; attention must be paid to the patency of the patient's air passage and vomiting should be prevented. For the preparation and use of artificial hibernation mixtures, see Chap. II.

3.5 Use of Urinary Retention Catheter

When the patient's hourly output of urine needs to be observed (in adults with burns to more than 40% of the BSA or third degree burns to more than 20% of the BSA), a urinary retention catheter should be used. If anuria, oliguria, or hemoglobinuria appear after the preburn residual urine has been emptied by catheterization, they must be treated (cf. Chap. II).

3.6 Debridement

At the time of primary debridement, blood volume deficit must be constantly kept in mind. That is to say, the management of the local wound must wait until shock has become stable and the patient has quietened down.

In the past, so-called radical debridement was used; however, since it could increase the severity of shock and injure the wound surface but not decrease infection of the wound, it was abandoned and replaced by simple debridement, the procedure of which is as follows:

1. Shave the hair of the burn area and its neighboring region. When the hands and feet are burned, nails should be trimmed using scissors.

2. Remove all of the loose epidermis and gently wipe the wound with 1/1,000 germicide, 1/2,000 Hibitane (chlorhexidine), or physiologic saline solution. If the wound is contaminated by dust, first irrigate with water or saline solution, then wash the skin surrounding the wound with soap and water, and finally paint the wound surface with 1/1,000 germicide or 1/2,000 Hibitane.

3. Debridement of Chemical Burn, cf. Chap. IX.

4. For superficial second degree burns with small blisters, no treatment is necessary. If the blisters are large, the contents may be emptied by draining from the dependent part. Blisters of deep second degree burns ought to be removed completely in order to prevent infection of the fluid in the blisters. The remaining epidermis on the third degree burn wound should be removed as far as possible, because it prevents evaporation of water, thus delaying drying of the eschar.

5. Circular constrictive eschars of the limbs may affect circulation of the distal extremities, while circular eschars of the chest and abdomen may effect respiratory movement. All constrictive eschars should be decompressed immediately; see Fig. I.7 for sites of decompression incisions.

The incision should reach the deep fascia, otherwise the object of decompression cannot be realized (cf. Fig. I.8). The wound surface following incision may be protected with iodoform gauze or silver sulfadiazine cream.

6. Depending upon the location, depth, and condition of the wound, Chinese herb medicine may be used for topical application, and the wound may be exposed or bandaged (cf. Chap. III).

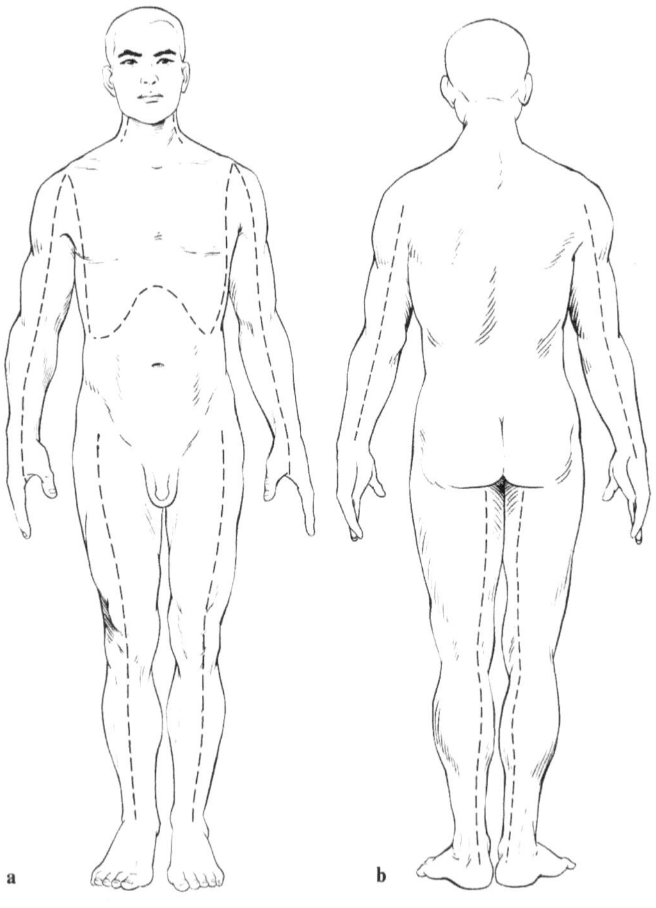

Fig. I.7. Proposed lines of incision for constrictive eschars

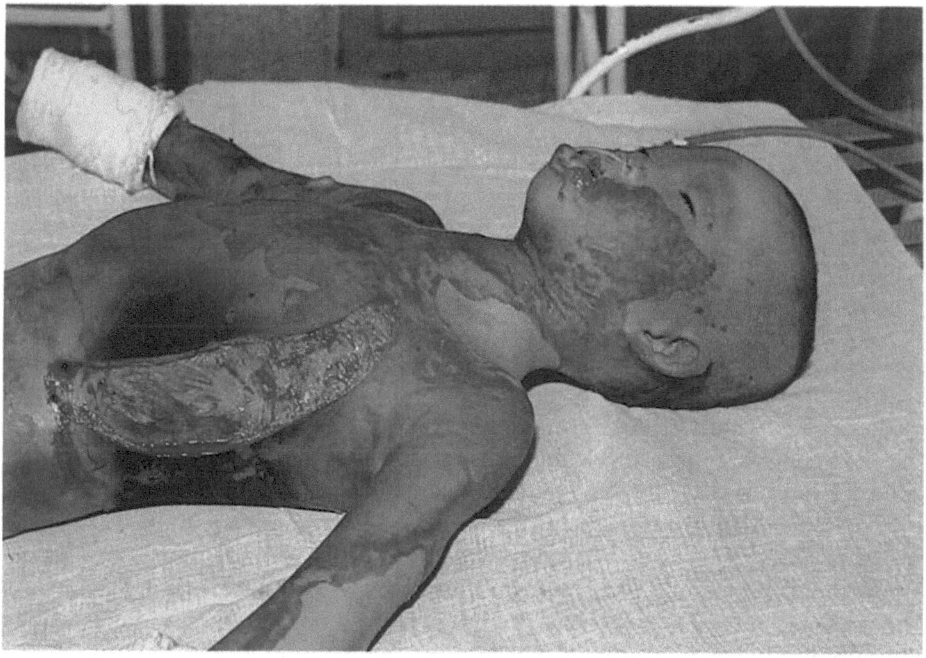

Fig. I.8. Six-year-old male with burns to 85% of the BSA; 68.5% of the BSA was affected by third degree burn. Constrictive trunk eschar was present, causing respiratory distress. Decompression incisions were made 4 h postburn. The edges of the incision parted, forming a gap of 4.5 cm in maximum breadth and exposing the necrotic intercostal muscles. Respiratory distress was thus relieved

3.7 Prevention of Tetanus and Hemolytic Streptococcus Infection

1. Tetanus antitoxin should be injected intramuscularly, 3,000 units for adults and 1,500 units for children. If the patient has electric burns or large pieces of muscle have been destroyed by burn, tetanus toxoids should be injected.

2. Prophylactic injection of antibiotics (see Chap. IV).

Chapter II Burn Shock

Hsu Wei-shia

Translated by Ling Li-li

After extensive burns, the chief manifestation of the early shock stage is the destruction of the semipermeable membrane characteristics of the capillaries in the burned area. A prodigious amount of plasma-like fluid thus leaks into the extracellular space and sequesters into the degenerative collagen resulting from the burn insult. The above-mentioned changes cause precipitous reduction of the functional extracellular space and the effective circulatory blood volume which eventually leads to hemoconcentration and hypovolemic shock, inadequate tissue perfusion, tissue anoxia, functional disturbance of myocardium, and decrease of cardiac output. During this period, besides shock, local swelling of the burned area and profuse weeping on the wound surface with formation of vesicles may be observed. In burns covering extremely large areas, especially in extensive third degree burns, there may be generalized reactive edema. Clinical manifestations during the shock stage are oliguria, tachycardia, poor peripheral perfusion, and restlessness, all of which are the symptoms of hypovolemia.

The fudamental solution to these problems is to maintain the capillary integrity and reduce the leakage. Research on the inherent causes of exudation from the wound surface and reduction of the exudates is still in the experimental stage. Therefore, at present the solution of these problems is mainly by the replacement of the fluid lost, in order to restore the effective circulatory blood volume and to improve the peripheral perfusion. The amount of electrolytes in the exudates of the burn is similar to that in the plasma, while the protein content is approximately half that of plasma. The majority of the proteins in the exudate are of a lower molecular weight and mainly consist of easily leaking albumin. The rate of exudation is at its fastest within 6–8 h postburn, after which it gradually slows down. The amount of fluid exudation usually reaches its maximum 24 h postburn; it then gradually slows down and ceases at 36 h–48 h. Therefore, we call the 48-h post-burn period the shock stage. If the wound is not severely infected, in the majority of cases resorption of fluids and electrolytes which have exudated into the tissue spaces will then begin to take place as shown by increases in urinary output and subsidence of edema. The more severe the burn, the later resorption begins and the slower edema subsides. Figure II.1 illustrates the ratio of fluid intake to urine output 1–10 days postburn in 12 patients with burns to more than 80% of the BSA and 39 patients with burns to 40%–60% of the BSA.

In patients with a total burn area approximating 50% of the BSA or third degree burns approximating 20% of the BSA, subsidence of edema starts about

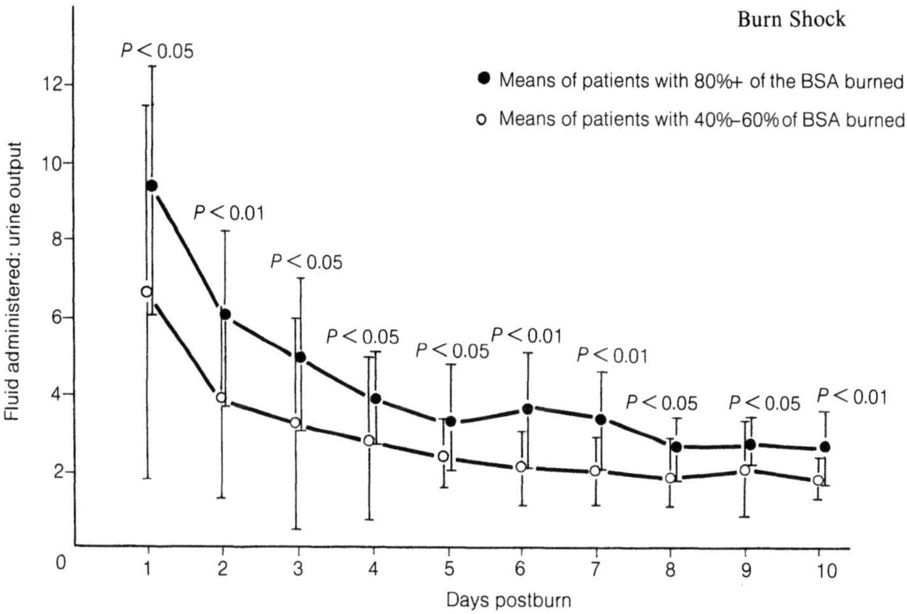

Fig. II.1. Comparison of the ratio of fluid intake to urine output in two groups of burn patients. *40%–60% BSA group:* Water release at about 48 h postburn and completion of reabsorption of edema at about 5 days postburn. *Above 80% BSA group:* Water release at about 5 days postburn and completion of subsidence of edema at about 10 days postburn

36–48 h post burn, and resorption is completed 5 days postburn. In patients with a total burn area of more than 80% of the BSA and third degree burns to more than 50% of the BSA, the completion of resorption of edema is often postponed to the 10th day postburn or thereabouts. In patients with extensive burns there will be signs of toxemia, such as high fever, delirium, shivering, and abdominal distension, within the 3–5 days following resorption of the edema, and blood leukocytes may be temporarily decreased to 6,000/mm^3. (After an extensive burn there is usually leukocytosis up to 10,000/mm^3.) The greater the burn area and the more extensive the third degree burn, the earlier shock appears. In patients with medium and extensive burns, shock generally occurs within 6 h–12 h postburn, while in patients with very extensive burns, there may be hypovolemic shock within 1 h postburn. Table II.1 shows the occurrence of shock in 93 patients with burns to more than 80% of the BSA who had not received fluid therapy prior to admission. From the table, it is obvious that the incidence of shock among those admitted later than 2 h postburn is as high as 50%–60%. Therefore, after a burn it is essential to give fluid immediately to patients requiring intravenous infusion. During intravenous infusion, it is important to keep the patient warm and to give him analgesics, etc.

In the majority of burn patients, the fall of blood pressure during the shock stage is mainly due to hypovolemia; therefore, it is necessary to increase the speed of infusion. Elevating blood pressure by vasopressors alone is not only useless but also deleterious. Patients may die of shock; besides, improper management of the shock stage will lead to cerebral edema, pulmonary edema, acute renal failure, and other complications. Patients who survive but have

Table II.1. Relationship between the time of admission (hours postburn) and the incidence of shock in 93 patients with total burn areas exceeding 80% of the BSA

Time of admission (hours postburn)	No. of patients	No. of cases of shock	Incidence of shock (%)
1	33	2	6.6
1–2	34	6	17.6
2–3	4	2	50
3–4	10	6	60
4–6	6	3	50
6–8	6	3	50

had a stormy shock stage are prone to develop early fulminating septicemia (cf. Chap. IV). Therefore, it is necessary to help the patient to pass the shock stage smoothly.

1 Method of Fluid Therapy

In adults with a superficial burn area of less than 15% of the BSA and in children with a superficial burn area of less than 10% (not including burns of the head and face), "oral electrolyte solution" may be given to replace the fluid lost. Intravenous infusion is usually not necessary. The composition of oral electrolyte solution is: sodium chloride 0.3 g, sodium bicarbonate 0.15 g, saccharin 0.04 g; add water to 100 ml.

The following points concerning oral administration of the solution should be noted:

1. Salt-containing solution should be given; intake of glucose solution alone is not permissible.
2. Small amounts should be given at frequent intervals. The amount given at one time should not exceed 200 ml in adults.
3. If the patient is suffering from gastric retention or vomiting, oral administration of fluid is contraindicated.
4. Symptoms of hypovolemia should be watched for closely.

1.1 Estimation of Amount of Fluid Required

During the past decades various formulas were advocated for budgeting the fluid requirements for the shock stage. Among which the Evans, Brooke, and Parkland formulas are universally adopted owing to their sound clinical and experimental basis, and thousands of patients were thus successfully resuscitated. For treating those extensive deep burns, we usually prescribed artificial hibernation drugs as a routine in their shock period, therefore we are of the opinion to give the patient a certain amount of colloids in the shock period, not only to secure the cardiac output but also to guarantee an adequate blood volume.

We summarized the fluid therapy during the shock stage in 600 patients without respiratory tract burn or other complications. These patients were admitted to the hospital within 8 h postburn, they passed the shock stage uneventfully, and the data concerning fluid intake and urinary output were complete. During the first 24 h postburn, for infants weighing under 15 kg and having an average urinary output of 5 ml–15 ml per hour, the average amount of colloid and electrolyte solutions given was 2.0 ml ± 0.58 ml per kilogram body weight for 1% of the burn surface area; for children weighing 15 kg–30 kg and having an average urinary output of 15 ml–25 ml per hour, the average amount of colloid and electrolyte solutions given was 1.80 ml ± 0.49 ml per kilogram for 1% of the burn surface area; for adults with urinary output of 20 ml–40 ml per hour, colloid and electrolyte solutions were given in amounts averaging 1.55 ml ± 0.37 ml per kilogram for 1% of the burn surface area. The ratio of colloid to electrolyte solution was about 1:1. The amount of fluid administered during the second 24 h was one-half of the amount given during the first 24 h.

On the basis of these findings, we suggest that during the first 24 h the following amounts of fluid are given: 1.5 ml colloid and electrolyte solutions per kilogram body weight for 1% of the burn surface area for adults, 2 ml for infants, and 1.75 ml for children. Half of the amount stated should be given within 6 h–8 h postburn, and the ratio of colloid to electrolyte solution should be determined according to the surface area and depth of the burn. For superficial burns of a medium or small area, electrolytes can be given alone; for patients with extensive burns, particularly when third degree, the ratio of colloid to electrolyte solution should be 1:1. In addition, for compensation of salt-free water lost, water may be given according to the daily requirement: 3,000 ml for adults, 70 ml–100 ml/kg body weight for children, and 100 ml–150 ml/kg for infants. The water should be given at regular intervals within 24 h. During the second 24 h, half of the amount of colloid and electrolyte solutions actually given during the first 24 h should be administered, while the amount of water is the same as that in the first 24 h. During the third 24 h, fluid therapy is determined according to the condition of the patient. For superficial burns covering less than 50% of the BSA there is no need to give colloid, only electrolyte solutions are needed; if the burn area exceeds 50%, an adequate amount of colloid may be given. Customarily 400 ml–800 ml whole blood or plasma are given. Oral intake of water starts at this time. The insufficient amount is supplemented by intravenous glucose solution. For extensive burns, and especially for extensive deep burns, intravenous administration of glucose solution is mandatory.

To give an example of the above instructions: In a patient with a body weight of 50 kg and deep second degree burns involving 60% of the BSA, the fluid replacement budget for the first 24 h is as follows:

Electrolyte solution	$50 \times 60 \times 0.75 = 2{,}250$ ml
Colloid solution	$50 \times 60 \times 0.75 = 2{,}250$ ml
Water	3,000 ml
Total fluid intake	7,500 ml

Name: C Sex: M Age: 20 Date of burn: 1972. 12. 7 Hospital number: 172756 Postburn day: 1
Admitted 1 h after burn

Weight: 54 kg

Total BSA burned: 85%

I° ___ %
II° 33%
III° 52%

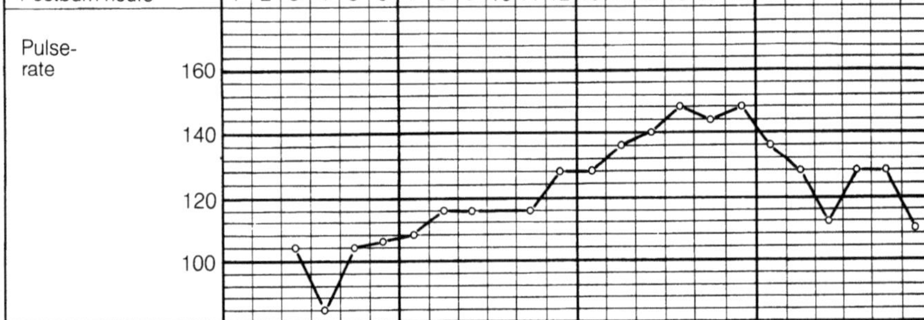

	Postburn hours	1	2	3	4	5	6	7	8	9	10	11	12	13	14	15	16	17	18	19	20	21	22	23	24	Total
Fluid intake	Blood				200			200			200				200					200		100	100	200		1400
	Plasma	200		200			200		150	50			200				200				400				100	1700
	Dextran	500																								500
	Normal saline	150																								150
	Balance salt solut.		650		250				100		100	300		200		80	120		450		200	550			300	3300
	5% sod. bicarbonate				200																					200
	5% glucose					300		50		300			200	150	50	250		300		100			100	200		2000
	20% mannitol				125										125											250
	Hibern. mixt. No. 4								70		55															125
Total intake																										9625
Urine		30	460	12	74	177	44	47	38	39	37	24	20	26	26	144	34	41	36	21	32	52	54	42	40	Total: 1546

a

Fig. II.2. Hourly recording charts for **a** the first 24 h and **b** the second 24 h postburn

Time distribution for fluid intake:

	First 8 h	Second 8 h	Third 8 h
Electrolyte solution	1,130 ml	560 ml	560 ml
Colloid solution	1,130 ml	560 ml	560 ml
Water	1,000 ml	1,000 ml	1,000 ml

The amount of colloid and electrolyte solutions replaced during the second 24 h is one-half of the amount during the first 24 h, i.e., electrolyte solution, 1,130 ml; colloid solution, 1,130 ml; salt-free water, 3,000 ml; total amount administered, 5,260 ml.

Case Illustration. Male, age 20, body weight 54 kg. Flame burn, 85% of the BSA affected, with third degree burns to 52% of the BSA. Figure II.2 illustrates the fluid intake, urinary output, and heart rate during the first and second 24 h post burn. The patient passed the shock stage uneventfully and survived.

From Fig. II.2 it may be seen that during the first 24 h postburn, the total colloid and electrolyte solutions given amounted to 1.5 ml per kilogram body weight for 1% of the burn surface area, the ratio of colloid to electrolyte solution was 1:1, the average urinary output per hour was 64 ml (250 ml of

Name: C Sex: M Age: 20 Date of burn: 1972. 12. 7 Hospital number: 172756 Postburn day(s) 2
Admitted 1 h

Weight: 54 kg
Total BSA burned: 85%
I° ____ %
II° 33%
III° 52%

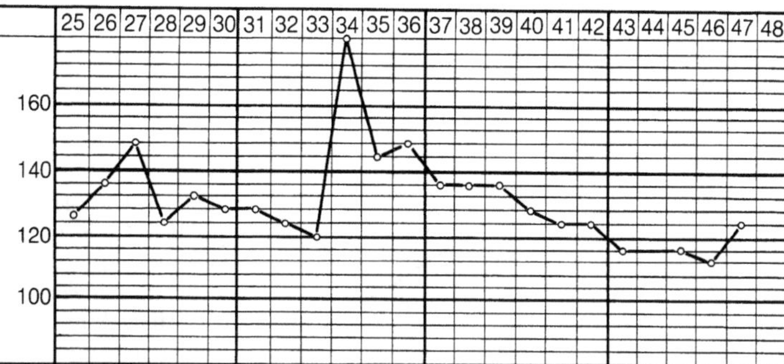

Postburn hours	25	26	27	28	29	30	31	32	33	34	35	36	37	38	39	40	41	42	43	44	45	46	47	48	Total
Fluid intake: Blood			200				200			150	50				200					150	50				1000
Plasma	100					200							200				150	50							700
Balance salt solut.		260		100	240			150			350			200	50								150	200	1700
5% glucose									50	50		300	100	100		200		200							1000
10% glucose	200		100	200		100		200	200							100	100		200	100	180	220	100		2000
Hibern. mixt. No. 4										100															100
Total intake																									6500
Urine	31	34	26	40	22	32	27	30	42	20	16	29	60	32	43	71	72	59	37	57	46	46	31	23	Total: 926

b

20% mannitol had been given), and hemoglobinuria ceased 10 h postburn. During the second 24 h, 0.74 ml colloid and electrolyte solutions were given per kilogram body weight for 1% of the burn surface area, the ratio of colloid to electrolyte solution was 1:1, and the average urinary output per hour was 38 ml; solute diuretics were not given.

It may be seen that after using 100 ml of hibernation mixture No. 4, heart rate increased from 120 min to 180 min, and urinary output decreased; after administration of additional colloid and sodium bicarbonate–physiologic saline solutions (cf. Chap. VI), the heart rate slowed to about 140/min, and urinary output increased. This indicates that additional colloids or electrolytes must be given to compensate the circulatory volume deficit due to lowering of the peripheral vascular resistance.

1.2 Points to Note in Fluid Therapy

1. Amounts of fluid intake should be calculated according to the actual BSA burned (excluding first degree).

2. The ratio of colloid to electrolyte solution should be determined by the surface area and depth of the burn. For medium and small burns, electrolyte solutions may be given alone; for extensive third degree burns, the ratio of colloid to electrolyte solution should be 1:2 or 1:1. If only electrolyte solutions are used during the first 24 h postburn, then colloids must be given right at the beginning of the second postburn day.

3. Usually, the colloids given are in the form of whole blood or plasma. Considering the nature of the fluid lost and the hemoconcentration soon after

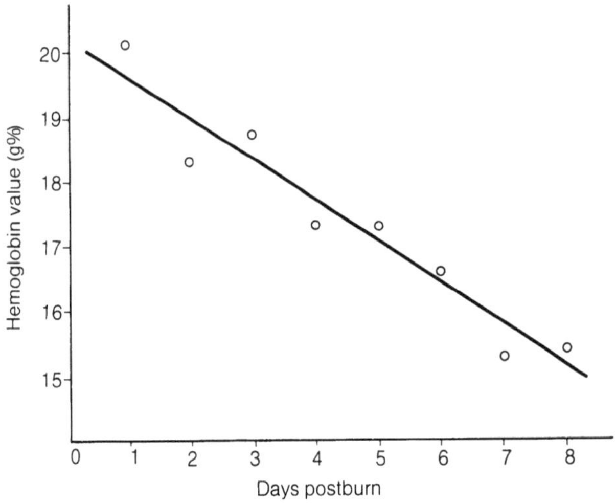

Fig. II.3. Changes in the hemoglobin value in 11 patients with burns to over 80% of the BSA, including third degree burns to over 50%. A progressive fall in hemoglobin value is seen, despite infusion of large quantities of whole blood

burn, it is better to choose plasma or 5% human albumin. However, for extensive third degree burns, plasma together with whole blood should be chosen instead. Among the plasma substitutes, dextran (average molecular weight, 75,000) solution containing 0.9% NaCl is most commonly used. If dextran solution is used, the amount should not exceed 1,000 ml per day. The ratio of whole blood to plasma is determined by the degree of hemoconcentration. In extensive third degree burns, the amount of red cell destruction is large and progressive. Eleven patients with more than 80% of the BSA burned and with third degree burns exceeding 50% of the BSA survived; during the first 8 days postburn each of them received 4,477 ml whole blood on average, yet their hemoglobin levels fell daily and approached normal only after 8 days had elapsed since burn (Fig. II.3). Therefore, for extensive third degree burns, it is necessary to give more whole blood.

4. Routinely, we use sodium bicarbonate-physiologic saline solution for supplying electrolytes. Two parts of physiologic saline solution and one part of 1.25% sodium bicarbonate solution are mixed to form a sodium bicarbonate-physiologic saline solution containing 150 mEq/liter of Na^+, 103 mEq/liter of Cl^-, and 48 mEq/liter of HCO_3^-.

It is necessary to keep the urine alkaline in cases of hemoglobinuria. In addition to sodium bicarbonate–physiologic saline solution, one should administer 250 ml of 5% sodium bicarbonate solution to adults with third degree burns to more than 20% of the BSA, and sodium bicarbonate solution to children with third degree burns to more than 5% of the BSA. In the case of children the strength of the the solution depends on the plasma standard bicarbonate content or CO_2 combining power monitored.

5. If there is extra loss of water, the amount of fluid supplied should be increased accordingly. For instance, when warm air therapy is employed, the amount of water needed in 24 h may reach 4,000 ml–5,000 ml. If feasible, water should be given according to the serum sodium level.

6. The colloids, electrolytes, and water should be given in alternation, and to avoid dilutional hyponatremia and the resulting hypotonicity it is especially

Table II.2. The administration of fluids to, and the urine output of, ten extensively burned patients within 48 h postburn

Case number	Age (years)	Body weight (kg)	Cause of burn	% of BSA burned (III°)	First 24 h postburn			Second 24 h postburn		
					Colloids and crystalloids (ml)	Colloids, crystalloids/1% of the BSA burned/kg (ml)	Average urine volume (ml/h)	Colloids and crystalloids (ml)	Colloids, crystalloids/1% of the BSA burned/kg (ml)	Average urine volume (ml/h)
1	38	48	Alkaline	27 (17)	2,500	2.09	39.0	1,100	0.85	60.0
2	28	51.5	Hot wine lees	80.5 (0)	7,140	1.72	39.0	1,670	0.40	64.9
3	38	55	Steam	98 (0)	6,760	1.07	39.3	3,150	0.58	44.7
4	35	58.5	Lime	34 (2)	3,100	1.15	52.0	1,250	0.63	34.0
5	30	57	Flame	60 (6)	5,175	1.51	46.5	2,400	0.70	34.5
6	33	44.5	Flame	81 (60)	5,310	1.47	35.7	2,800	0.77	32.9
7	41	55	Flame	90 (65)	5,700	1.10	52.9	2,400	0.47	73.3
8	36	61	Flame	98 (90)	4,200	0.70	48.0	1,300	0.21	37.0
9	41	43	Steam	87 (1.5)	7,700	2.05	34.9	3,550	0.95	38.7
10	17	58	Flame	99 (94)	5,420	0.94	68	3,840	0.67	70

important not to give large amounts of glucose solution within a limited period. Since diffusion of sodium ions through the blood-brain barrier is slow, if the osmotic pressure of body fluid falls precipitously, water will be transferred rapidly to the brain tissue, causing cerebral edema (cf. Chap. VI).

7. If the patient is in shock on admission, the amount of colloid and electrolyte solutions needed is usually more than the budget estimation. Tissue anoxia will further reduce the functional extracellular space and the effective circulatory blood volume; therefore greater amounts of colloid and electrolyte solutions are needed to ensure maintenance of the effective circulatory volume.

If the patient had a severe shock stage due to insufficient fluid replacement during the first 24 h, the amount of fluid given should be increased accordingly during the second 24 h.

8. This budget can only be used for reference and preliminary calculation of fluid replacement. Individual variations are marked (Table II.2), and additional factors, such as cause of burn, depth of burn, age of patient, variations in cardiovascular compensatory function, time of starting fluid therapy postburn, and distance of transportation of the patient, will influence the amount of fluid replacement. For instance, the amount of fluid replacement needed in acid burn is less than that in thermal burn (cf. Chap. IX). It is also less in superficial burn than in deep burn. Fluid replaced should be more in children with burns to the head and face – in individual cases the colloid and electrolyte solutions needed may be as high as 3 ml–4 ml per kg for each percent of the BSA burned.

Case Illustration. Male, aged 4, body weight 18 kg. The burn was caused by hot congee (the water in which rice has been boiled) and involved 20% of the BSA, including third degree burns to 3%. The boy was admitted 3 h postburn. Prior to admission, 250 ml of 5% glucose–physiologic saline solution were given. On arrival at hospital, the patient was quiet, with warm extremities and a pulse rate of 138/min. Colloid and electrolyte solutions were given according to calculation. However, hypovolemic shock appeared clinically with manifestations of tachycardia, feebleness of radial pulse, weakness of heart sounds, pallor of limbs, coldness, and oliguria. After speedy infusion, shock was alleviated. Altogether, 500 ml colloid and 500 ml electrolyte solution were given within the first 24 h postburn; this totals 3.6 ml per kilogram body weight for each percent of the BSA burned, which is double the amount needed ordinarily.

1.3 Clinical Guidelines for Adjustment of Fluid Volume Administered

Fluid replacement therapy is at present the fundamental measure for the prevention and treatment of burn shock. If the amount of fluid replaced is insufficient and hypovolemia is not corrected, shock may ensue; on the other hand, fluid in excess will lead to such complications as pulmonary and cerebral edema. If there is massive local edema after excessive fluid administration, toxemia in the resorption stage and wound infection will be more serious and will have a significant bearing on the prognosis. Therefore, it is necessary to adjust the amount of fluids according to the following guidelines so that the patient may pass the shock stage smoothly with the maintenance of an effective circulatory blood volume.

1.3.1 Main Guidelines

1. *Urinary output.* With a normal renal function, the amount of urine indirectly mirrors the blood volume, and decrease in urine volume often precedes fall in blood pressure. Therefore, urinary output per hour is an important, simple, sensitive, and reliable guide for judging the adequacy of blood volume.

In an analysis of the data concerning 600 clinical cases, we found that in 218 during the first 24 h the average urinary output per hour in infants was about 10 ml (5 ml–15 ml), in children about 20 ml (15 ml–25 ml), and in adults about 30 ml (20 ml–40 ml). All except one patient, who had burns to 92% of the BSA with third degree burns to 76% of the BSA, passed the shock stage uneventfully. There were 311 patients with average urinary output per hour higher than the upper limit cited above (in infants 15 ml, in children 25 ml, and in adults 40 ml); 4 of these 311 died of shock. There were 71 patients with urinary output below the lower limit (in infants 5 ml, in children 15 ml, and in adults 20 ml); 20 of these 71 died of shock. Therefore we are of the opinion that, in cases in which solute diuretics are not used, if urinary output per hour can be evenly maintained at 10 ml in infants, 15 ml in children, and 30 ml in adults, the majority will maintain an adequate blood volume and pass the shock stage smoothly. Urinary output below that level is a sign of insufficiency of fluid replacement, and it is necessary to increase the quantity and speed of fluid administration. Urinary output above that level is a sign of excessive fluid replacement, and it is necessary to decrease the speed and quantity of the fluid given.

For elderly patients and those with heart disease or the complications of respiratory burn or brain injury, the standard urine volume should be set lower: 20 ml/hour for adults is enough. In adults with hemoglobinuria the standard should be set higher, at about 100 ml/hour, which may be achieved by increasing fluid intake and administering diuretics. A retention catheter should be inserted for the observation of hourly urine output.

2. *Restlessness.* Adequate fluid replacement can keep the patient quiet. Restlessness is a sign of insufficient replacement.

3. *Pulse rate.* During the shock stage the pulse rate usually rises to around 120/min in adults and 140/min in children. Pulse rate exceeding the above-mentioned figures usually denotes inadequate fluid administration.

4. *Peripheral circulation.* If peripheral circulation is poor, fluid administration should be increased. Good peripheral circulation is shown by warmth of the terminal parts of the extremities, rapid refilling of capillaries, and strength of pulsation of the dorsal artery of the foot.

The clinical guidelines given above are those we used commonly; of them, the most sensitive is urinary output.

1.3.2 Criteria for Reference

1. *Blood pressure.* Maintenance of systolic pressure above 90 mm Hg. The decrease in blood volume in burn is not as rapid as in acute hemorrhage. Therefore the blood pressure may be normal or even slightly elevated during the compensatory phase of shock stage; consequently, generally speaking it cannot reflect promptly and accurately the condition of shock. If the blood pressure is low and urine scanty, inadequacy of blood volume is evident and colloids and electrolytes should be supplied. If the blood pressure is normal and urine scanty, it is possible that renal factors are responsible.

2. *Hematrocrit:* Ideally, the hematocrit value should be kept below 50%–55% in adults and 45%–50% in children. However, in extensive burns, and especially in extensive third degree burns, it can hardly be kept below 60% even with the use of plasma alone for the colloids. Therefore, this criterion is of little value.

3. *Central venous pressure.* Measuring of the central venous pressure provides a rough estimation of the blood volume and mirrors the pressure of the right atrium. It can be used for reference if there is suspicion that fluid replacement has been excessive. For the aged, patients with prior cardiac or renal diseases, and patients with burn of the respiratory tract or accompanying cerebral injuries, the safety range of fluid therapy is small, and central venous pressure may serve as an important criterion for reference in controlling strictly the amount of fluid supply.

The normal value of central venous pressure is 6 cm–12 cm water column. A low central venous pressure (0 cm–6 cm H_2O) and oliguria indicate hypovolemia, and the rate of fluid replacement should be increased. If the central venous pressure is obviously elevated (15 cm–20 cm H_2O) with a large urinary output, the fluid replacement may be excessive. If the central venous pressure is high, urinary output scanty, blood pressure normal, and peripheral circulation and cardiac function satisfactory, then the oliguria may be due to renal factors. If the amount of urine remains small or is increased only slightly after speeding up the fluid supply, while the central venous pressure keeps on rising, cardiac insufficiency may be present; the rate of fluid therapy should not be increased blindly.

2 The Clinical Significance and Management of Common Symptoms in the Shock Stage

1. *Thirst.* This is an early symptom indicating hypovolemia. This kind of thirst cannot be relieved by drinking water, and the patient may become more thirsty the more he or she drinks. The degree of thirst parallels the severity of burn. Severely burned patients should not be allowed to drink continuously, otherwise gastrointestinal dysfunction, such as vomiting or acute dilatation of stomach, or even hypotonicity of body fluids and resultant cerebral edema will ensue.

2. *Restlessness.* If restlessness is not relieved after intravenous injection of an adequate amount of analgesic (morphine 10 mg or Dolantin 100 mg in adults), it is then also a common manifestation of hypovolemia and cerebral anoxia. The rate of fluid administration should be increased, especially the supply of colloids. In patients with severe burns of the head and face or burns of the respiratory tract, the appearance of restlessness should be considered as a symptom of anoxia due to obstruction of the respiratory tract. If there is obstruction, immediate tracheotomy is indicated.

3. *Oliguria or anuria.* First of all, the urinary catheter should be examined to exclude obstruction, kinking, or slipping out. If the catheter is found to be in proper condition, insufficiency of fluid intake or impairment of renal function should be distinguished. If the amount of fluid supplied is less than or almost equal to the estimated volume, the symptom may be caused by hypovolemia due to insufficient fluid supply, and speedy fluid therapy is necessary. If there is still oliguria after increasing the rate of infusion, the administration of solute diuretics, mannitol or sorbitol at doses of 0.5g/kg–1 g/kg body weight is advocated (4 g/kg many be used within 24 h).

The infusion should be completed within 15 min. If the solute diuretics used give a poor result, they should be administered in combination with ethacrynic acid (Edecrin) or furosemide (Lasix) (Fig. II.4).

In the event of renal vascular spasm, a "diuretic mixture" comprising procaine 3 g, vitamin C 3 g, caffeine 1.5 g, and 10% glucose 1,000 ml is recommended. The dosage is 250 ml–500 ml per dose for adults and 50 ml–125 ml for children, and administration is by intravenous infusion.

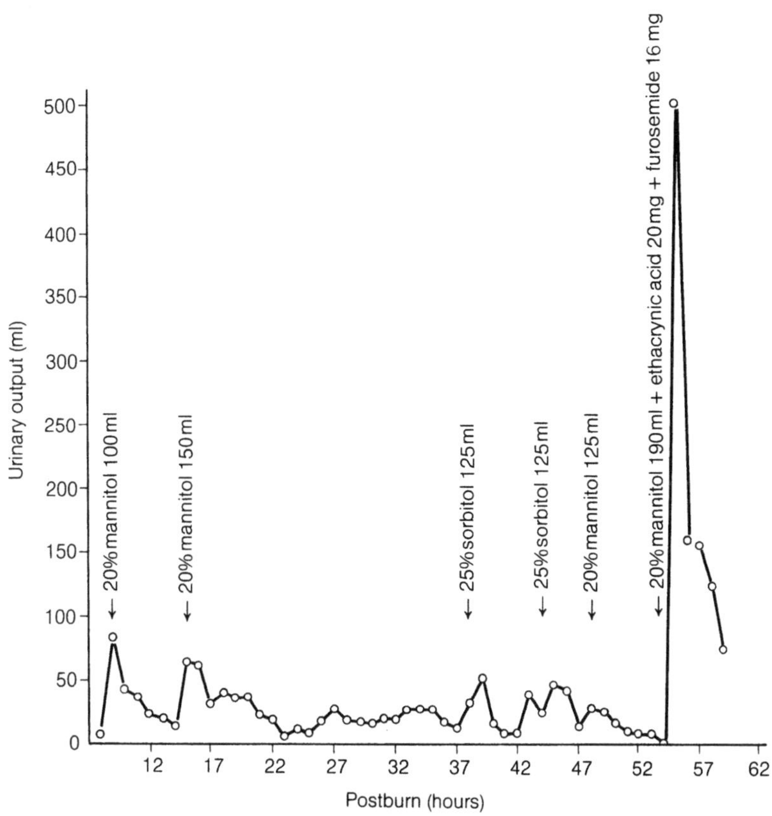

Fig. II.4. The influence of diuretics on urinary output during the early postburn period

If the urine volume is still not increased after the administration of diuretic mixture, solute diuretics, ethacrynic acid, or furosemide, then central venous pressure monitoring is mandatory. If the pressure is high and cardiac function normal, acute renal insufficiency should be considered and treated accordingly (cf. Chap. XI).

4. *Hyperthermia, coma, and convulsions.* These are commonly seen in children, especially when there are deep burns of head and face with a stormy shock stage. Overuse of water or administration of large amounts of salt-free water will result in hyponatremia and eventually lead to hyperthermia, coma, and convulsion.

Treatment consists of artificial hibernation drugs to lower body temperature in combination with anticonvulsive measures such as intravenous amobarbital sodium (sodium amytal), 5 mg/kg per dose in children and 0.5 g in adults.

For removal of the excessive water 20% mannitol 1 g/kg body weight is administered by rapid intravenous infusion. Hydrocortisone 50 mg–100 mg or dexamethasone 2.5 mg–5 mg by intravenous infusion may be beneficial.

In cerebral edema due to dilutional hyponatremia (serum sodium below 125 mEq/kg), 2.5% hypertonic saline solution administered by intravenous infusion is indicated. For hyperthermia, coma, and convulsions in children with deep burns of the head and face, hypertonic saline solution is contraindicated.

5. *Vomiting.* This is commonly seen in patients who have had an eventful shock stage. Vomiting may occur in hypovolemia, burns after a big meal, or premature oral feeding in the shock stage, before recovery of gastrointestinal function. Therefore, fasting is necessary for patients who have large area burns and are in the shock stage.

6. *Delayed refilling of capillaries.* This may occur in the compensatory phase of shock and is an early sign.

7. *Thready and rapid pulse.* Most of the patients with extensive burns have a rapid pulse, exceeding 100/min. But if the pulse rate reaches 140/min or more in adults and the strength is weak it is usually a sign of hypovolemia which should be promptly corrected.

8. *Pulmonary edema.* If there is difficulty in breathing, continuous coughing, or a large amount of frothy sputum, pulmonary edema should be watched for. At the beginning of pulmonary edema, there may be only scattered or localized wheezing sounds or moist rales shown by auscultation. Later, moist rales may be heard all over both lungs. Diagnosis of pulmonary edema is established if large amounts of pinkish, frothy, serous sputum gushes out.

Pulmonary edema is commonly seen in burns of the lower respiratory tract or in inhalation of irritating or corrosive chemicals. Fluid overload during the shock stage or too rapid infusion may also provoke pulmonary edema, especially in patients with cardiac disease prior to injury or in old people.

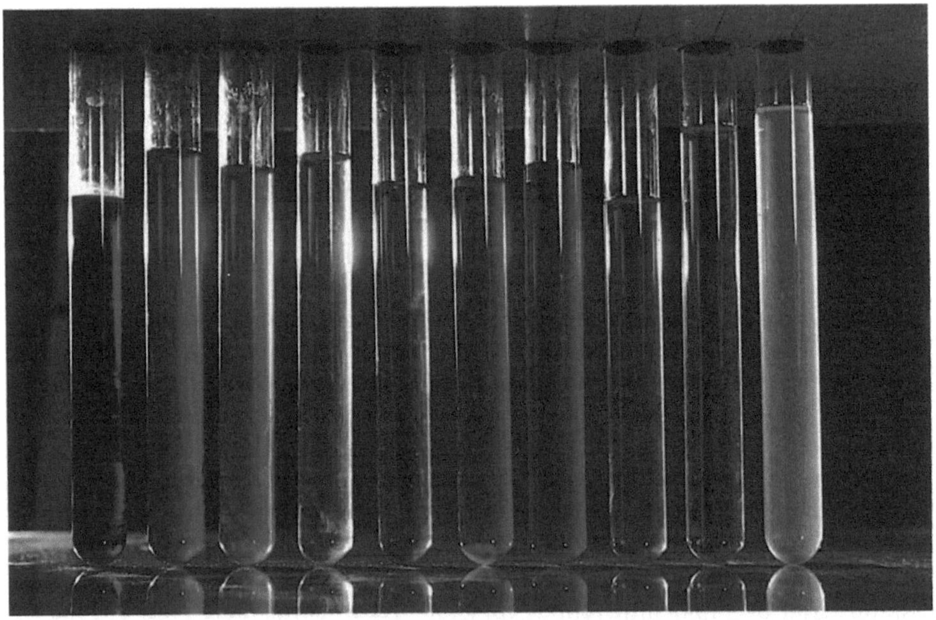

Fig. II.5. Six-year-old boy with burns to 85% of the BSA, including third degree burns to 68.5%, with the bulk of the muscles burned off. *From to left right:* **a** on admission, intense hemoglobinuria; **b–e** increased output of urine after administration of solute diuretics; **f–g** urine decrease, hemoglobinuria intensified; *j* normal coloration at the end of the first 24 h

The first thing to do in cases with pulmonary edema is to establish the cause, so that appropriate measures may be undertaken.

9. *Hemoglobinuria and myohemoglobinuria.* In extensive deep burns, the red blood cells are destroyed in large amounts and the hemoglobin liberated is excreted through the kidneys, causing hemoglobinuria. Extensive destruction of muscles (as in electric injuries) liberates free myohemoglobin, which is excreted through the kidneys, causing myohemoglobinuria. The injury to kidneys and clinical manifestations are the same in both conditions. The free hemoglobin and myohemoglobin will cause spasm of the renal vessels, and may be precipitated out in acidic urine, causing mechanical obstruction of renal tubules. The clinical feature is soy-color urine, and the deeper the color, the more serious the hemoglobinuria or myohemoglobinuria. If the amount of urine is increased after using solute diuretics, the grossly visible hemoglobinuria will diminish gradually and the urine becomes clear (Fig. II.5). Acute renal failure may result if the hemoglobinuria or myohemoglobinuria is not treated promptly. In extensive third degree burns or electric injuries, if the catheterized urine is clear on admission, it means that the urine obtained is the residual urine. In cases of anuria due to hypovolemia after burn, it is necessary to give fluid rapidly and to inject mannitol intravenously until hemoglobinuria shows up in the catheterized urine. The disappearance of hemoglobinuria or myohemoglobinuria in extensive third degree burns or electric injuries is indicated by gradual change of urine to a lighter color. If the color of urine changes suddenly from soy-color to clear, or the amount decreases suddenly, it is a sign of impending acute renal failure and is a bad omen.

The managements include increasing the amount of fluid supply or speeding up the rate of infusion and using solute diuretics to maintain the hourly urine output at above 100 ml. 2.5% sodium bicarbonate may be used. It will take time for hemoglobinuria or myohemoglobinuria to disappear. By summarizing the data concerning ten patients who survived burns exceeding 80% of the BSA and third degree burns to more than 50% of the BSA, we found that with the above management, the grossly visible hemoglobinuria or myohemoglobinuria disappeared about 20 h postburn.

3 Administration of Artificial Hibernation Drugs

Artificial hibernation drugs cannot act as a substitute for fluid replacement therapy in the prevention and treatment of burn shock. Indeed, they may even make the condition worse by their hypotensive side effect. Yet artificial hibernation drugs have the effects of relieving pain, hypnotization, and lowering body temperature. They inhibit overexcitation of the central and sympathetic nervous systems and improve the function of sphincters of the microvasculature. The tissue perfusion is thereby improved, basal metabolic rate lowered, and oxygen consumption lessened. Furthermore, artificial hibernation drugs help to improve the various excessive neurohormonal reactions during the early stage of shock. Therefore, for seriously burned patients, artificial hibernation drugs may be used providing blood volume is sufficient. In experimental burn of guinea pigs,

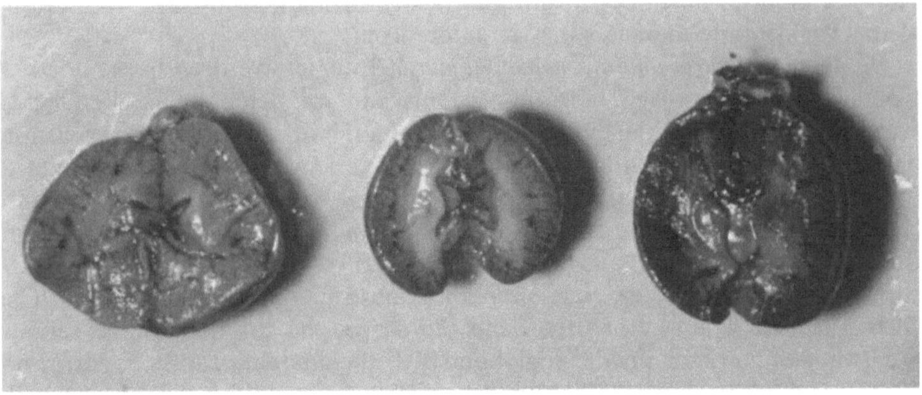

Fig. II.6. Protective effect of artificial hibernation drugs on the guinea pig kidney. *Left:* Burn, without use of artificial hibernation drugs. No injected pigment can be seen in the cortical region. *Center:* Control kidney showing normal cortical circulation. *Right:* Burn, after administration of artificial hibernation drugs. The kidney is swollen, but good cortical circulation is maintained

the use of artificial hibernation drugs prevented contraction of splanchnic blood vessels and inadequate perfusion of tissues. Following injection of colored substance into the arteries of guinea pigs 2 h–4 h postburn, blue color was seen evenly distributed in the renal cortex, which is a sign of improvement in circulation (Fig. II.6). The same results were seen when observing the vasculature of the small intestine (Fig. II.7). In another experimental burn of guinea pigs, renal tubular necrosis and gastrointestinal lesions in the artificial hibernation group were milder than in controls.

Artificial hibernation drugs have the action of dilating vessels and increasing the fluid requirement during burn shock. If artificial hibernation drugs are administered before correction of hypovolemia, they may cause a sudden fall in blood pressure and increase the seriousness of shock, leading to cardiac arrest and even death. During their administration, transportation of the patient may cause orthostatic hypotension. Therefore, these drugs should not be used before correction of blood volume in shock stage (which is usually kept at a low level due to increased permeability of capillaries during burn shock), and a patient under artificial hibernation drugs should not be transported.

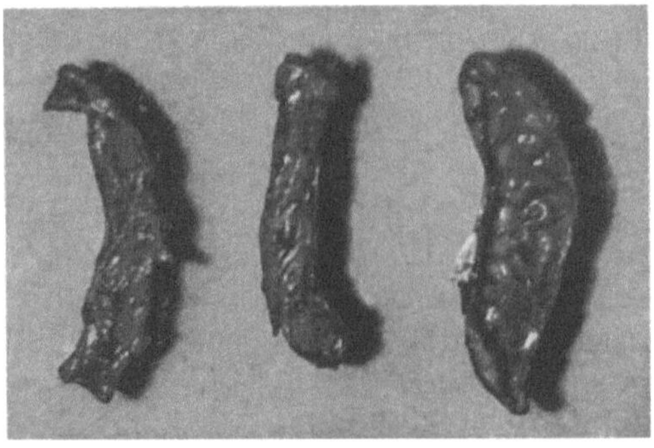

Fig. II.7. Protective effect of artificial hibernation drugs on the guinea pig intestine. *Left*: Burn, without administration of artificial hibernation drugs. Severe vasoconstriction is seen. *Center:* Control intestine showing injected pigment. *Right:* Burn, after administration of artificial hibernation drugs. There is excellent filling of the intestinal microvasculature by the pigment

To summarize, the use of artificial hibernation drugs in burn shock is beneficial, but attention must also be paid to their harmful aspects.

3.1 Pharmacologic Actions and Composition

Different kinds of artificial hibernation drugs have different sites of action and different pharmacologic features, and the mixtures are mutually reinforcing. We chiefly use dolantin and promazine groups.

1. *Dolantin* has a strong analgesic effect and can inhibit overexcitation of the parasympathetic nervous system. Its inhibitory effect on the central nervous system is weaker than morphine, and it may replace morphine in the treatment of burn patients. It has a mild action in lowering blood pressure. Overdosage will reduce the respiratory rate to less than 10/min. When used alone, it has a mild histaminelike action. Therefore, it is better to use it in combination with Phenergan. Prolonged usage will cause addiction. The dosage is 1 mg–2 mg/kg, and the total daily dose is 200 mg–400 mg in adults. There are usually no ill-effects. It should be given intravenously during the shock stage.

2. *Chlropromazine hydrochloride* is the chief drug with hibernation effect. It enhances the inhibitory action and reduces the excitatory action of the cerebral cortex, resulting in quietness and drowsiness. Its inhibitory action on subcortical centers is manifested by lowering of body temperature and lowering of basal metabolic rate (BMR). It depresses the sympathetic nervous center, blocks the sympathetic ganglia and vasoconstrictive action of adrenaline, dilates the peripheral vessels, and improves the splanchnic circulation in the early stage of shock. All of these actions help to prevent anuria, gastrointestinal ulceration, and pulmonary edema. It inhibits the vomiting receptor and prevents vomiting. Our customary method of administration is as a hibernation mixture by intravenous infusion.

The side effects of chlorpromazine include anorexia, jaundice, constipation, drug rash, agranulocytosis, orthostatic hypotension, and thrombophlebitis.

3. *Acetylpromazine maleate*, which has a weaker action and milder side effects than chlorpromazine hydrochloride, can be used in the latter's place. The dosage is 0.4 mg/kg–0.5 mg/kg for one dose. It can be made into hibernation mixture and given by intravenous infusion.

4. *Promethazine hydrochloride*. Besides its strong antihistamine action, if administered in large doses it also restricts vomiting and causes central sedation, hypnotization, hypothermia, and lowering of the BMR. The dosage is 0.5 mg/kg–1 mg/kg for each dose. It may be given orally, intramuscularly, or intravenously.

In cases of bronchial spasm caused by toxemia or wound sepsis, large doses of promethazine by intravenous injection (200 mg per dose) may be helpful.

The composition of the commonly used artificial hibernation mixtures is:

No. 1. Chlorpromazine 50 mg, promethazine 50 mg, Dolantin 100 mg, 5% glucose solution or physiologic saline solution 500 ml. This is one dose for intravenous drip.

No. 4. Acetylpromazine 20 mg, promethazine 50 mg, Dolantin 100 mg, 5% glucose solution or saline solution 500 ml. This is also one dose for intravenous drip.

For restriction of fluid administration, the mixture may be concentrated to half of the original volume to make a dose of 250 ml (concentrated mixture). In children and infants, the above mixtures should be modified. Dosages of chlorpromazine, promethazine, and Dolantin should all be 1 mg/kg body weight (acetylpromazine 0.4 mg/kg), and the daily dose of each of the aforementioned drugs should not exceed 2 mg/kg. The concentration of mixtures is similar to that used in adults (chlorpromazine and promethazine 10 mg/100 ml each). Dolantin is contraindicated in infants under 1 year of age.

The analgesic action of mixture No. 1 is stronger than that of No. 4, and the hypothermal effect is also better. The adverse effect of No. 4 on circulation is smaller than that of No. 1: it has less effect in increasing heart rate and lowering blood pressure.

3.2 Methods of Administration and Precautions

1. Artificial hibernation drugs should be used on the basis of an adequate blood volume. On admission, patients should first be supplied with colloids or electrolyte solutions, not artificial hibernation drugs. This is very important and must be emphasized. Artificial hibernation drugs will dilate blood vessels. If they are used in the presence of hypovolemia, blood pressure will fall suddenly; shock may be aggravated, and even sudden cardiac arrest may occur.

After admission, 400 ml–1,000 ml crystalloids or colloids should be administered rapidly, according to the surface area and depth of burn. When the blood volume is sufficient, artificial hibernation mixture may be given. Thereafter, before the artificial hibernation drug is given each time, a certain amount of colloid or electrolyte solution should also be supplied.

2. Rate of infusion: 30–100 drops/min.

3. There are individual variations in sensitivity to the artificial hibernation drugs, and the drug should be discontinued whenever the patient quietly falls asleep.

Usually, after intravenous infusion of half to one dose of artificial hibernation mixture, the patient will be in the artificial hibernation stage: respiration becomes slower and deeper with excellent gas exchange, body temperature drops to below 37° C (usually 35°–36° C), and pulse rate increases temporarily, usually 160/min. In deeper artificial hibernation, the pulse rate slows down, and buccal and lip mucosa, nailbeds, and auricles appear pinkish.

If necessary, administration of the artificial hibernation mixture can be repeated every 4 h–6 h. The total daily dosage is two to four doses.

4. During artificial hibernation, a special attendant is required to observe pulse, temperature, respiration, blood pressure, and urinary output. Particular attention should be paid to pulse and urinary output. If the patient shows an obvious rapid but weak pulse and diminished urinary output after administration of artificial hibernation mixture, hypovolemia is evident, and speedy administration of colloids is necessary. The pulse then slows down and becomes stronger, and urinary output is also increased.

5. After using artificial hibernation drugs, to prevent orthostatic hypotension it is imperative not to elevate the head or to turn over the patient.

6. Individual patients may be sensitive to artificial hibernation drugs, even very small amounts causing a drop of blood pressure. If this is the case, the drugs should be discontinued immediately and colloids infused quickly. If this is ineffective, noradrenaline should be given by intravenous drip as an emergency measure.

7. In some patients, the use of artificial hibernation drugs may cause retraction of the tongue, leading to respiratory obstruction with interference of gas exchange. Patients should be kept under close observation and an airway should be inserted if necessary.

8. Artificial hibernation drugs may cause aspiration of the vomit into the respiratory tract due to poor laryngeal reflex. Therefore, they should be used with care in patients who have recently had a heavy meal.

9. Artificial hibernation drugs are acidic and may cause chemical irritation to blood vessel walls, leading to phlebitis. Dripping should be done after dilution.

4 Administration of Diuretics

After burn the renal vessels contract, leading to diminished renal blood flow. Decrease in glomerular filtration rate will thus be caused, and with the additional factor of oversecretion of antidiuretic hormone, urinary output is markedly decreased in burn shock. The hemoglobin and myohemoglobin produced after destruction of erythrocytes and muscles may also cause vasospasm of the kidneys, further aggravating the ischemic state. In extensive burns, the ratio of fluid supply to urinary output is usually raised to 10:1 or even to 16:1 within 24 h postburn, indicating that the urine output cannot be increased markedly by the supply of large amounts of fluid. Prolonged renal ischemia will lead to tubular necrosis and obstruction by hemoglobin and myohemoglobin, and acute renal failure may be caused. Therefore, simultaneously with the correction of blood volume in seriously burned patients, appropriate vasodilators should be used to increase renal blood flow. Solute diuretics should be employed to counteract the action of antidiuretic hormones on distal convoluted tubules and collecting tubules. Furosemide should be administered to inhibit tubular resorption of sodium and water. All of these measures are valuable in the prevention of acute renal failure.

4.1 Indications for the Use of Diuretics

1. Appearance of hemoglobinuria or myohemoglobinuria after extensive deep burns or after bulky muscle involvement.
2. When blood volume is sufficient but urinary output is still scanty.
3. Burns complicated with cerebral or pulmonary edema.

4.2 Choice of Drugs and Methods of Use

1. *Solute diuretics* will reduce the resistance of renal vessels and thereby increase the renal blood flow. The solute diuretics used clinically are not absorbed

by renal tubules; therefore while traversing the tubules they will carry out water and dilute the toxic substances, serving as the so-called mechanical flushing action and preventing obstruction of renal tubules by hemoglobin and myohemoglobin. Solute diuretics are commonly used in burn shock and are particularly indicated for patients with hemoglobinuria, myohemoglobinuria, and chemical intoxication. The commonly used diuretics are 20% mannitol and 25% sorbitol. The dosage is the same for both, 0.5%–1 g/kg for each dose given rapidly, and may be repeated every 6 h–8 h if necessary. The action of solute diuretics commonly lasts for about 3 h, a factor which should be remembered in fluid administration. The urinary output during this period no longer reflects the blood volume. The total amount of urine within these 3 h should exceed the amount of the solute diuretics given. If it does not, it is possible that acute renal failure has occurred. On the other hand, if brisk diuresis has occurred, extra water must be given to compensate the urinary loss.

2. *Diuretic mixture* for composition and dosage, see p. 32. The procaine in the diuretic mixture has the action of vasodilatation and can relieve renal vasospasm. The mixture has a definite effect on oliguria caused by renal vasospasm. Sometimes it may be effective in cases refractory to mannitol or sorbitol. The rate of intravenous infusion of procaine should not be too rapid, 500 ml as one dose should be infused within 2–3 h. Rapid infusion of procaine may induce convulsions and vomiting, which can be combated by barbiturates.

3. Ethacrynic acid and furosemide will prevent resorption of sodium and water by the proximal convoluted tubules and Henle's loop. The diuretic action is strong and will quickly relieve cerebral or pulmonary edema. They are usually not used in the shock stage of burn and are only resorted to when solute diuretics and diuretic mixtures fail to act. Ethacrynic acid is given in doses of 25 mg–50 mg, and furosemide in doses of 20 mg–40 mg. Both are given intravenously.

Case Illustration. Male, aged 78. The patient had flame burns to 60% of the BSA, including third degree burns to 40%. The amount of urine was below the normal level within 48 h postburn. The effect of solute diuretics was not obvious. During the first and second 24-h periods, the urine volumes were 624 ml (average amount of urine, 26 ml per hour) and 588 ml (average amount of urine, 24.5 ml per hour) respectively. The amount was further decreased 50 h after injury and continued to decrease for 4 h, being 10, 7, 7, and 0 ml per hour. Ethacrynic acid 25 mg and furosemide 20 mg were added to 20% mannitol and infused quickly with the result of marked increase of urine to 502 ml in 1 h. The urine volume rose to 1,690 ml within 18 h.

Chapter III Management of the Burn Wound

YANG CHIH-CHUN, XIAO YU-RUI, and LI YING-YU

Translated by NYI PAO-CHUN and YANG CHIH-CHUN

Generally speaking, the changes occurring in the burned surface are reflected by the condition of the human body as a whole. During the treatment of burns, careful and systematic observation of the wound is of great importance in order to judge the changes occurring there and to decide upon the course of treatment. Proper management will not only prevent local infection but also hasten repair of the wound, shorten the period of hospitalization, and minimize deformity, thus securing success of the treatment. Indeed, treatment of the burn wound is the main determinant of success or failure in the entire course of treatment. It is necessary to avoid paying attention only to systemic treatment and overlooking the local treatment of the burn wound. The inclination to use a good deal of internal medication and yet to do nothing for the wound is erroneous. Even in the shock stage, much attention should be paid to the treatment of the burn wound.

1 Principles of Management

Management of the burn wound must vary according to (a) the general condition of the patient, (b) the extent, depth, and location of the burn and (c) the severity of infection. Restrictions are, however, imposed by the particular time and place of treatment.

1. *First degree burn:* Maintain cleanliness of the burn wound and decrease pain.
2. *Superficial second degree burn:* Prevent infection, decrease pain, and promote healing.
3. *Deep second degree burn:* Prevent infection, protect the remaining epidermal elements, promote healing, and minimize scar formation.
4. *Third degree burn:* Prevent infection, maintain the entity and dryness of the eschar, and remove the necrotic tissues when necessary. Third degree burns of small areas will heal spontaneously by scarring, but in extensive third degree burns, skin (autograft, allograft, xenograft, or artificial skin) should be transplanted as soon as granulation tissue begins to appear in order to avoid exposure of the raw surface.

Ideally, treatment involves:

1. Simple, economical, and practical methods
2. Facilities for nursing care
3. Rapid healing
4. Absence of scar or, in third degree burns, reduction of scar formation to a minimum

2 Methods and Choice of Treatment

The choice of treatment should be based upon the general condition of the patient, the extent, location, and depth of the burn, the severity of infection, the season of year, and the availability of equipment and manpower. Flexibility of application of methods should be kept in mind.

2.1 Treatment by Bandaging (Fig. III.1)

2.1.1 Purpose

The bandage provides adequate protection of the burn wound, facilitating the use of topical medication. It also keeps the body warm and ensures immobilization, aiding transportation and nursing care.

2.1.2 Method

A layer of petrolatum-impregnated gauze is first placed on the burned surface; on it are laid sterilized gauze and cotton, and a bandage is then applied with gentle pressure. The dressing materials must possess good water-absorbing properties in order to absorb exudates, maintain dryness of the wound, and facilitate drainage. The dressings should be sufficiently thick to prevent wetting of the outermost layer by exudates or purulent fluid. Of course, the necessary thickness varies with different stages of the burn process. After debridement, at the time of the first bandaging, the dressings should be 3 cm–5 cm thick as the wound is in the exudation stage. After that, the thickness should vary according to the amount of purulent exudate present. If there is heavy infection or medicaments are being used for the removal of the eschar, and consequently a large amount of purulent exudate is present, then the dressing should be thicker.

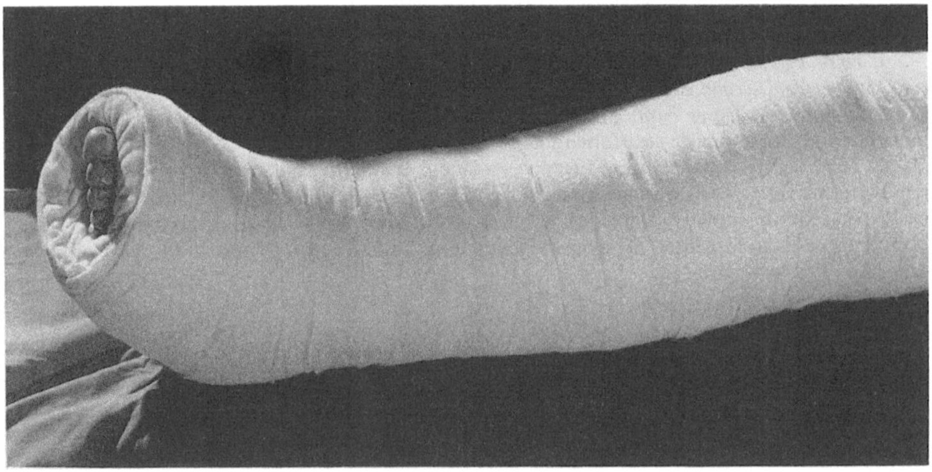

Fig. III.1. Treatment by bandaging

If infection is light and the wound is dry, then it may be thinner. After the transplantation of skin, dressings should be somewhat thicker in order to immobilize the skin grafts.

When bandaging is used as a treatment, topical medicament may be impregnated in the gauze or applied on the inner layer of gauze. If topical medication and petrolatum-impregnated gauze can not be used, bandaging must consist of many layers of dry gauze – so-called dry bandaging. This method is suitable for the bandaging of third degree burns during transportation.

2.1.3 Indications

1. Slightly infected or clean second degree burns of the extremities and small burn wound of the torso;

2. For transportation of patients;

3. In the presence of insufficient air conditioning;

4. For bandaging the donor areas of the extremities;

5. For fixation of the skin grafts after transplantation, and immobilization of the joints of the recipient area;

6. For the protection of the granulation wound or after the use of local medicaments.

2.1.4 Points for Attention

1. When bandaging, the force used should be even and suitable. If the dressing is too loose it may be cast off and the purpose of obtaining good drainage may not be realized. And, if too tight, it may cause circulatory disturbances.

2. Each layer of the dressing must be spread smoothly.

3. The content of petrolatum in the impregnated gauze should be small. In its preparation, a suitable amount of liquid paraffin may be added to the vaseline used.

4. Bandaging should be smooth and the bandaged area should exceed the wound surface area.

5. When bandaging the extremities, the procedure should begin from the distal end of the limb. When it is necessary to observe the condition of digital circulation, fingertips and/or toes should be left exposed. The distal end of the affected extremity should sometimes be included in the bandage in order to prevent edema.

It is important to attend to and examine the circulation of the distal end of the extremities, expecially after the removal of the eschar and after the transplantation of large sheets of allografts, as it is often necessary to apply pressure bandages to achieve hemostatic effects. When the eschar of the extremities is excised with its subcutaneous fat, the buffer effect of the fat pad against pressure is lost. Therefore, if the force used in bandaging is not even, the extremities may suffer from uneven circular pressure and circulatory disturbances or even necrosis of the extremities may result.

6. On bandaging, the joints of the extremities should be placed in functional positions: for the knee joint, extension in 150°; for the ankle joint, dorsiflexion

in 90°. When the hand is burned, in order to prevent occurrence of the clawhand deformity the thumb should be kept in opponens, with interphalangeal joints extended and the metacarpophalangeal joints flexed 80°. We usually term this the "reasonable" position of the hand, since the collateral ligaments of the MP and IP joints are at their full length, thus preventing contractures. The fingers should be separated by a layer of petrolatum-impregnated gauze. The wrist should be dorsiflexed.

7. The dressings should be kept clean and dry. Observe frequently whether any exudate has seeped through the dressings. If so, the dressings should be changed. If the outer layers are soiled, then only the soiled layers need to be changed.

8. When bandaging is used after debridement as an early treatment and dressings are changed on the 3rd day after injury, dry dressings should be used to replace the exudate-soiled dressings in order to dry the wound. If, when changing the dressings, the inner layer is dry and adherent to the wound surface, it indicates that there is no serious infection, and the inner layer does not need to be removed; it is only necessary to change the outer layers. If there is a small area of accumulated pus under the inner layer, a small pieces of gauze may be cut off with scissors (the area cut off should be equivalent to the size of pus accumulation). The pus is then absorbed off, and only a small piece of fresh gauze needs to be replaced. As it is not necessary to remove all of the inner layer, trauma or spread of infection may be avoided.

9. When bandaging is used as a method of treatment, all the dressings should be changed and the wound examined in the following cases, which are highly suggestive of severe infection: complaints by the patient of continuous pulsating pain, seeping of exudate or pus through the outer layers, presence of a foul odor, and high fever with abnormally high or low white blood cell count.

10. Special attention is necessary if severe infection of the wound surface is already present when bandaging is reapplied. If proper treatment is not given, the aftereffects might very serious. To give an example: A patient with deep second degree burns to 61% of the BSA, was admitted to the hospital on the 2nd day after injury. At the time of admission, his general condition was fair, but the wound was already heavily infected. After routine simple debridement in the emergency room, the wound surface was dressed with petrolatum-impregnated gauze. (*Note:* the surgeon had used neither Sulfamylon nor silver sulfadiazine, although they were highly indicated). When the dressings were changed on the 3rd day after admission, the wound was found to be heavily infected with *Pseudomonas aeruginosa* and had an appearance of patchy necrosis. The condition of the patient rapidly deteriorated and finally, in spite of various emergency measures, the patient died. Therefore, if a patient with heavy infection of the wound is admitted into the hospital more than 24 h after injury, the wound surface should in principle be treated by full exposure and suitable topical antibacterial agents, such as 10% Sulfamylon cream, 1% silver sulfadiazine cream, should be used. (In deep burns we prefer Sulfamylon, in superficial burns, silver sulfadiazine. In children with very extensive burns we recommend silver sulfadiazine.)

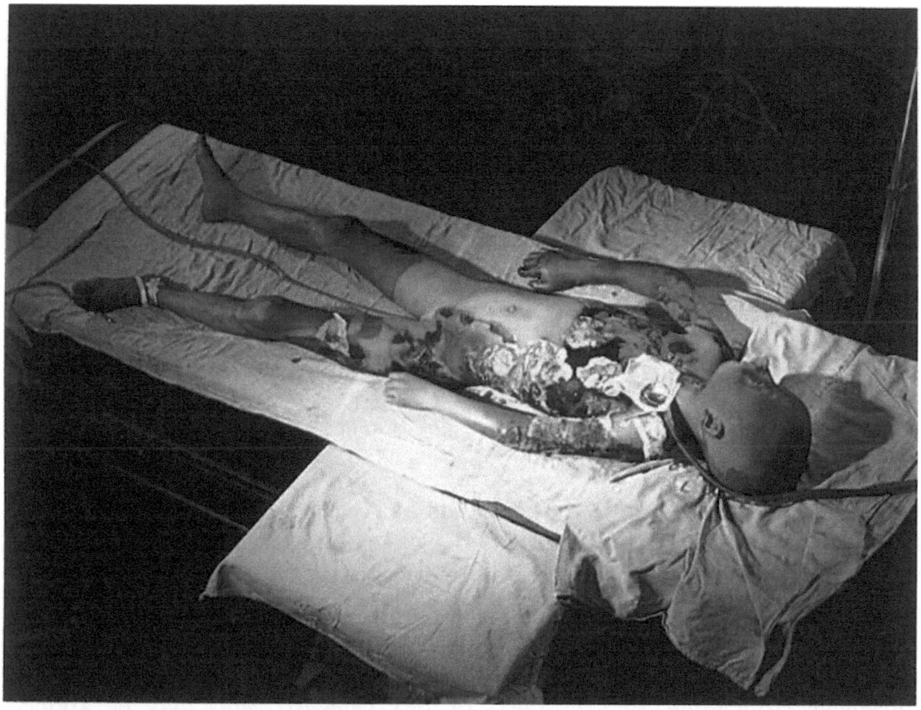

a

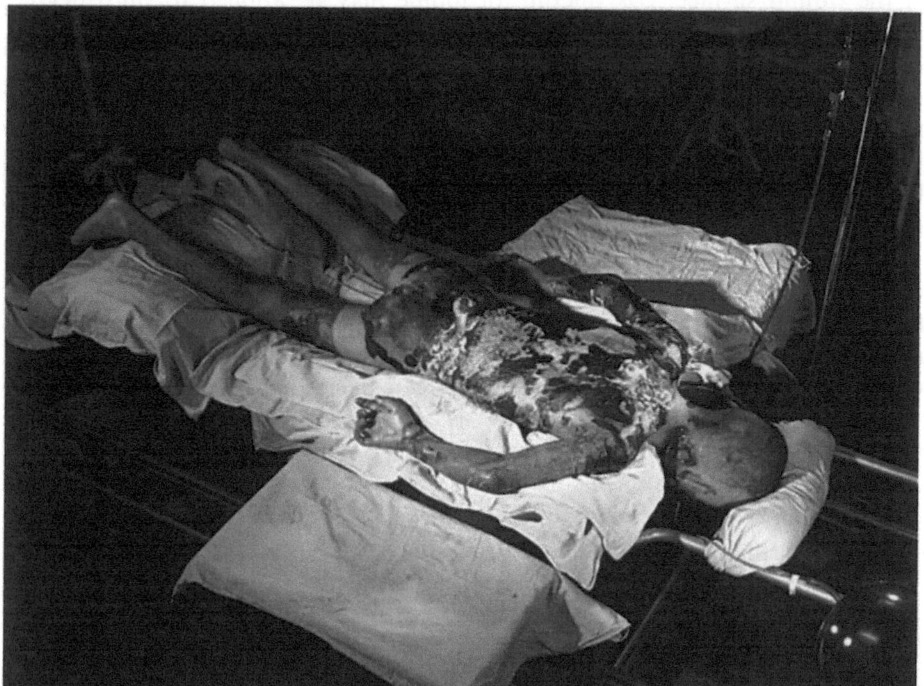

b

Fig. III.2. Treatment by exposure. This patient was seriously injured by lightning, but survived

2.2 Treatment by Exposure (Fig. III.2)

If the condition permits, it is usually best to employ exposure treatment.

2.2.1 Purpose

The principal purpose is to cause rapid drying of the wound and formation of a layer of dry eschar, thereby decreasing the growth of pathogenic bacteria. After the wound surface has been treated properly with exposure, sometimes even a deep second degree burn will achieve subeschar healing, and a third degree burn wound surface may become covered with an integral desiccated eschar.

The advantage of this method is that it facilitates observation of the wound.

2.2.2 Method

After debridement the patient is laid upon a foam plastic mattress with a layer of sterile gauze, and warm air is blown underneath, enabling the wound surface to be directly exposed to warm, dry, clean air. In order to avoid certain parts of the wound under pressure becoming moist, the patient should be turned, to expose these parts periodically by the use of a turning frame. To promote rapid formation of crust or eschar, certain Chinese herb escharotics such as *Polygonum cuspidatum* Sieb. et Zucc. or *Ilex chinensis* Sims may be applied on the wound surface. 2% tincture of iodine may be applied to third degree or deep second degree burns; it can dehydrate the tissue, promoting drying of the wound surface. In order to hasten the formation of eschar on deep second degree and third degree burn wound surfaces, at the time of initial treatment the loosened layer of epidermis should be peeled off, because the stratum corneum of the epidermis prevents evaporation of the exudate and thus delays drying of the necrotic tissue under the epidermis and eschar formation.

During the shock stage (especially when complicated by other injuries), warm dry air ventilation may be used to promote drying of the wound surface if the patient cannot be turned to expose the back. For this purpose the patient may be put upon a mattress made of spongy plastics with large pores on which a single layer of sterile gauze has been placed in advance. The source of dry heat and a ventilating apparatus (electric fan) are placed under the mattress, thus ventilating and drying the wound surface on the patient's back.

In patients with deep burns of the head and/or neck on whom tracheotomy has not been performed and in patients under artificial hibernation in the shock stage, this method makes it possible to dry the back without turning the patient. Any possible accident due to turning is thus avoided.

2.2.3 Indications

1. Wounds of head and face, neck, trunk, buttocks, and perineum;
2. Deep dermal or full-thickness burns;

3. Early severe contamination of wound surfaces with inadequate debridement;

4. Burn wounds infected by gram-negative bacilli (particularly *P. aeruginosa*);

5. Wounds infected by fungi.

2.2.4 Points for Attention

1. Exposure must be full and thorough. The wound surface should not be covered with dressing, clothing, or any other covering.

2. To gain the full benefit of drying, the wound surface should not be submitted to pressure; if any, it should be as light as possible. Therefore, the position of patients suffering from circumferential burns should be changed from time to time in order to expose those parts under pressure. The best methods are to place the patient on a turning frame or to dry the back with warm air ventilation. In principle, the patient ought to be turned to prone position as early as possible, but is imperative to avoid edema of the larynx, which causes asphyxia. In general, the patient may be turned to the prone position when the shock stage is over (in the case of extensive burns, 48 h postburn). The patient should not be left in the prone position too long during the first few times of turning. Intent observation must be maintained by medical personnel. In cases of burns of the head and neck, it is safer to perform tracheotomy in advance if danger of suffocation in the prone position is expected. If the surface of the back becomes moist "mushy", or severely infected or petechial hemorrhages are present, which indicates that the back can no longer bear pressure, ways and means of earlier turning of the patient should be found, because it is profitable to achieve for short durations, even during the shock stage. But, before turning the patient, adequate blood volume should be assured.

3. If absolutely no facility for turning the patient exists, warm air ventilation or periodic changing of dressings (usually 3–4 times a day) may be employed in order to maintain dryness of the part of wound surface under pressure. At the same time as the dressings are changed, the condition of the wound surface of the back must be examined.

4. It is necessary to limit the motion of the patient's body or to employ immobilization in order to avoid further trauma of the wound. If motion of the body is not suitably limited, the eschar may be cracked, and, as a result, bacteria may invade the tissue through the cracks. This is especially important in the case of burned children. If the eschar has been broken, the exposed wound may be covered with iodoform gauze to prevent the spread of infection.

5. If there is no serious infection, the exposed wound surface will usually gradually become dry during the first 24 h after injury. After about 48 h–72 h, a dry crust will be formed on the surface. During this stage, exudates from the wound should be carefully and meticulously wiped off with sterile cotton swabs. If escharotics are used, the crust may be formed earlier than usual.

6. Before the crust is formed, the patient may suffer from pain. Suitable analgesics may be given to alleviate it.

7. On third degree burn eschar, 2% tincture of iodine may be applied 3–6 times per day.

8. If fungi infection is found on the wound surface, 1% clotrimazole in propylene glycol 400 solution or 2% tincture of iodine may be painted on.

9. It is necessary to observe whether there is any accumulation of pus under the crust. If accumulated pus is found, then the crust at that point should be scissored off and the pus removed in order to secure re-formation of the crust. If there is a large amount of pus and the re-formed eschar remains purulent, it is advisable to abandon the exposure method in favor of bandaging.

The exposure method should not be used for wounds with large amounts of pus. Wet dressings should be used or 1% silver sulfadiazine or 10% Sulfamylon cream may be applied. When infection has been controlled, the surface may again be exposed.

Granulation wounds should not be exposed, otherwise the superficial layer of the wound may become dry and necrotic.

2.3 Treatment by Semiexposure

2.3.1 Purpose

The principal purposes are to aid crust formation of deep second degree wound and to immobilize split-skin grafts.

2.3.2 Method

A single layer of Physiologic saline gauze, petrolatum-impregnated gauze, or gauze containing antibiotic solution is cut to suit the size of the wound and then laid on tightly.

2.3.3 Indications

1. Comparatively clean wounds of deep second degree burn, after the sloughing of necrotic tissue.

2. Deep second degree burn, from which the accumulated pus has been removed after exposure treatment. If there is little purulent exudation, the semiexposure method may be used to aid re-formation of a "healthy" crust.

3. For wounds with *P. aeruginosa* infection, a single layer of gauze impregnated with solutions containing 1:500 gentamicin, 1:1,000 polymyxin B, or 10% Sulfamylon may be applied. It is necessary to moisten the gauze from time to time with the above-mentioned solution.

4. Those wound surfaces which, after skin grafting, are not suitable for bandaging, e.g., the trunk, shoulder, axilla, inguinal region, buttocks,

5. Donor areas where bandaging is infeasible.

2.3.4 Points for Attention

1. The semiexposure method should not be used on wounds with a large amount of pus without adequate drainage.

2. In order to avoid the accumulation of pus, the gauze should be applied tightly to the wound surface, no space being left between them.

3. In deep second degree burn wounds with re-formation of the crust after the use of the semiexposure method, pressure should be totally avoided during the following 24 h; if this is impossible, only very slight pressure is permissible. The exposed single-layer wet gauze may gradually dry by evaporation and become adherent to the wound surface. Thus the single layer of gauze forms the outer layer of the crust and the inner layer is dry necrotic tissue. In such instances it is sometimes possible to secure "subcrust" healing.

4. The "crust" formed by the gauze and the exudate should be examined frequently to see if there is any accumulation of pus under it. If there is, the gauze should be removed; one should either apply fresh gauze or employ alternative measures.

It is necessary to note that sometimes when the semiexposed wound surface appears dry, there is actually pus underneath the crust. Therefore, when pus accumulation is suspected several small openings should be made with scissors for scrupulous examination.

5. Semiexposure is used to immobilize split-skin grafts on the granulating surface. If pus has accumulated in the interspace, then the semiexposure gauze should be changed. If there is a good deal of pus, then the gauze may need to be changed several times a day when the patient is turned.

6. If pus has accumulated under the "crust" formed after semiexposure, the gauze should be changed at a time when the surface has just been subjected to pressure for a relatively long period (e.g., semiexposure gauze on the back should be removed when the patient is turned into the prone position). This is because the "crust" becomes moist after pressure and is then easy to remove, thus reducing bleeding, trauma, and pain. Alternatively, the gauze may be moistened with wet dressing or softened by the use of liquid paraffin and then removed.

2.4 Treatment with Wet Dressing

2.4.1 Purpose

The principal purpose of this method is to clean away exudation, purulent crust, and necrotic tissue in order to decrease infection and to hasten sloughing of the crust.

2.4.2 Method

Three to six layers of gauze with good absorbent qualities are wetted with physiologic saline solution (or any other antibiotic solution) and then squeezed fairly dry before being laid smoothly on the wound. Bandages are applied.

2.4.3 Indications

1. Wounds with comparatively large amounts of purulent exudate.
2. Wounds with purulent crust formation after exposure treatment.
3. Granulation wounds in preparation for skin grafting.

2.4.4 Points for Attention

1. Usually, wet dressings should be changed twice a day. However, when infection is serious and there is a larger than average amount of pus, the gauze should be changed more often.

As the infection is being brought under control, the interval between dressing changes may be decreased accordingly. If antibiotic solutions are used in the wet dressing, it needs to be changed only once or twice a day.

2. When necessary, the antibiotic solution used for wet compressing may be selected on the basis of the species of bacteria cultured from the wound. Frequently 1:6,000 furacilin, 1% neomycin, 0.1% Hibitane, 10% Sulfamylon, 0.2% gentamicin, or 0.1% polymyxin B are used. When such a solution is used, two layers of gauze are sufficient.

3. For wounds with large amounts of necrotic tissue, Dakin's solution may be selected.

4. For edematous granulating wounds, wet compressing with 2.5%–4% physiologic saline solution and pressure bandaging may be used.

5. For the parts suitable for bandaging, such as extremities and face, wet dressings may be kept in place by pressure bandaging, in order to prevent slipping and to promote drainage.

6. Whenever the wound with a large amount of necrotic tissue is heavily infected by *P. aeruginosa*, wet dressing should not be used (Sulfamylon or gentamicin wet dressings are also contraindicated) since it may aggravate the infection and endanger the patient's life.

2.5 Treatment by Immersion

2.5.1 Purpose

Treatment by immersion cleans the wound surface, decreases the number of infective bacteria and amount of toxin, promotes the separation of eschar, and facilitates drainage of pus accumulated beneath the eschar.

2.5.2 Method

Immersion of the whole body or part of the body. The wound should be immersed thoroughly in tepid physiologic saline solution.

2.5.3 Indications

1. Infected wound of extremities.

2. In the stage of separation of the eschar.

3. Extensively burned patients in the late stage of hospitalization with remnant small, heavily infected wounds.

2.5.4 Points for Attention

1. Before the first immersion, the attending physician or nurse must take steps to free the patient's mind of all misgivings concerning the method of treatment.

2. The immersion fluid may be a solution containing 0.9% table salt.

3. The patient's opinion with regard to the temperature of the water may be taken into consideration. Generally, it should be 1° C warmer as compared to the patient's body temperature. During the process of immersion, the temperature of the fluid should be kept constant.

4. Immersion should not last too long; it is advisable not to exceed 30 min.

5. After the bath, dry the patient quickly with dry gauze use heat or warm air to prevent the patient catching cold.

6. If bandaging treatment is used, after the removal of the outer layers, the inner layers may be immersed for a certain time. When they become loose, they are removed slowly while still in the fluid to lessen bleeding and pain. At the same time, the softened separated parts of the eschar may be scissored off.

7. When the whole body is immersed, care must be taken to observe the general condition of the patient. Immersion should be stopped immediately if pulse and respiration accelerate and the patient appears pale with signs of collapse.

8. As to the number of immersions as well as the time interval between them, a decision may be made in accordance with patient's condition and general reaction. When there are heavily infected wounds, immersion should take place once a day.

9. Usually after whole body immersion of an extensively burned patient, the body temperature is elevated, the pulse quickened, and the patient feels tired. After a few hours rest, recovery will gradually take place.

10. After skin grafting, the grafted area may be immersed within 48 h–72 h. The donor areas, however, should usually be kept dry for 1 week.

11. For those patients with remnant small, heavily infected wounds in the late stage of extensive burns, soap should be used at the time of immersion to clean thoroughly the skin surrounding the wounds as well as other parts of the body.

12. After immersion, treatment by exposure, semiexposure, wet compressing, or bandaging may be used, according to the condition of the wound.

13. After immersion, all the utensils used should be disinfected with 3%–5% cresol and soap solution and kept dry in order to eliminate cross infection.

3 Application and Choice of Chinese Herb Medicine

Chinese medicine and pharmacology is a great treasure house. For many years we had a fixed belief that escharotics containing tannins are very toxic to the liver and might be lethal, and that they should therefore not be used on burns. Thus we abandoned the use of Chinese escharotic herb medicine in treating burns simply because it contains various amounts of tannin.

Recently we have again investigated Chinese escharotic herb medicine containing tannin. From the laboratory data concerning the hepatic toxicity of seven tannins extracted from Chinese herb medicine, we gained the impression that the hydrolyzable group of tannins possesses strong toxicity while the condensed group has either only minor reversible toxicity or no hepatic toxicity at all. Tannins extracted from commonly used Chinese herb medicine belong either to the hydrolyzable group or to the condensed group. Therefore, concrete analysis and categorization of these tannins is necessary.

We used 10% *Polygonum cuspidatum* on up to 70% of the BSA, and no damage to the liver was seen. When *P. cuspidatum* solution is painted on to the wound surface after debridement, eschar formation is rapid. In certain second degree burns, primary healing under the eschar has been obtained.

The experimental data on hand show that with the use of 1:100 tincture of *P. cuspidatum* for in vitro bactericidal experiments, the following gram-negative bacilli may be killed: *B. pseudomonous*, *Proteus*, and E. coli, as well as the following gram-positive cocci: *Staphylococcus aureus*, *Streptococcus faecalis*, *Streptococcus pyogenes*, and *Monilia albicans*. By the application of the commonly used astringent Chinese escharotic herbs, we found that not only is exudation of the wound decreased, but also infection.

Many kinds of Chinese herb preparations are used for topical application in burn injuries. In general, they may be divided into three groups:

1. Crust-forming drugs with astringent effect;
2. Eschar-removal drugs with properties of promoting separation of necrotic tissue;
3. Wound-healing drugs with properties of promoting the growth of epidermis.

All three groups have specific indications as well as points for attention. The requirement for treatment varies with different kinds of wounds. It is not permissible to use invariably one certain drug for all wounds irrespective of the depth of burn and presence or absence of infection.

3.1 Crust-Forming Drugs

3.1.1 Purpose

The purpose of the use of these drugs is to promote rapid formation of pressure-bearing dry crust, thereby avoiding or lessening infection, and to secure healing under the crust. They are suitable for second degree wound surfaces.

3.1.2 Points for Attention

1. One must constantly pay attention to the possible existence of accumulated pus under the crust. If pus is found to be present, the eschar should be removed and drainage established.
2. These drugs should be used immediately after debridement, before the wound becomes infected.

3. Whether it is possible to secure the good result of primary healing under the eschar depends upon the amount of necrotic tissue or the amount of remaining dermal elements as well as upon factors related to infection. If, on the deep second degree wound, few dermal elements are left and much necrotic tissue is present, then the rate of infection under the crust is bound to be high. It would therefore be rather difficult to secure primary healing under the crust.

4. On the basis of the data on hand, the condensed type of tannins contained in *P. cuspidatum* Sieb, et Zucc., *Ilex chinensis* Sims, and *Loropetalum chinense* Oliv. are the principal substances with astringent function. These tannins have little toxic effect on the liver.

5. A suitable amount of *Asarum sieboldi* Mig, *Alpinia officinarum* Hance or large dosage of *dl*-borneol may be added to these crust-forming drugs to lessen pain arising from the stimulation of wound surfaces by these drugs.

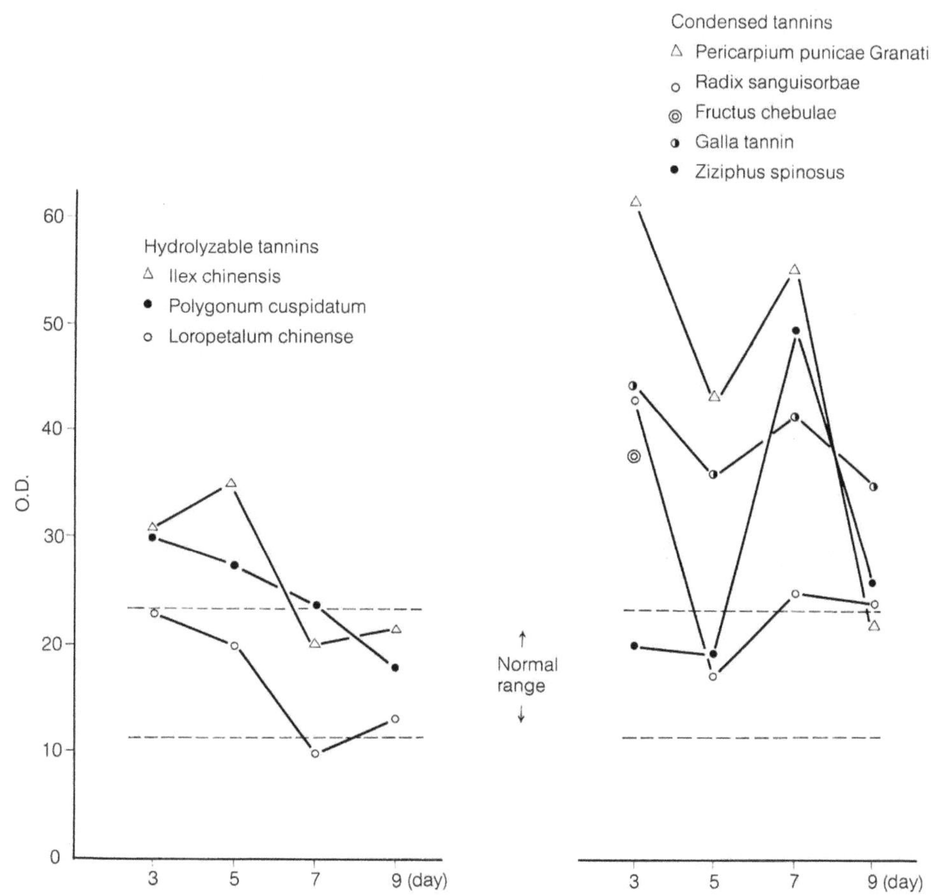

Fig. III.3. The effects of condensed and hydrolyzable tannins on the SGPT of albino mice. *O.D.*, optic density of spectrophotometer

3.1.3 Choice of Drug

Polygonum cuspidatum Sieb. et Zucc. preparations: This category of escharotics is suitable for superficial second degree wounds. The preparations may be spread on the wound surface as a powder, painted on as a paste formed by mixing with sesame oil or water, or used as 10% tinctures.

1. Frequency of application: After debridement, apply to the clean wound surface twice with intervals of 2 h. If there is a large amount of exudation, the number of applications should be increased.

2. Experimental observation: In regard to the chemical structures, tannins may be divided into two groups, the hydrolyzable type and the condensed type. Hydrolyzable tannins contain ester or glucosidic bonds. When reacting with acids they are readily broken down into substances no longer possessing any tannin effect. We choose pericarpium *Punicae granati,* fructus *Chebulae,* radix *Sanguisorbae, Ziziphus spinosus* bark, and *Galla chinensis* (usually called medical tannin) as the sources of experimental hydrolyzable tannin (confirmed by colorimetric determination).

The molecular structure of the condensed type contains only one single carbon skeleton and the benzene nuclei which build up these molecules are linked by carbon-carbon bonds. When reacting with strong acids, the molecules immediately condense into an amorphous red precipitate – tannin red. Tannins from *P. cuspidatum* Sieb. et Zucc., *Loropetalum chinense* Oliv., and *Ilex chinensis* Sims belong to the condensed type.

Corresponding tannin concentrations of the above-mentioned herbs were adjusted using 0.5% *Galla* tannin (conventional medical tannin) as standard

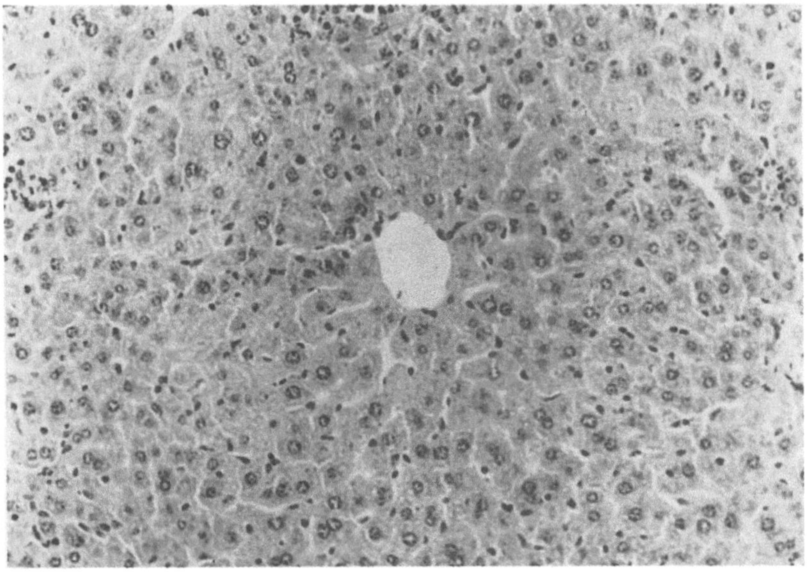

Fig. III.4. The regularly arranged hepatic cords of a normal albino mouse

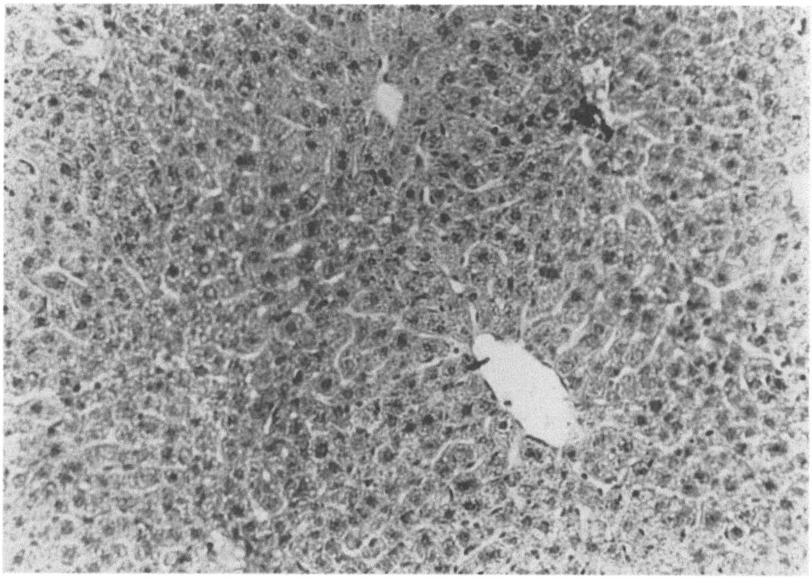

Fig. III.5. After injection of *P. cuspidatum* extract in an albino mouse, hepatic cords are seen to remain regular. Degeneration of hepatic cells and inflammatory cell infiltration are mild

and injected subcutaneously for a certain number of days to groups of mice. Serum SGPT determinations and histologic examinations of the liver were made. Figure III.3 shows the SGPT values within 9 days after administration of the tannins. Those of the condensed type, i.e., *P. cuspidatum* Sieb. et Zucc., *Ilex chinensis* Sims, and *Loropetalum chinense* Oliv. were normal or nearly normal, whereas the hydrolyzable tannins from pericarpium *Punicae granati,* radix *Sanguisorbae, Ziziphus spinosus,* and fructus *Chebulae*, and *Galla* tannins caused consistently elevated SGPT values (*Galla* tannin) or elevated values at the early stage (*Pericarpium punicae* Granati and Radix *sanguisorbae*) or the late stage (*Ziziphus spinosus*) during the 9-day period.

In regard to histologic changes in the liver, in the *P. cuspidatum* tannin group of mice no significant gross changes were observed, and only a few animals presented a swollen, pale liver. Microscopically the hepatic cords were arranged regularly, with integral cells, homogeneous cytoplasm, and distinct nuclear contents. A few specimens showed varying degrees of degenerative changes, vacuole formation, and minimal inflammatory cell infiltration, but no significant hepatic cellular necrosis was found, even at the late stage. These findings denote that the toxicity was low. In the *Galla* tannin group of mice, histologic examination of sections of the livers after the same or even smaller doses showed central necrosis, loss of cellular structure, vacuolation, acidophilic staining, infiltration of large amounts of inflammatory cells, pyknotic nuclei, and derangement of hepatic cords. A few animals had scattered focal necrosis. At the late stage, degenerative changes and focal necrosis of the hepatic cells still persisted despite a certain recovery (Figs. III.4–III.6).

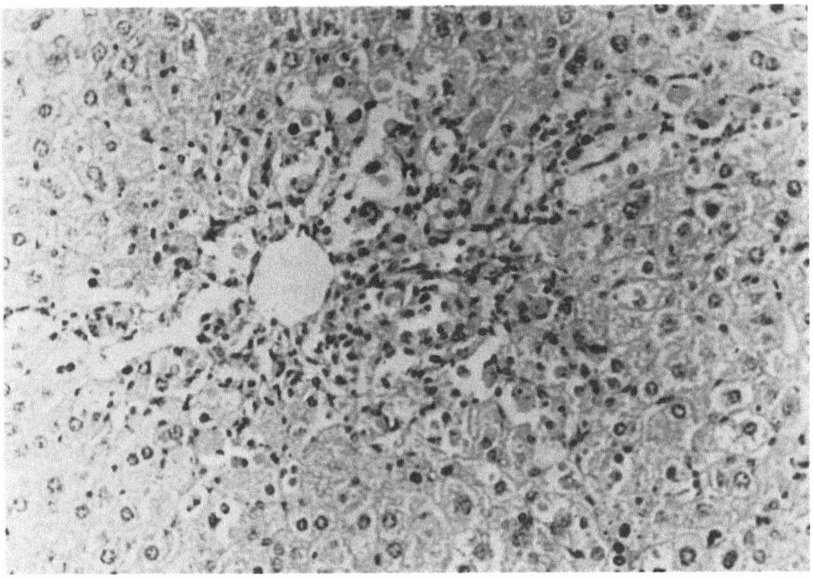

Fig. III.6. After injection of *Galla* tannin, the liver of the albino mouse showed central necrosis, degeneration of hepatic cells, and massive infiltration by inflammatory cells

3.2 Eschar Removal Drugs

3.2.1 Purpose

The purpose of the use of this category of medicament is to promote separation of the necrotic tissue and formation of fresh granulation tissue and to secure coverage of the wound at an early date after skin grafting. These drugs are also used for drainage of the wound. They are suitable for use on third degree wounds or on infected deep second degree wounds.

3.2.2 Points for Attention

1. During treatment with these drugs there is a large amount of purulent exudation, especially when the necrotic tissues are about to separate. This is a normal phenomenon and no cause for concern.

2. If a certain degree of general reaction, such as high fever, loss of appetite, and increase of thirst, occurs and is accompanied by large amounts of local purulent exudation, then supportive treatment must be given. The stronger the function of the eschar removal drugs, the more evident the general reaction will be.

3. The number of days required for the sloughing of eschar is related to the condition of the necrotic tissue when the drugs are applied. The later the drugs are used, the fewer the medication days required, because the eschar

already has the tendency to separate. Vice versa, the earlier the drugs are used, the more medication days are needed. Therefore, in order to obtain the removal of eschar as early as possible on the one hand, and to restrict the amount of time that drugs are applied on the other, it is proper to begin using the drugs 5–7 days after the injury.

4. In order to avoid the separation and removal of the entire eschar all at once, which would leave too large an area of exposed granulation tissue and no means of covering it with allografts or xenografts (because immediately after the sloughing of the eschar there is usually some infected dead tissue adhering to the wound, and time is needed to prepare the wound for grafting), it is necessary to control the amount of eschar separation within a certain defined degree. This amount should be established on the basis of the size of the patient's total burn area, the area covered by third degree burns, and the patient's general condition. Usually removal of an amount of eschar of up to 10% of the BSA is sufficient at one time. When the burn area is large, stage removals should be performed.

5. A number of islets of skin may sometimes be seen after the castoff of the necrotic tissue. They must not be mistaken for necrotic tissue and removed mechanically.

3.2.3 Choice of Drug

3.2.3.1 Wound Healing Ointment No. 10

This ointment is suitable for the removal of eschar of third degree wound.

Preparation. 1,000 g calcined smithsonite, 800 g calcined gypsum, 800 g calcined mirabilite, 800 g *Pteria margaritifera*, 20 g *dl*- borneol, 10 g ethylparaben, 5,000 g Vaseline, 1,000 g lanolin, and quantum sufficit of liquid paraffin.

Method of Application. With a sterilized tongue depressor, paint the ointment on sterilized gauze to a thickness of 1 mm–3 mm over an area a little bigger than the wound surface. The gauze is placed directly over the wound and bandaged with a certain amount of dressings. At the time of separation of the necrotic tissue, the dressings should be thicker owing to the presence of large amounts of purulent fluid. Generally, the dressings are changed every other day but if there is an abundance of purulent fluid, then they should be changed once a day. Every time that the medicated gauze is changed, all of the already separated necrotic tissue should be gently scissored off, avoiding bleeding if possible; the exudates are then gently sponged off with sterilized physiologic saline gauze, and fresh medicated gauze applied. When the necrotic tissues have been removed and after the appearance of fresh granulation tissue suitable for skin grafting, this medication is discontinued and the wound surface is dressed with physiologic saline or antibiotic solution to prepare it for skin grafting on the next day. Alternatively, after a short period of physiologic saline wet dressing, skin grafting is done right away. After skin grafting, Wound Healing Ointment No. 10 is no longer required.

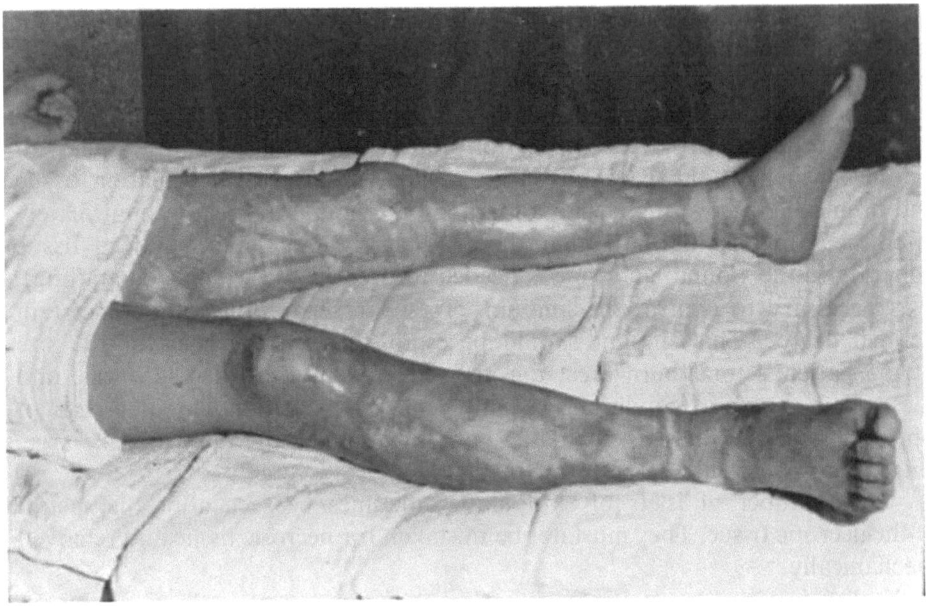

Fig. III.7. Twenty-year-old male with flame burns to 30% of the BSA, including third degree burns to 20%. The photograph was taken on the 2nd day postburn, prior to local application of Wound Healing Ointment No. 10

Clinical Observations. We have observed the results of the use of this ointment on the wound surface in 33 cases, as follows: medication area 3%–5% of the BSA, 7 cases; 6%–9% of the BSA, 10 cases; above 10% of the BSA, 16 cases (among them 3 involving medication to over 20% of the BSA). At the time when the medication was used, the wounds had already formed a dry eschar with various degrees of infection. When medication was used within 7 days after injury, usually most of the necrotic tissue had separated 3–8 days later, and after preparation, skin might be grafted on the next day or even on the same day. When Wound Healing Ointment No. 10 was used for eschar removal, the granulations on the wound surface were fresh, and the percentage of take of grafted skin was high. With the use of Wound Healing Ointment no. 10, maturation of the granulation tissue under the third degree eschar as a rule took place at least about 1 week earlier than spontaneous separation (Figs. III.7, III.8). Consequently, the wound was covered earlier than usual. On the dorsum of the foot, ankle, and the front of the tibia, where only a

Fig. III.8. a Same patient as in **Fig. III.7,** 16 days postburn and 8 days after the application ▷ of Wound Healing Ointment No. 10. Most of the eschar is sloughed and fresh granulation tissue is seen. **b** Same patient, 20 days postburn and 12 days after the application of Wound Healing Ointment No. 10. All the necrotic tissue has sloughed off. The granulation tissue is fresh and ready to accept a graft

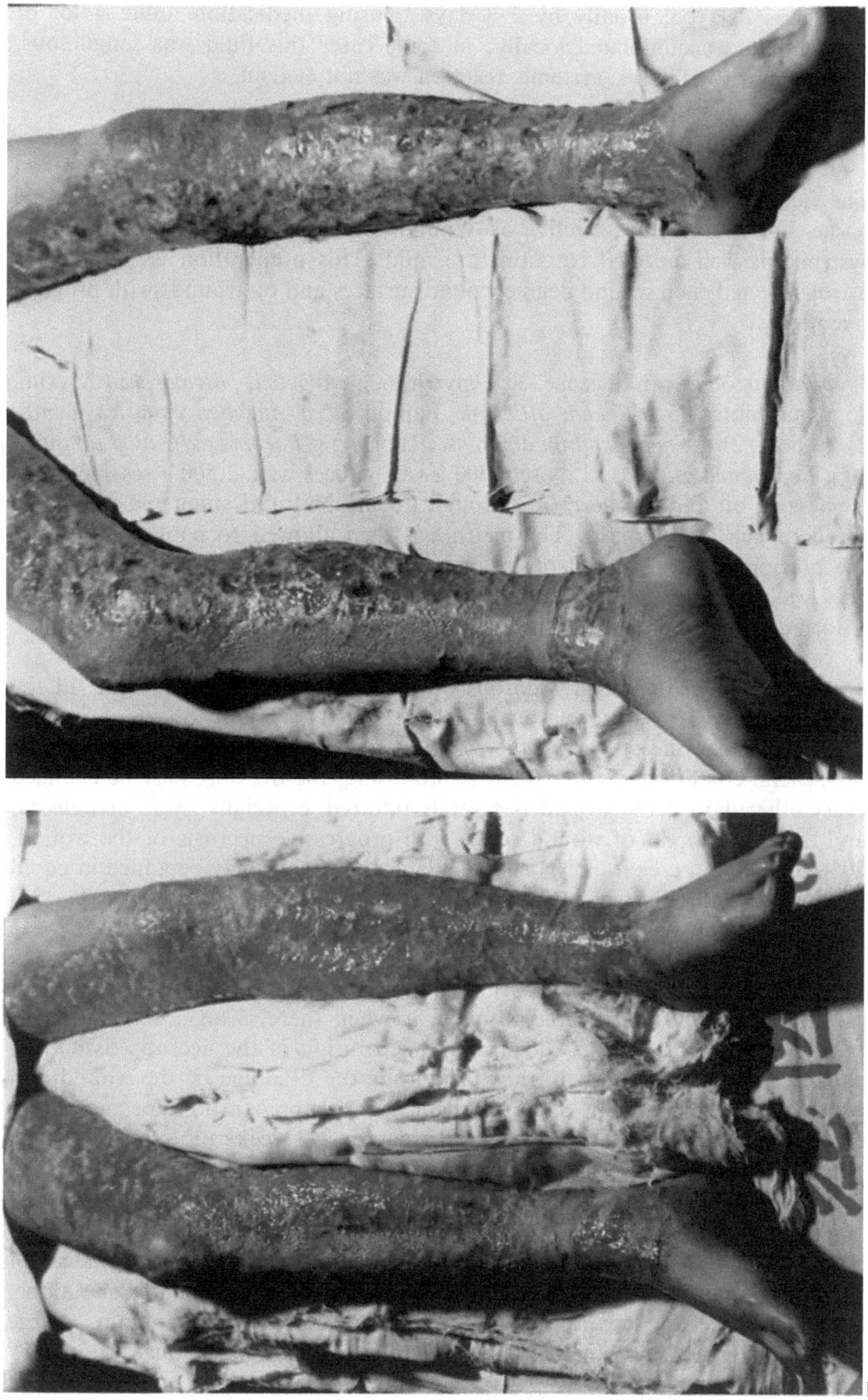

a

b

very small amount of subcutaneous fat is present, separation of the necrotic tissue was delayed, usually by 2–3 days. During medication, quite a lot of purulent fluid accumulated locally; in some cases this fluid was sanguinous. In the majority of cases, systemic reaction was not evident.

3.2.3.2 Burn and Scald Ointment

The function of this ointment is also to promote the separation of necrotic tissue, but it is not as effective as Wound Healing Ointment no. 10. Again, systemic as well as local reactions are mild. This preparation is suitable for use on infected deep second degree wound surfaces and on wounds with progressive necrosis.

Preparation. 30 g frankincense, 30 g myrrh, 60 g *Angelica polymorphea* Maxim, 45 g mirabilite, 45 g *Rheum officinale* Baillon, 45 g *Angelica dahurica* Benth, 21 g Lacca, 21 g *Pnellodendron amurense* Rupr, 45 g *Paeonia suffruticosa* Andr., 90 g *Rehmannia glutinosa* Libosch, 300 g yellow bees wax, 1,500 g sesame oil.

Sesame oil and the herbs are brought to the boil and simmered until they are homogeneously mixed. The mixture is then allowed to cool slightly, and the precipitates are filtered off using a stainless steel sieve. Chips of yellow bees wax are then added, and the mixture stirred until it is well mixed. It is then allowed to cool naturally, and forms a homogeneous brown ointment.

Method of Application. Stir vigorously with a sterile tongue depressor till the ointment turns to a thin paste and then spread it evenly on sterile gauze. Place the gauze directly over the wound, and secure it with a bandage. If the general condition of the patient is promising, the dressing may be changed every other day. If the wound is severely infected, especially by *P. aeruginosa*, and there is a threat of wound sepsis with progressive necrosis of the wound, 20% Sulfamylon cream or 2% silver sulfadiazine cream may be added in equal portions into the ointment; the dressing should then be changed every 6–12 h until the patient's general condition improves.

Clinical Observations. Burn and Scald Ointment may be considered for purulent eschars of deep second degree wounds or when there is an accumulation of pus under the crust, because it promotes separation of the necrotic tissue and enhances granulation growth, thus facilitating the drainage of the wound and protecting the remnants of epidermal elements. This preparation does not accelerate re-epithelization: as a rule, it will require 2–3 weeks (about 16–17 days) before the generation of new epidermis. At that time fever will show a marked drop. Complete healing of the wound will require another 5–10 days.

When wound sepsis appears, 10% Sulfamylon cream or 1% silver sulfadiazine may be added to the Burn and Scald Ointment. The drainage effect of the latter is much better than that of Sulfamylon or silver sulfadiazine alone. It can promote the separation of the necrotic tissues (which contain a large amount of bacteria) from their base, manifesting first as gradual "floating" and then as casting-off, leaving a fresh granulating surface.

3.3 Wound-Healing Drugs

3.3.1 Purpose

The purpose of using this kind of preparation is to stimulate the growth of the epidermis. Indications for the use of drugs of this group are not always the same: some are indicated in superficial second degree burns, while others are suitable for use on small remnant granulation wound appearing at the late stage. Nevertheless, all of them possess the function of stimulating the growth of epithelium, and they are therefore included in the same group.

3.3.2 Points for Attention

1. As a rule, drugs of this group possess no bacteriocidal or bacteriostatic effect, and if they do have such an effect, then it is very weak. Therefore they are not to be used on seriously infected wounds with a copious amount of purulent exudate. These drugs will give good results only after infection has been adequately controlled.

2. For preparation, oil base is preferred.

3. When smearing a layer of the preparation on to the gauze or preparing impregnated gauze, care should be taken not to block the mesh of the gauze, in order to facilitate drainage.

3.3.3 Choice of Drugs

3.3.3.1 Lacca Ointment

This ointment is indicated for superficial or deep second degree wounds and donor areas.

Preparation. 30 g lacca, 30 g *Lonicera japonica* Thunb, 30 g *Angelica dahurica*, 30 g *Rheum officinale* Baill, 45 g sesame oil, 30 g yellow wax.

Heat the sesame oil slightly. Add lacca, *L. japonica* Thunb, *A. dahurica*, and *R. officinale* Baill. Heat until the *A. dahurica* becomes brown (at about 30 min), and then filter off the residues. Melt the yellow bees wax in the filtrate while heating, and let it cool naturally.

Method of Application. When gauze impregnated with this ointment is used for uninfected or only slightly infected wounds, it needs to be changed only every 3–4 days. For seriously infected surfaces with a large amount of pus, it should be changed daily.

Clinical Observations. This preparation has anti-inflammatory and analgesic properties, as well as the function of stimulating the growth of the epidermis. After the application of this ointment on superficial or deep second degree wounds, the patient feels quite comfortable owing to its local soothing effect. It also has the advantage that the inner layer of the dressings usually remains dry and the rate of infection is low.

3.3.3.2 "Duet Ointment"

Duet ointment is indicated for the small granulation wounds present at the late stage of the healing process.

Prepation. 9 g lead tetroxide, 0.9 g *dl*-borneol, 30 g calcined gypsum, 30 g boric acid, 9 g lead monoxide. Grind and then mix evenly with Vaseline.

Method of Application. The ointment may be smeared on a piece of sterilized gauze by the use of a sterilized tongue depressor, or ready-made gauze impregnated with the preparation may be used. When impregnated gauze is being prepared, one should wear sterilized gloves. The ointment should be thoroughly soaked into the gauze so that it is distributed evenly into the latter. Light pressure should be applied when bandaging. If the wound surface is heavily infected with large amounts of pus, this preparation should not be used until the infection has been controlled since it possesses no bacteriocidal or bacteriostatic properties.

Clinical Observations. For more than twenty years of observation, our practical experiences have shown that Duet Ointment has a proposed function of accelerating the extension of creeping epidermis on the periphery of the granulation wound. Nevertheless, in the case of heavily infected wounds, due to the presence of plenty of pus, the result will be interfered with.

4 Treatment of Third Degree Eschar

The treatment of third degree burn wounds includes the removal of the eschar and transplantation of skin. In this section, the problem of removal of the eschar is discussed. In principle, there are two ways of removing the eschar: by spontaneous separation (including removal by medication) and by operative measures. In clinical practice, we should use both methods, without favoring one and neglecting the other.

4.1 Spontaneous Separation (or Withering Away) of Eschar by "Silkworm Bite"

After the self-dissoluted necrotic tissue of third degree eschar is separated from the new growth of granulation tissue, the already separated and loosened eschar should be scissored off immediately. The maneuver must be conducted gently, so as to avoid bleeding if possible. If the granulation tissue appears fresh and healthy after the casting-off of the eschar, grafting – using small stamp-sized autografts – should be done immediately to cover the wound surface, even if some remains of necrotic tissues are still present. This is due to the fact that at this time the ability of the wound to accept skin graft is at its maximum; delay may cause a valuable opportunity to be missed. The longer the granulation tissue is exposed, the greater is (a) the chance of infection and (b) general debilitation. Therefore, after the eschar has been cast off, the principle of "graft-

Table III.1. Details concerning autografting in three extensively burned patients who survived (burns exceeded 80% of the BSA, including third degree burns of more than 50%)

Case number	Age (yrs)	Percentage of BSA burned/III°	1st autograft operation (days postburn)	Interval between two autograft operations (days)	No. of autografts	Amount of autografts harvested each time (cm^2)	Total amount of autografts harvested (cm^2)	Ultimate coverage of wound (days postburn)
1	33	81/60	20	2–15[a] (5.9)	9	20–800[a] (215)	2,150[b]	74
2	28	98/81	16	1–7 (3.5)	18	12–277 (95)	1,707	79
3	44	80/52	20	2–8 (3.6)	12	30–100 (82)	985	64

[a] Average figures are in parentheses
[b] Stamp-sized autografts were used

ing as much as possible" should be adopted to ensure that the wound is covered with autografts or allografts in time. In the case of extensive burns, coverage with skin should be done as soon as the granulating wounds are exposed. Since all granulation tissue is infected, culture for bacteria will always be positive; therefore there is no need to wait for a negative culture before skin is grafted. Generally speaking, apart from hemolytic *Streptococcus* and hemolytic *Staphylococcus aureus,* no other bacterium influences the take of skin grafts. Nevertheless, if the wound is seriously infected with the presence of large quantities of purulent exudate unfavorable to the take of the skin grafts, then before skin grafts are transplanted one should treat the wound (usually for 1–3 days) until the local infection is adequately controlled.

In the case of more extensive and deep third degree burns, removal of a large area of eschar all at once would be liable to induce sepsis. Therefore one should protect one part of the eschar while causing another part to separate earlier. To "protect" the eschar means to protect its integrity and dryness, and to minimize pressure bearing. Chinese herb medicine with astringent properties may be used to this end. On the other hand, in order to promote the separation of the eschar, the best technique is to moisten it. For this purpose, dressings with Chinese herbal ointment may be applied (cf. Sect. II.2).

In order to secure immediate coverage in extensively burned patients after spontaneous separation of the eschar, numerous operations are needed. However, since the time required for each operation is short and no deep anesthesia is necessary, patients usually come through the operations quite well.

Table III.1 shows the condition of autografting in three patients with burns of more than 80% of the BSA, including third degree burns to more than 50% of the BSA, and spontaneous separation of eschar (all three patients survived).

Sometimes it is not necessary to wait for complete separation of the third degree eschar, since debridement may be done when the patient's condition permits (Fig. III.9). Between the 2nd and 3rd week after injury, when there is already a new growth of granulation tissue under the eschar, we place the patient under general anesthesia and "help" to separate the eschar by trimming

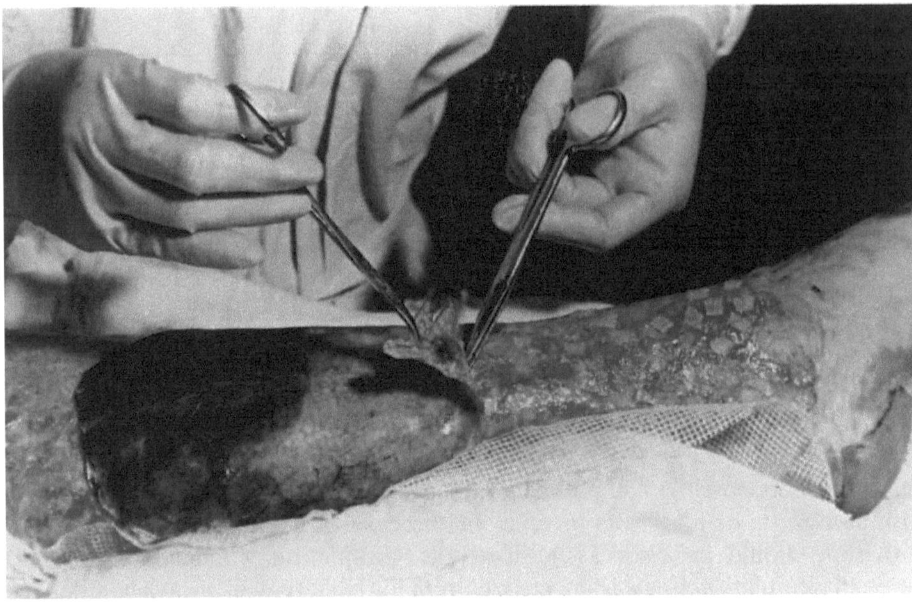

Fig. III.9. Debridement using scissors. The granulation bed is suitable for skin grafting

the wound with scissors or a knife. Skin grafting may be done after the use of wet dressing or bandaging until the necrotic tissue further casts away (after 2–3 days). Debridement, however, must be avoided before the eschar has the tendency to separate spontaneously, the reason being that at this time its base is formed by necrotic tissue, and skin grafting could not be performed within a short period after debridement. Moreover, the ability of the adipose tissue to resist infection is weak; consequently it is liable to be infected when exposed and serious consequences may ensue.

4.2 Surgical Removal of Eschar

4.2.1 Indications for Tangential Excision

1. For deep second degree and third degree burns, especially deep second degree burn of functional parts.

2. For wounds soiled with absorbable poisonous substances (emergency tangential excison may be considered in such cases).

Before the operation, the depth of the burn must be estimated by experienced surgeon in order to avoid an excision which is too shallow or too deep. If the excision is too shallow, necrotic tissues may be left behind and subsequent skin grafting may end in failure; if too deep, the remnants of the epidermis may all be excised and a deep second degree wound for which autografting was not needed originally may thus be turned into a third degree wound. It is not easy for an inexperienced surgeon to achieve an ideal depth at the first attempt. The technique of tangential excision is essentially similar to that of obtaining split-thickness skin grafts. On the extremities, tangential excision may be carried out with the use of a tourniquet (nevertheless, a tourniquet renders it comparatively difficult to judge the depth). As a rule, for deep second degree burns excision should reach a silvery, shiny surface, resulting in a surface which is devoid of thrombosed capillaries. For third degree eschar, excision should reach normal adipose tissue. After careful hemostasis, skin grafting is performed and a pressure bandage applied. In recent years, we have also used porcine skin for the coverage of the wound after tangential excision of deep second degree burns.

When the tourniquet is not used, it is comparatively easy to judge the depth of excision. For deep second degree burns, when excision is extended to the depth of normal tissue, active pinpoint bleeding points can be seen. As stated above, for third degree burns excision must reach the normal adipose tissue, which shows shiny yellowish fat with active bleeding points and is devoid of thrombosed vessels. After hemostasis, the wound is covered with grafts and a pressure bandage is applied. For deep second degree burns, allografts, thin sheets of xenografts, or artificial skin substitutes may be used in place of autografts. However, some autografting is often necessary in order to obtain good functional results. After the wound has healed, allografts, xenografts, or artificial skin will drop off spontaneously. For third degree burns, thin sheets of autografts intermingled with allografts are transplanted.

4.2.2 Eschar Excision

For deep third degree burns, excision of the eschar in combination with skin grafting may be used. It is possible to cover the wound at an earlier date, thereby shortening the course of treatment and avoiding various complications. For third degree burns located on the hand or functional parts of the joints, after eschar excision and grafting of large sheets of skin, contracture may be reduced to a minimum and the recovery of function is satisfactory. Therefore, comparatively speaking, this is an ideal method.

4.2.2.1 Indications

1. Localized third degree wound surfaces on the extremities and the trunk, especially when charred subcutaneous fat and muscles are present.
2. Infected wounds which seriously threaten the life of the patient (foci of wound sepsis).
3. Very extensive third degree burns, especially when it is difficult to obtain autografts.
4. Deep burns of functional parts of the body, e.g., neck, hand, and joints. With a view to the optimal recovery of function, eschar excision may be performed in combination with the use of large sheets of autograft or mesh graft.
5. Contaminated burn surfaces with the possibility of absorption of poisonous substances (such as inorganic phosphorus burn).

4.2.2.2 Timing

The timing of excision should be determined by the patient's general condition, the total burned area, and the extent of third degree burn.

1. For minor burns with small third degree burns, third degree eschar may be excised immediately after injury if the general condition of the patient permits.

2. For extensive burns with third degree burns, it is necessary to wait until the patient has smoothly passed the shock stage before excising the eschar. Eschar excision may be done 3–14 days after injury, depending upon the patient's general condition, and may be performed all at once or in several stages. In extensive third degree burns, one should strive to excise the eschar as soon as possible, since when excision is performed at an early date, infection is slight and the rate of take of skin grafts is high. The time of the first excision operation should, as a rule, be about 5 days after injury. At this time the patient has already passed the shock stage, edema has essentially been reabsorbed, and the patient is in a relatively stable condition. After the shock stage, when edema is being resorbed, symptoms of toxemia or even sepsis may appear. Some patients will have a reduced white cell count and lowered resistance against infection. Therefore, if the timing of the first operation is selected before the resorption of edema, then the reaction to the operation will coincide with toxemia or sepsis and the patient will not usually survive. Nevertheless, if the wound is seriously infected and there is onset of severe sepsis, the first operation may be advanced in order to excise the foci of infection.

Case Illustration. Male, aged 3. The patient had burns to 50% of the BSA, including third degree burns to 39%. He was admitted 18 h postburn. After shock was rectified, the patient became extremely irritable and restless. His pulse was above 200 per minute; respiration was 46 per minute, with cogwheel breathing. The wound was heavily infected, and the patient was in critical condition. Fifty-two hours after injury and on the 5th postburn day we excised third degree eschar covering 34% of the BSA during two operations and transplanted immediately with large sheets of allografts. After the operations, the patient's deteriorating condition was checked. The wound was covered with autografts 33 days after injury.

As a rule, eschar excision operations are not to be done later than 3 weeks after injury, since the major part of the eschar has then already dissolved and new growths of granulation tissue are already present, which may render the operative procedure difficult. There may be a good deal of bleeding, and skin grafting will often result in failure due to the presence of hematoma under the skin or infection. Nevertheless, if the integrity of the eschar has been maintained and it is dry, excision may still be considered even 3 weeks after injury. One of our patients had burns to 98% of the BSA with third degree burns to 90% of the BSA. In this case good results were obtained by performing eschar excision in stages: the first operation was on the 18th day and the last on the 28th day.

4.2.2.3 *Size and Location of Excision*

In recent years we have analyzed a total of 56 eschar excision operations for third degree burns of more than 30% of the BSA on patients who are still living. In the majority of cases the area excised was 15%–20% of the BSA, the largest area excised being 38%.

As to the selection of locality, as a rule the extremities were chosen first and the trunk of the body afterwards, the principal reasons being:

1. On the extremities, eschar excision may be performed with the use of a tourniquet, so that there is only a small amount of bleeding and the operative procedure is easy.

2. If decompression incisions have been made during the early stage of shock, the sites of incision are often liable to become infected; therefore eschar excision should be performed at an early stage at these sites.

3. Burns of the extremities are often deeper than those of the head and trunk, and may be accompanied by muscular necrosis or even charring of the limb involved. These complications should be treated at the same time.

4. After the excision of the eschar together with the burned subcutaneous fat, the circumference of the extremity is reduced considerably, so that the area which needs to be grafted is decreased accordingly.

For the above-mentioned reasons we prefer to excise the eschar of the extremities first. But if the constricted chest eschar becomes infected, then it is advisable to excise it first. Furthermore, if the infected eschar has become foci of infection or necrosis of bulks of musles are detected, these sites should be given priority to be excised.

4.2.2.4 *The Interval Between Two Excisions*

As a rule, the interval is about 3 days. If the general condition of the patient is stable, then it may be suitably shortened. It is necessary to make good use of the 2 weeks postburn for opearation, since this is the most opportune time.

4.2.2.5 *Preparation for Excision*

1. For patients with extensive burns, allografts or xenografts of good quality should be prepared beforehand.

2. The personnel of the surgical team should be well organized. For very extensive burns, the operation may be done by two, and occasionally three, teams at the same time. It is best to complete the operation within 2 h.

3. Intravenous lines should be established and blood for transfusion should be on hand. In analyzing 56 eschar excision operations for patients with third degree burns exceeding 30% of the BSA, we found that for the first operation the amount of blood transfused was 51.7 ml ± 36.7 ml per 1% of eschar excised. For the following operations, for every 1% eschar excised, an average amount of 88.9 ml ± 44.7 ml blood was transfused. The reason why the amount of blood transfused in the successive operations was larger than in the first operation

is that, as a rule, successive eschar excisions are always accompanied by skin harvesting and autografting. (The above figures include the amount of blood needed daily for the extensively burned.)

The amount of blood loss is often underestimated, especially when necrotic muscles are excised simultaneously. This is because on such an extensive blood-exudating surface the amount of blood loss is sizable, and there may still be a certain amount of oozing after the operation. These factors must be fully appraised.

Case Illustration. Female, aged 21. This patient, with burns to 95% of the BSA, including third degree burns to 90% of the BSA, died on the 10th day after injury from wound sepsis. The patient had an uneventful shock stage. Tangential excision of eschars on both lower extremities and buttocks was performed on the 4th day after injury. The eschar excised amounted to about 39% of the BSA. Bleeding was profuse during the operation, and 3,200 ml whole blood were transfused. Before the operation the hemoglobin was 19.2 g%, while at the end of the operation it was 10 g%; blood pressure was 80/30, and another 800 ml blood were quickly given. Two hours later hemoglobin was found to be 9 g%, and a further 1,000 ml whole blood were given. Hemoglobin rose to 12.5 g%, and blood pressure became steady at 110/70. It is evident that the amount of blood loss during and after tangential excision is tremendous.

After the operation, blood pressure and hemoglobin should be checked from time to time to estimate the amount of blood to be transfused. In order to guarantee the safety of the operation, two reliable intravenous lines should be established, one for blood transfusion and other for medicaments, such as anesthetics and antibiotics.

To prevent the flare-up of infection, sensitive antibiotics, based on the microbes isolated from the wound, should be selected for use both before and after the operation.

4.2.2.6 Anesthesia (cf. Chap. XV)

4.2.2.7 Method

1. Routine preparation of the operative field.

2. For operation on the limbs a tourniquet may be applied. It should be noted that burn wounds are often infected; therefore driving of blood from the distal end of the limb should not be permitted.

3. Incisions. On the extremities, a circular incision is made both at the upper and at the lower end. A longitudinal incision is made on the front of the limb, connecting the two circular incisions (Fig. III.10). In the case of the trunk, we prefer to start with a median incision. Since the bleeding points are located under the eschar, which is hard and does not give way, there is no way to ensure hemostasis when making a long incision. Therefore, incision should not be made all at once. A small vertical incision should first

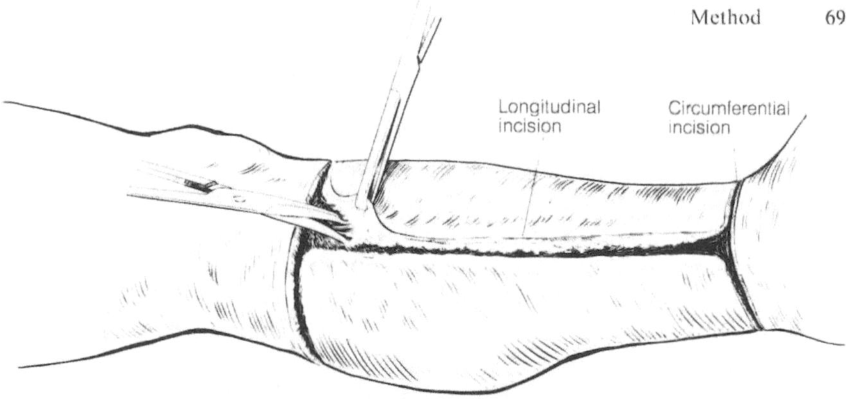

Fig. III.10. Method of raising flap in excision of eschar on the extremities

be made at the point of intersection of the planned circular and longitudinal incisions; a triangular flap of eschar with subcutaneous fat may then be raised, and the transectional surface is turned outward. In this manner, the bleeding points can be clearly exposed and hemostasis may be secured with ease. The flap can then be extended gradually till the whole eschar is excised.

4. To establish the line of cleavage of the deep fascia is an extremely important step (Fig. III.11), since this will reduce bleeding to a minimum. When the line of cleavage is found, dissection is carried out along the surface of the deep fascia. Since the blood vessels supplying the skin and the subcutaneous

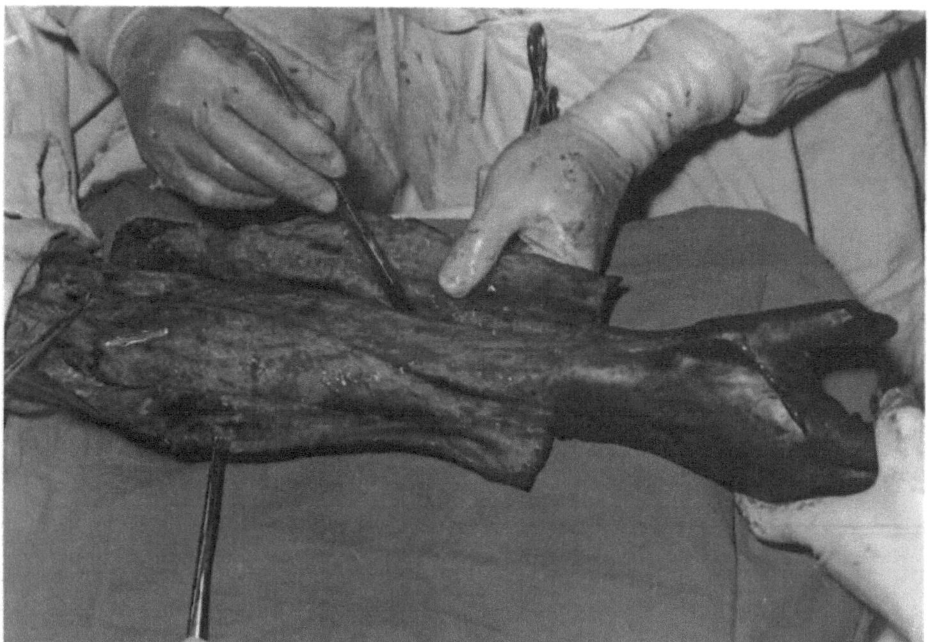

Fig. III.11. Establishment of the line of cleavage of the deep fascia – an extremely important step in excision of third degree eschar

tissue lie perpendicular to the longitudinal axis of the body, blunt dissection should be employed. Dissecting in this manner, blood vessels can be ligated with ease. All necrotic tissues must be excised. Skin grafts should never be placed on any necrotic tissue, since severe infection is liable to occur. When excising eschar along the deep fascial plane, one is liable to excise too deeply over the Achilles tendon, the popliteal space, and along Hunter's Canal; therefore care must be taken to leave some subcutaneous fat at these regions (Figs. III. 12–III. 14).

5. If necrotic muscle are found during the operation, they should be excised at the same time.

6. After excision, pressure gauze bandage, with the gauze presoaked in warm physiologic saline solution containing adrenaline (500 ml normal saline containing 1 ml 1:1,000 adrenaline) should be applied. The tourniquet is then released. The bandage is then released section by section, and hemostasis is secured with ligatures or electrocoagulation. Hemostasis should be done meticulously, because subcutaneous hematoma is a frequent cause of failure of the graft to take. After careful hemostasis, large sheets of autografts, allografts, or xenografts should be applied. For the trunk semiexposure is used while on the extremities pressure bandage is applied.

7. If blunt dissection of the eschar is performed and the vertical perforating blood vessels are carefully ligated, one may delay release of the tourniquet until skin grafting is completed and pressure bandage applied. The advantage of this method is to decrease blood oozing when the tourniquet is released,

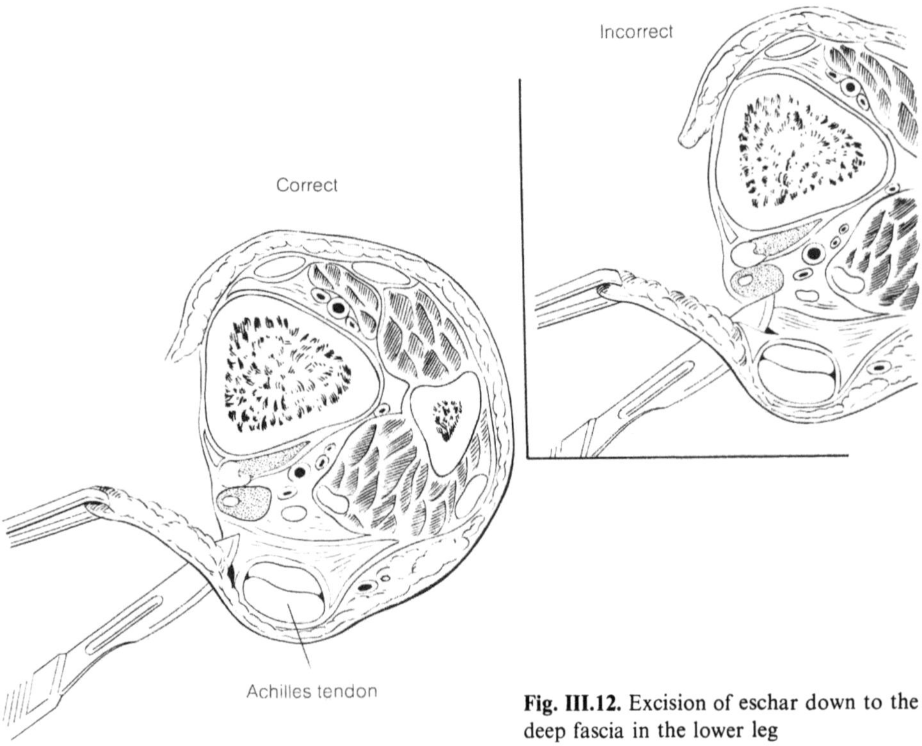

Fig. III.12. Excision of eschar down to the deep fascia in the lower leg

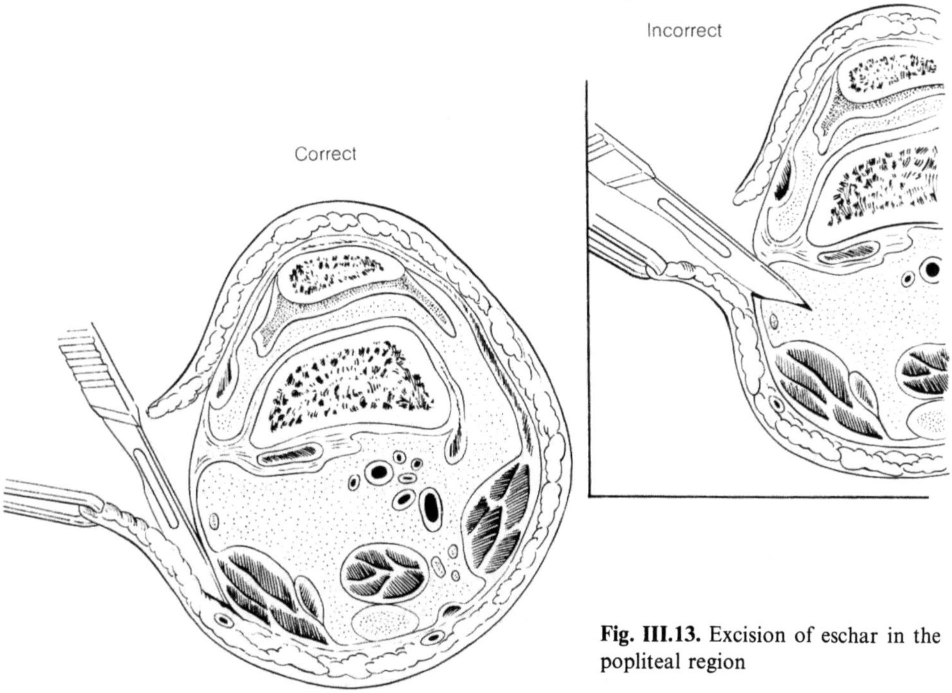

Fig. III.13. Excision of eschar in the popliteal region

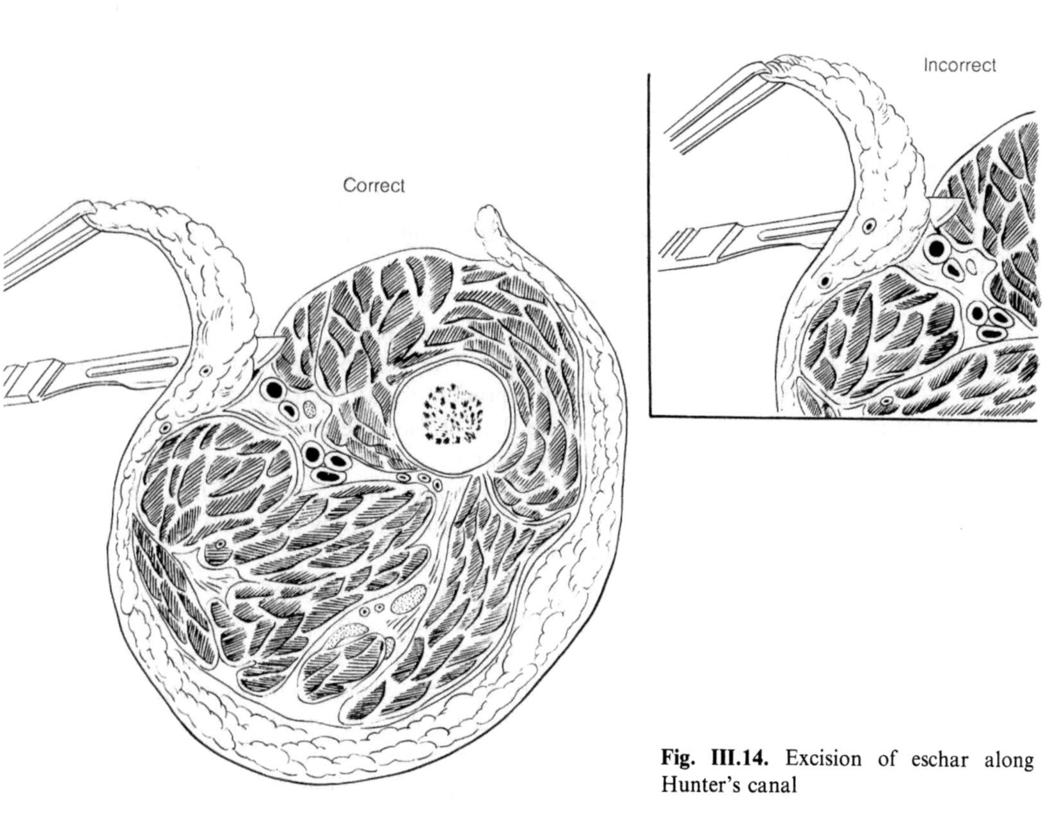

Fig. III.14. Excision of eschar along Hunter's canal

thus lessening the amount of blood lost. This method does, however require much skill and can be performed only by an experienced surgeon. The operation must be completed within 90 min (including the time needed for skin grafting and bandaging). Furthermore, it is crucial that bleeding points should be ligated one by one and hemostasis assured, otherwise large hematomas may be formed under the grafts, resulting in failure.

4.2.2.8 Use of CO_2 Laser

In 1971, Stellar first introduced continous Laser scalpel into the field of burn treatment by performing successful excisional operations and immediate grafting on pigs. In 1974 Levine employed the same sort of instrument in clinical practice with promising results. We did not adopt the use of CO_2 laser until 1977. In regard to the reduction of blood lost during the operation and the percentage of graft taking, our data show results similar to Fidler's, thus justifying further investigation.

Instrumentation. The equipment (Fig. III.15) consists of three main parts: the CO_2 laser tube, the power supply, and the mechanical revolver or transmission system.

1. CO_2 laser tube: A closed intracavity tube is used. The length of the discharge tube is about 1.8 m. The wavelength (10.6 μm) of the coherent beam is within the infrared spectrum, with multiple modes. The output power created is greater than 80 W, with a photospot diameter of 6 mm–7 mm.

2. Power supply: Direct current is used. The primary voltage of the high-tension transformer is regulated by controlled silicon (variable transformers can also be used). The high voltage of secondary rating direct current is 40 kV and the current rated is 40 mA. Silicon stack bridge rectifier is used. Through the L-type filter, high voltage direct current is generated at the two ends of the laser tube.

3. The light transmission system consists of mechanical revolving articulated arms (MRAA) which have six pyramidal glass refractory blocks and are joined together by adaptors of different lengths. The refractory mirrors are made of plain glasses which are coated with golden foils; their refractory rate to 10.6 μm infrared light amounts to more than 97%. The entire articulated arms are under strict and refined optical adjustment.

The length of the articular arms is 943 mm, and their maximal maneuverability is about 300 mm–400 mm. There is an approximately 17%–20% "decay" of the laser beam during transmission.

The handpiece comprises a mirror house, a cone-shaped outcoat, and a germanium lens for focusing (Fig. III.16). For cutting purposes the germanium lens is so adjusted as to give a focal distance of 80 mm, spot size 0.2 mm. A power density of 2×10^4 W/cm^2 is thus created. Suction and blowing devices are incorporated in the handpiece for sucking off the smoke formed by the vaporized tissue and for blowing nitrogen gas simultaneously to cool the lens and the spot surroundings in order to lessen tissue damage during cutting.

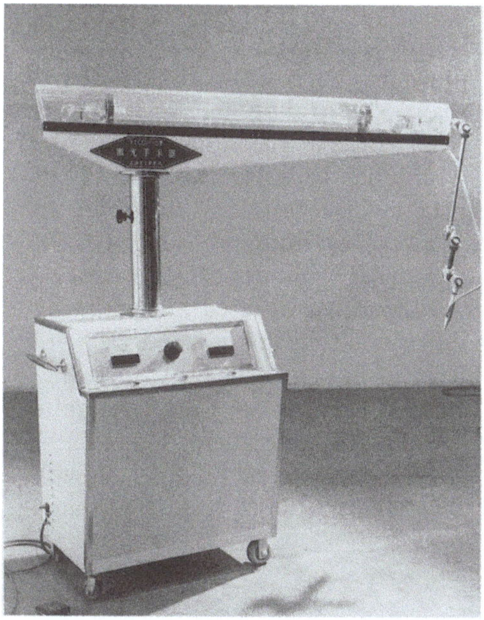

Fig. III.15. CO_2 laser, supplied by the Laser Laboratory, Shanghai Second Medical College

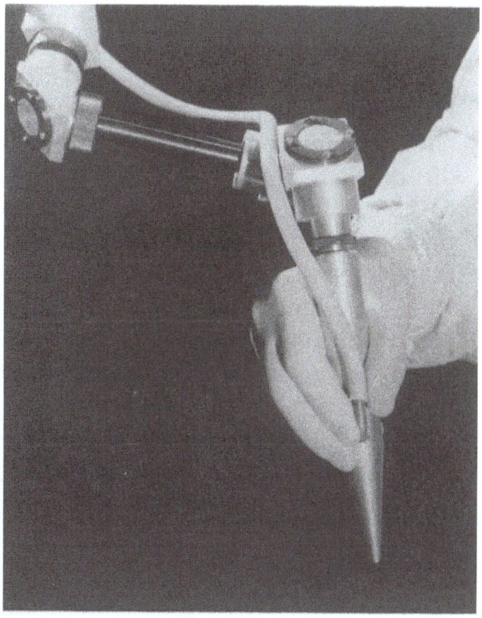

Fig. III.16. Handpiece of a CO_2 laser scalpel

Clinical Application. If the eschar is excised within 1 week postburn, there is still quite a large amount of sequestered fluid beneath it. This can greatly reduce the heat surrounding the light spot by absorption during vaporization. Therefore in the case of late excision (we used to arrange the second or third stage excisions after 1 week postburn), physiologic saline is infiltrated under the eschar in order to lessen the tissue damage further.

Finer vessels (veins less than 2 mm in diameter, arteries less than 1 mm) are sealed while cutting with a laser scalpel. Consequently blood loss is much less than when an ordinary surgical scalpel is employed. (For instance, the blood loss per square centimeter of eschar excised by laser scalpel is 0.88 ml $\pm$ 0.12 ml, whereas when an ordinary surgical scalpel is used it is 4.18 ml $\pm$ 2.85 ml; $P < 0.05$.) The rate of take of the skin grafts is above 90%. CO_2 laser is especially indicated for those severely infected wounds which are submitted to excision. Sealing of the finer vessels will prevent further spreading of the badly infected foci.

After the eschar has been excised the wound must be irrigated with physiologic saline and the edge of the incision lightly rubbed using wet physiologic saline swab before grafting is performed.

When the laser is operating, no metallic instruments are allowed within the operating field; the wearing of glasses is compulsory in order to protect the operator's eyes from the reflecting beam.

4.2.2.9 Excision of Eschar of Extensive Third Degree Burns

In 1958, when we began to practice excisional operations, we were not able to obtain satisfactory results in patients with burns to more than 50% of the BSA, including third degree burns to more than 25%. At that time two problems remained unsolved: Firstly, the problem of coverage of the wound; secondly, the problem of the source of autografts. In order to solve the problem of coverage, in 1959 we began to use large sheets of fenestrated allografts. In the fenestrations, we transplanted postage stamp-sized autografts (Fig. III.17). Inspired by the work of Mowlem and Jackson, in 1961 we adopted their method with some modifications. Instead of alternating strips, we used a bricklaying pattern of autografts and allografts (Fig. III.18). Using this method we were able to save the life of a patient with burns to 81% of the BSA, including third degree burns to 60%. In 1963, we began to use large sheets of allografts with small punctured holes in which small autografts were inlaid (Fig. III.19). In 1966, on the basis of past practice, we combined the above method with staged excision of the eschar and utilized the scalp as a donor site for repeated

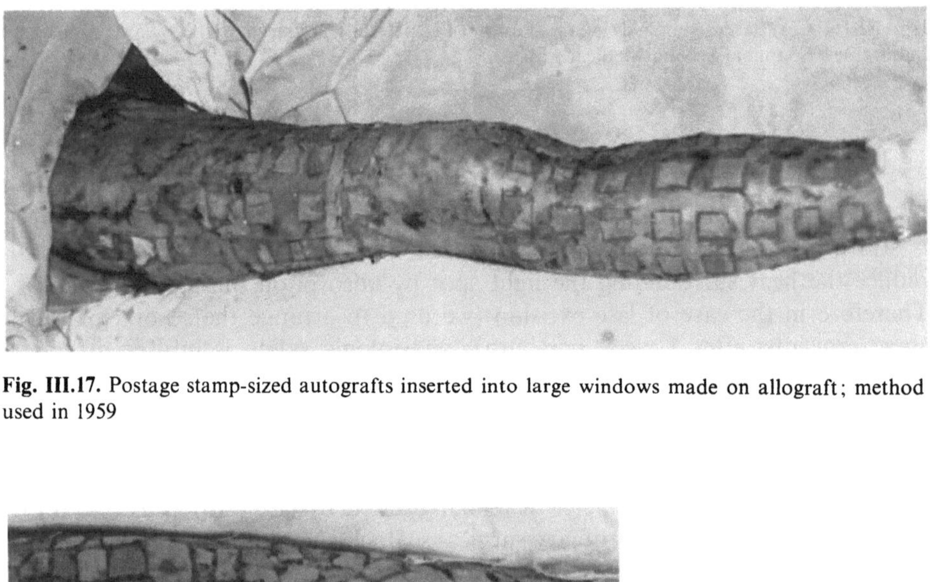

Fig. III.17. Postage stamp-sized autografts inserted into large windows made on allograft; method used in 1959

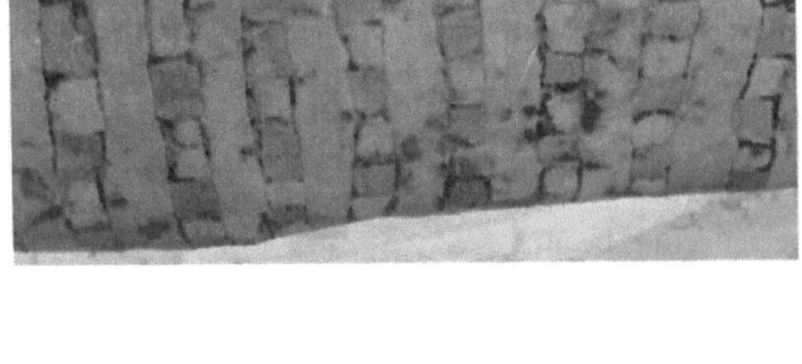

Fig. III.18. Bricklaying pattern of autografts (deep colored) and allografts (light colored); method used in 1961

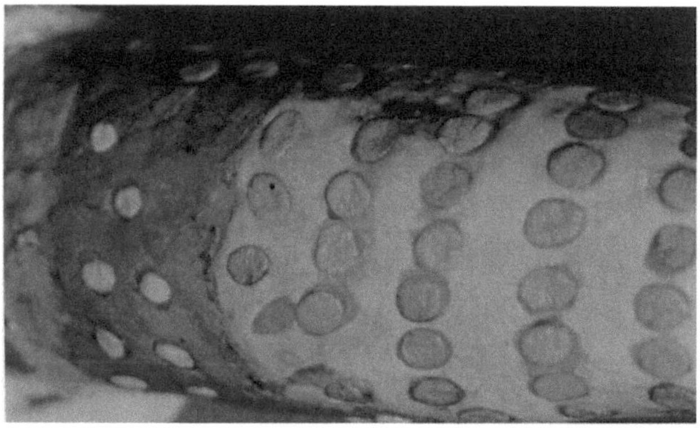

Fig. III.19. Small autografts inlaid in a large sheet of allograft (the dark-colored piece is a lyophilized allograft); method used in 1963

harvestings of autografts. In this way we were able to treat successfully a patient with burns to 98% of the BSA, including third degree burns to 90% (Figs. III.20–III.22). This technique paved the way for treatment of the eschar by staged excision and intermingled transplantation of allo- and autografts. The advantages of this method are as follows:

1. Spontaneous separation of the eschar will inevitably cause the growth and multiplication of microorganisms in the dissoluted necrotic tissue, and septicemia or wound sepsis is liable to develop. If the eschar is excised in stages and covered immediately with autografts or allografts, then the deleterious effect and threat of sepsis are greatly reduced.

2. With the use of the above-described method, i.e., covering the wound after surgical excision with large sheets of punctured allograft inlaid with small pieces of autograft which will gradually expand, the wound surface will finally be completely covered by autografts. By this means, when the allografts have temporarily survived and the autografts are inlaid, this part of wound is permanently sealed, so to speak. When this method is used, there is no need to

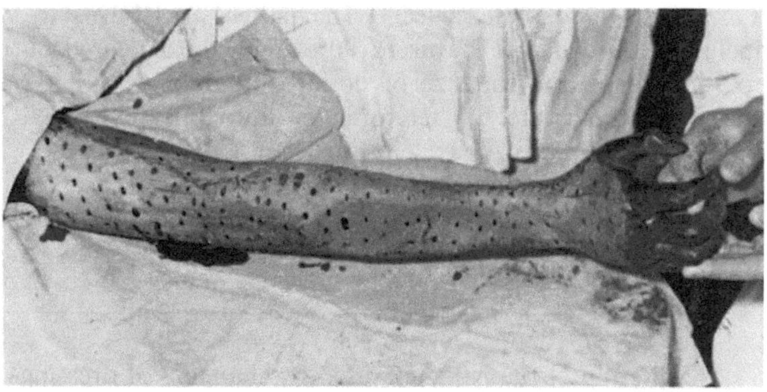

Fig. III.20. After excision of the eschar, a large sheet of punctured allograft is transplanted and small pieces of autograft are later inserted into the holes

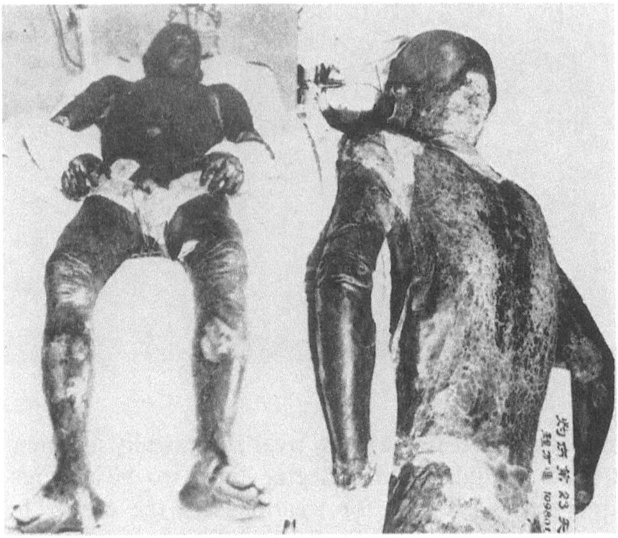

Fig. III.21. Patient admitted in 1966 with burns to 98% of the BSA, including third degree burns to 90%. The prone view is shown after bilateral disarticulation through the wrists

wait for the "ripening" of the granulation tissue, and autografts may be directly laid on the wound surface immediately after eschar excision. Statistics concerning a large number of patients show that autografting of skin after staged excision of eschar is performed 10 days earlier than after natural separation of the eschar. In patients with extensive third degree burns, when the donor area of autografts is very limited, the above method is very important for the success of treatment.

3. The amount of autografts needed is decreased. When the above-mentioned method is used the autografts will expand by seven times or more.

Case Illustration. Male, age 33. The patient had burns to 98% of the BSA, including third degree burns to 90%. The third degree burn area amounted to 15,635 cm^2, and the size of donor autografts was 1,132 cm^2. The wound was healed completely. Therefore, the autografts expanded to more than 13 times their original size.
Expansion index of autograft (EI)

$$EI = \frac{\text{BSA } (cm^2) \times \text{third degree burn } (\%)}{\text{Area of autograft cropping } (cm^2)}$$

---

4. Suffering of the patient caused by changing of dressings is decreased.

On the basis of our experience we may state that if one can master the principle and procedure of the above-mentioned method of eschar excision,

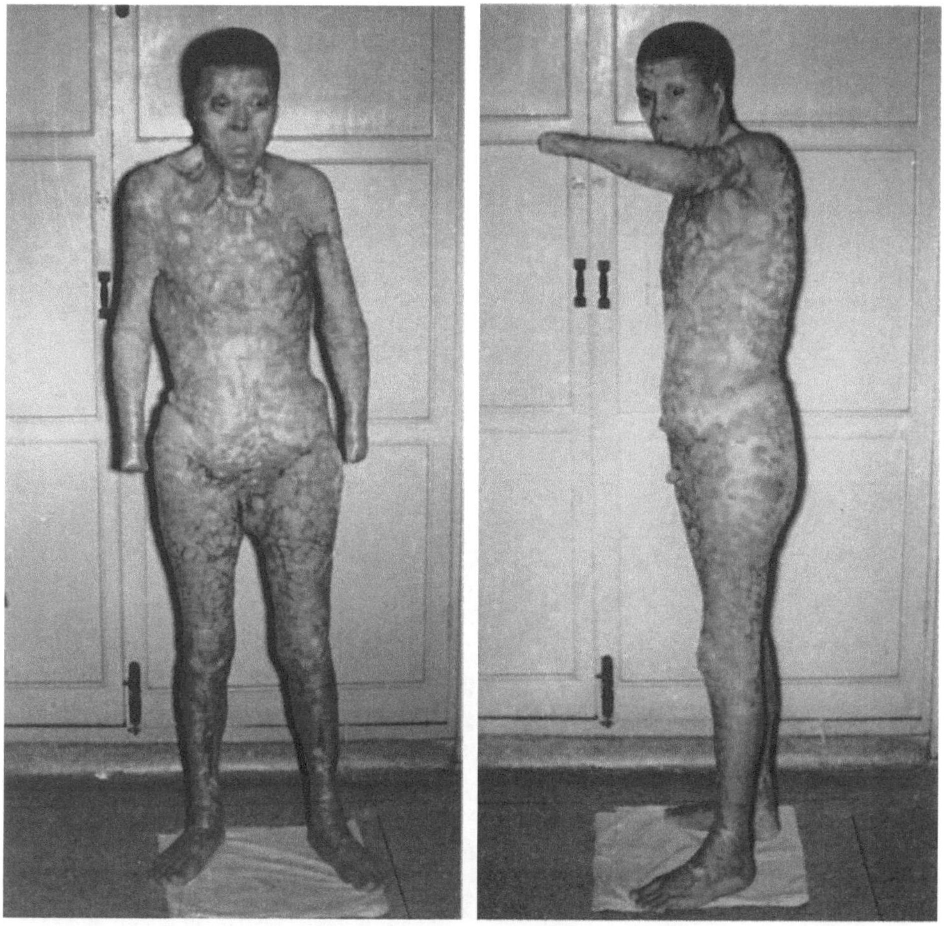

Fig. III.22. Same patient as in **Fig. III.21**, 2 years postburn. A pedicle flap was raised from the back and transferred to the chin for correction of the everted lip

and the allografts are of good quality, then it is possible to raise the survival rate of patients with extensive third degree burns.

From January 1966 to December 1978 we admitted and treated 68 patients with burns to more than 80% of the BSA, including third degree burns to more than 50%; of these patients, 26 have survived, including one with burns to 100% of the BSA, with third degree burns to 94% (Figs. III.23–III.26). Out of the above-mentioned 68 cases, in 57 treatment of the eschar consisted of staged excision and grafting followed by in-laying of small autografts into premade openings in a large sheet of allograft in combination with natural separation of the eschar and the use of a patchwork of autografts and allografts. General data concerning the 24 patients who survived when this method was used are presented in Table III.2.

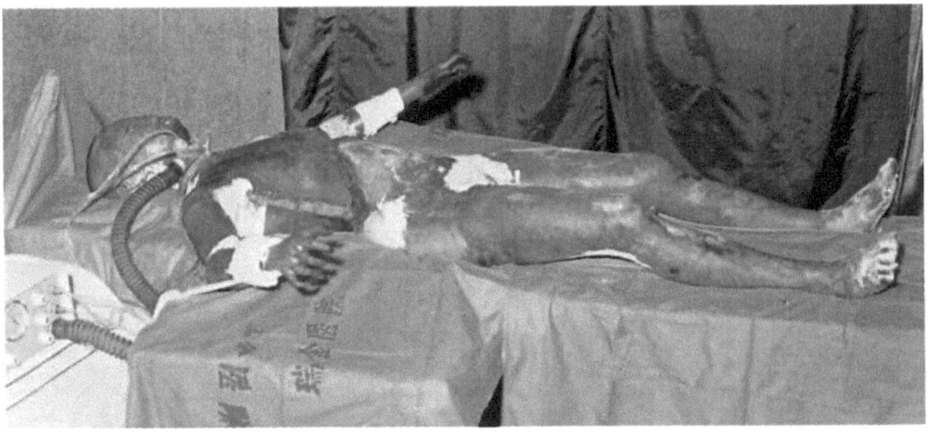

III.23

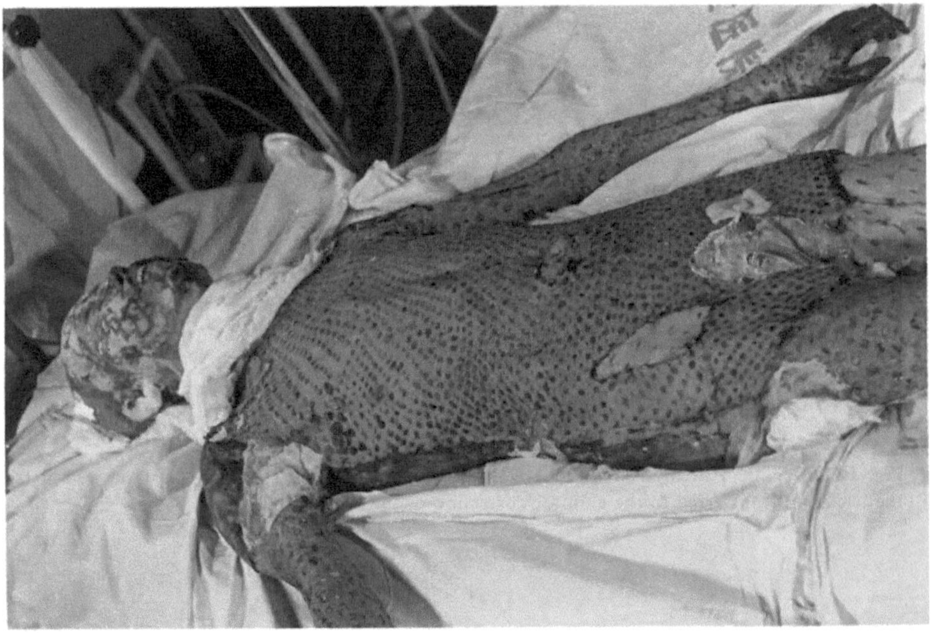

III.24

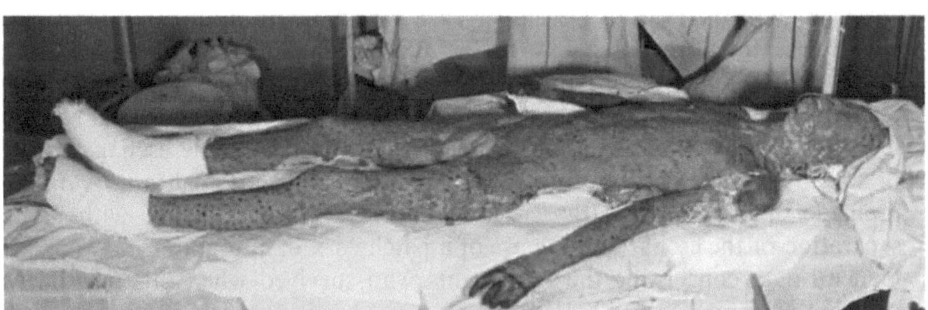

III.25

◁**Fig. III.23.** Thirty-five-year-old female with flame burns to 100% of the BSA, including third degree burns to 94%. Forty-eight hours postburn. Owing to respiratory burn and constrictive trunk eschar, a respirator was employed for 6 days

Fig. III.24. Same patient as in **Fig. III.23**, 13 days postburn. Two thousand holes are punctured in the allograft on the chest and abdomen

Fig. III.25. Same patient as in **Fig. III.23**, 21 days postburn. Three major operations involving eschar excision and intermingled transplantation of the trunk and limbs have already been performed

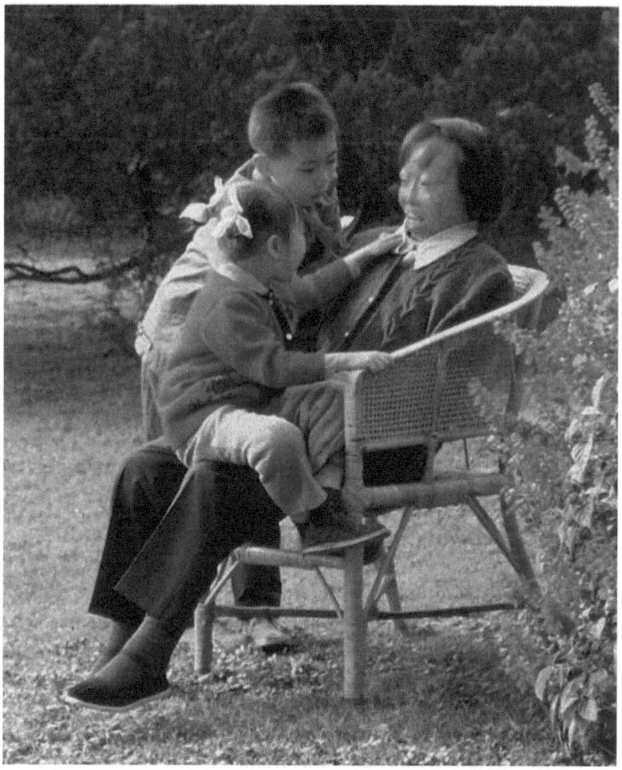

Fig. III.26. Same patient as in **Fig. III.23**, $2^1/_2$ years postburn, chatting with her son and daughter

It is evident from Tables III.3 and III.4 that the above-described method is effective in patient with extensive third degree burns. Therefore, we propose that for this category of patients, especially when the muscles are involved, it is possible to excise the third degree eschar by stages starting from the 5th postburn day (occasionally it can be done as early as the 3rd day after injury) and to cover the wound immediately with large sheets of punctured allograft (or xenograft) and inlays of autograft in the punctured holes, in combination with the method of covering the third degree wound surfaces after natural separation of the eschar, as well as the granulation surface, with alternating pieces of autograft and allograft. In third degree burns, the burn sometimes reaches the bones (most frequently at the anterior aspect of the tibia); after

Table III.2. General data concerning excisional operations on 24 patients (who survived) with burns exceeding 80% of the BSA including third degree burns exceeding 50%

Case number	Age (yrs)	Percentage of BSA burned (III°)	No. of excisions	First excision (days post-burn)	Interval between excisions (days)	Sites of excision[a]	Amputation	Area excised (%)[b]
1	33	98 (90)	3	18	3, 5	LL, RL, RUE, LUE, LT, RT	[c]	46
2	8	80 (60.5)	2	9	4	RLE, C		20
3	33	91 (72)	2	5	7	RUE, LUE, RLE, LLE		35
4	41	87 (50)	1	15	–	RUE, LUE		14
5	35	93.5 (71.5)	2	14	8	RUE, LUE		14
6	22	80 (50)	1	9	–	LL, RL		14
7	36	82.5 (75)	3	5	12, 2	RLE, LLE, C, LFA, RFA		25
8	17	99 (94)	3	10	3, 3	RLE, LLE, LFA, RUE		40
9	31	88 (68)	3	6	4, 6	LLE, RLE		32
10	26	88 (61)	3	10	7, 5	RUE, LUE, LLE, C		27
11	22	85 (52)	3	5	3, 3	LLE, RLE, RUE		38
12	6	85 (68.5)	3	4	3, 4	C, Ba, A, Bu, RUE, LUE, LT, RT		56
13	42	99 (71.5)	2	5	10	RLE, LLE, C, A		37
14	19	98 (90)	2	7	4	RUE, LUE, C, RLE, LLE		59
15	26	90 (51.5)	1	9	–	LL, RL, RF		15
16	35	90 (60)	1	19	–	RUE, LUE		11
17	43	85 (62.5)	2	8	4	RUE, LUE, RLE, LLE		35
18	35	100 (94)	3	7	4, 6	C, A, RUE, LUE, RLE, LLE		62
19	49	80.5 (53)	2	6	10	RUE, LUE, RLE, LLE		36
20	30	90 (60)	1	9	–	RLE, LLE		25
21	21	96 (83)	3	3	4, 3	C, RUE, LUE, RLE, LLE		46.5
22	48	94.5 (67)	4	5	4, 4, 9	RUE, LUE, RLE, LLE, A		50
23	42	89.5 (65.5)	4	8	7, 2, 8	RUE, LUE, RLE, LT, C	[d]	41
24	44	88 (62)	3	4	15, 4	RUE, LUE, LT, RT, C, A F, N, Bu	[e]	30

[a] *Abbreviations:* A, abdomen; Bu, buttocks; C, chest; F, face; N, neck; LT, left thigh; RT, right thigh; RF, right foot; RUE, right upper extremity; LUE, left upper extremity; LLE, left lower extremity; Ba, back; RLE, right lower extremity; LL, left leg; RL, right leg; LFA, left forearm; RFA, right forearm

[b] Area excised does not include the disarticulated or amputated portion

[c] Disarticulation through both wrists

[d] Disarticulation through knee joint

[e] Amputation of left lowerlimb at mid-thigh level and of right lower limb at the level of the lower third of the thigh

the necrotic tissue has been cleared away, the bone is exposed. Such a condition may be attended to at a later stage. However, in many patients with extensive third degree burns the above-mentioned method still ended in failure, demonstrating that many problems concerning the method remain to be solved. Some patients showed serious reactions to extensive excision of the eschar and skin grafting, including postoperative retention of water and sodium, repeated general edema, aggravation of general and local infection, and the appearance of inflammatory infiltration around the wound surface.

Table III.3. Comparison of results obtained in the treatment of eschar in extensively burned patients (burns to more than 80% of the BSA, including third degree burns to more than 50%) during different periods and using differing methods

Period	Method	No. of cases		Average percentage of BSA burned (III°)	No. of survivors		No. of deaths		Survival rate	
1958–1965	Natural separation	33		92.2 (75)	1[a]		32		3%	
1966–1978	Natural separation	68	11	92.1 (59.3)	26	2	42	9	38.2	18.1
	Combination of staged excisions and natural separation		57	89.9 (70.2)		24		33		42.1

[a] Total BSA burned was 81%, including third degree burns of 60% of the BSA. After natural separation of eschar the granulation wounds were covered by panelling of allo- and autografts

Table III.4. Summation of results given in Table III.3 according to method alone

Method	No. of cases	Average percentage of BSA burned (III°)	No. of survivors	Survival rate
Natural separation	44	92.2 (71.1)	3	6.8%
Combination of staged excisions with natural separation	57	89.9 (70.2)	24	42.1%

Case Illustration. Male, aged 46. The patient had burns to 82.5% of the BSA, including third degree burns to 75%, Circular constrictive eschar was present on the extremities. Longitudinal decompressive incisions were made immediately after admission. Six days after injury, excision of the eschar and skin grafting were performed on both lower extremities. The postoperative course was stormy with retention of water and sodium, evident general edema, large amounts of exudation from the incisional sites, and inflammatory infiltration around the wound. The patient's tongue was cherry red and dry. The abdomen was distended and the patient was very irritable and restless. After various treatments, the patient's general condition showed a tendency to become stable on the 6th day after operation. After further operations the patient was finally cured, although varying degrees of postoperative reaction again appeared (Fig. III.27).

Some patients, especially the aged, bore the operations very poorly. After the excision of large areas of the eschar, allografts failed to take, and general condition deteriorated, even ending in death.

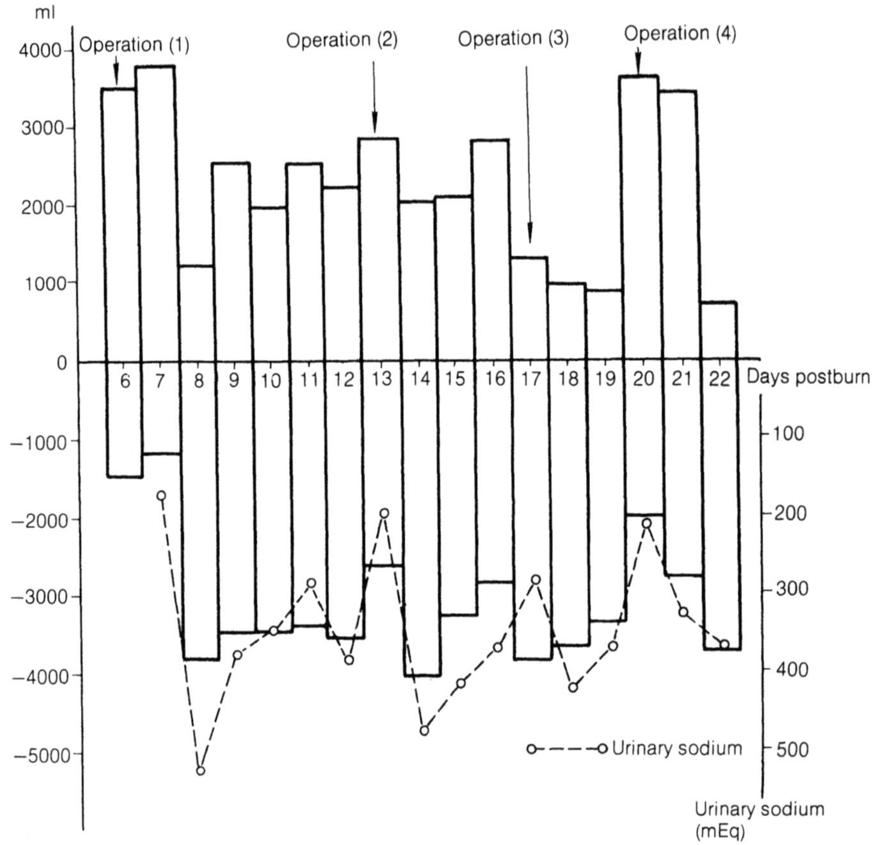

Fig. III.27. Fluid intake, urine output, and urinary sodium in a patient with extensive third degree burns. Marked sodium and water retention is seen on the day of operation; their release occurred within 24 h

As to the selection of site and the timing of eschar excision, further investigations and improvements are needed with regard to assessment of the condition of the necrotic tissue under the eschar, speed of qualitative and quantitative determination of the subeschar bacteria count, selection of anesthesia, operative technique, etc.

5 Skin Grafting

With regard to third degree burns, minor burns may heal by cicatrization of the wound with the epidermis "creeping" from its periphery, but large wounds will never heal by themselves, and autografting is necessary.

There are various methods of skin grafting. Depending on the condition of the wound, they may be divided into grafting on the granulating surface and grafting on the eschar excision surface. On the basis of their size and shape grafts may be classified as large or small split-thickness grafts or as mesh grafts. With respect to the relationship between autografts and allografts or xenografts, one can distinguish between intermingled transplantation, submerged grafts, and transplantation with alternating pieces. Finally, treatment after skin grafting may be divided into exposure and bandaging of the graft.

Large sheets of skin grafts should be used on the face and functional regions, but on account of the scarcity of donor sites in patients with extensive burns, even on the functional parts small grafts or meshed grafts need to be employed. When large sheets of skin graft are applied on the granulating surface, the wound should be sufficiently prepared: no necrotic tissue should be allowed to remain. If the necrotic tissue has not all sloughed off and is mingled with the granulation tissue, then small grafts ought to be used.

5.1 Requirements for the Take of Skin Grafts

1. The wound surface should be fresh, and without any remains of necrotic tissue.
2. Autografts should be freshly procured or stored at 4 °C in an icebox for no more than a week.
3. No serious infection should be present on the surface to receive the graft (especially hemolytic *Streptococci* or hemolytic *Staphylococci aureus*).
4. Hemostasis should be meticulous; subcutaneous hematoma must be avoided.
5. The grafts should be fully immobilized for 5 days after transplantation.

5.2 Preoperative Preparation for Skin Grafting

5.2.1 General Preparation

Before the operation, every effort should be made to ensure that the patient is in a comparatively good physical condition. By "comparatively good condition" we mean that anemia, hypoalbuminemia, water and electrolyte disturbances, and acidosis have been adjusted and that pulmonary infection is controlled, etc. The burn surface, especially the third degree burn surface, is the fundamental cause of the development of a series of pathologic changes of the human body. Every opportunity to cover the wound with skin grafts must be grasped, for only then will the general condition of the patient improve. Sometimes skin grafting should be performed without hesitation despite a poor general condition of the patient, with persistence of high fever or even wound sepsis. Passive waiting may cause aggravation of the infection and the general condition of the patient will get worse. Often a vicious circle is formed and only by extinguishing the wound with grafting will it be possible to interrupt the vicious circle and pave the way for the patients' recovery.

5.2.2 Preparation of the Surfaces to Receive Grafts

Skin grafting on the eschar excision surface: When the eschar has been excised, the necrotic tissue entirely removed, and complete hemostasis obtained, skin grafts may be laid right away. If it is not certain whether the necrotic tissue has been entirely excised, skin grafting may be delayed provided the size of the excised surface is not large.

Skin grafting of the granulating surface: As a granulation wound is an infected surface, bacteria are bound to grow, but with the exception of hemolytic *Streptococcus* and hemolytic *Staphylococcus aureus*, bacteria do not exert much influence on the take of the grafts. As long as the granulations are comparatively "firm," "healthy," and of a fresh red color, there is a good, ready recipient area. If there is a large amount of purulent fluid, wet dressings with physiologic saline solution, bacteriocidals, or antibiotics are indicated; skin grafting may be done when the amount of pus has decreased. As a rule, it is sufficient to apply wet dressings once during the night before operation and again during the operation. If positive culture of hemolytic *Streptococci* is reported, penicillin or other sensitive antibiotics should be prescribed for systemic as well as for topical use. If hemolytic *Streptococci* and penicillin-resistant hemolytic *Staphylococci aureus* coexist, then penicillin together with isoxazolyl penicillins or other sensitive antibiotics should be employed. If the granulation tissue appears edematous, wet dressing with 2%–3% physiologic saline solution in combination with pressure bandaging may be used. When there is an overgrowth of granulation tissue, it should be trimmed during the operation. The old granulated surfaces should be scraped off with a knife until a fibrous base is reached; there is a comparatively better chance of success of skin grafting when the grafts are laid on a "healthy" base.

5.2.3 Harvesting the Skin

There are many methods for harvesting the skin and various instruments are used.

5.2.3.1 Simple Method

The donor area should be held stretched, maintaining the skin in a flat surface. Sometimes 0.25%–0.5% procaine solution or physiologic saline may be evenly injected subcutaneously. We recommend the use of a Humby knife for harvesting. The sharp edge of the knife should be held at an acute angle (almost parallel while cutting thin grafts) to the skin surface. The graft is then cut with a gentle to-and-fro sawing motion of the knife while pushing the blade forward slowly; the width of the sawing motion should not be big. The thickness of the graft is dependent upon (a) the angle between the blade and the surface of skin and (b) the pressure used. The bigger the angle and the greater the pressure, the thicker will be the graft, and vice versa. In the process of taking the graft the angle and pressure may be adjusted in accordance with the required thickness of the graft. Whether the edge of the graft is smooth or not depends upon the width of the sawing motion; if the width is small, the edge of the graft will be comparatively smooth and vice versa.

The distance between the rotating axis and the blade can be adjusted according to the thickness demanded. When this instrument is used, large sheets

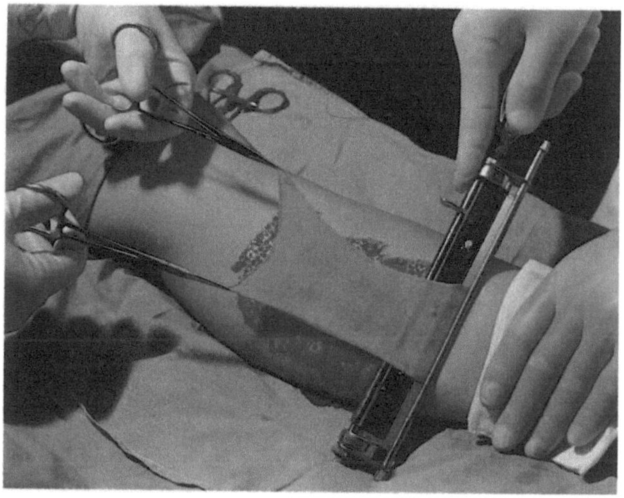

Fig. III.28. Harvesting of a large sheet of partial-thickness graft by means of a Humby knife

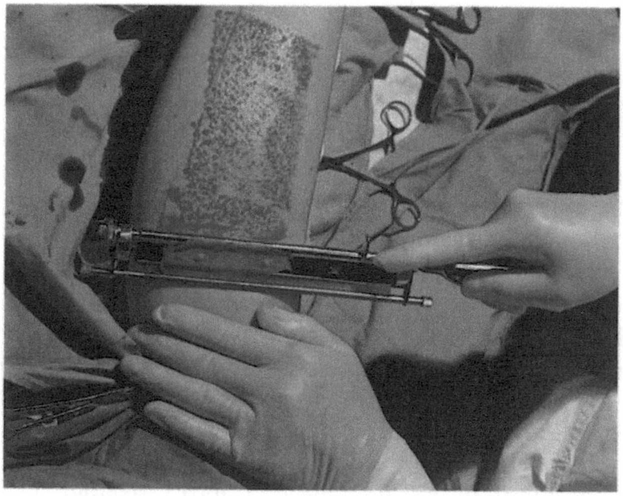

Fig. III.29. Pearl-like bleeding points are seen after harvesting of a partial-thickness graft

of grafts may be taken from certain parts of the body (such as the thigh, the buttocks, and the back) (Fig. III.28) suitable for the grafting of large surfaces or for mesh grafts. The donor area presents pearl-like bleeding points (Fig. III.29).

When there is a lack of donor sites, the grafts taken by the free hand method are small, such as those taken from the dorsum or sole of the foot or from the scalp. If the skin of the toes is to be taken, we use a razor blade held by a hemostat. This method can be easily managed and is commonly used.

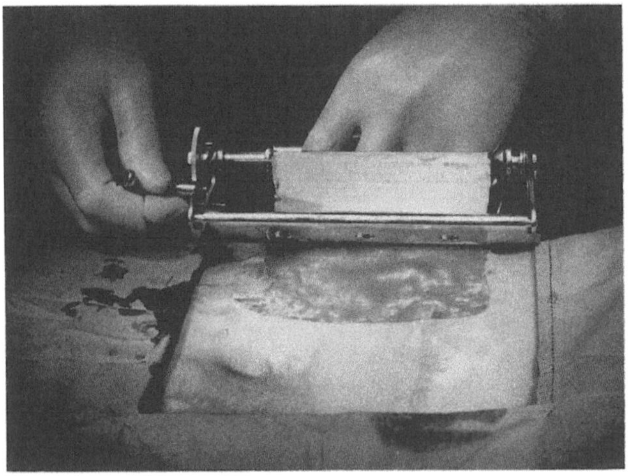

Fig. III.30. Harvesting skin by means of a Padgett dermatome

5.2.3.2 Cropping with a Drum Dermatome (*Padgett dermatome;* Fig. III.30)

This dermatome produces larger grafts with uniform thickness and smooth edges; the grafts are suitable for transplantation on the face, neck, hands, and other functional parts of the body.

The drum dermatome consists of four parts, namely drum, axis, knife, and adjustment screw. The calibre for the required thickness of the graft should be adjusted first: a medium thickness of 0.3 mm–0.4 mm is often used. The drum and the donor skin should be wiped with ether, and then glue (rubber cement) is applied evenly on the drum and the skin of the donor area. It is necessary to wait for a few moments until the glue is dry, after which the leading edge of the drum is pressed down firmly on the donor area and held in place, under some pressure, until the drum has firmly adhered to the donor skin. The drum is then lifted slightly, and the skin will come up with the front edge; at that moment, the knife can be put in place and to-and-fro cutting motions are commenced. As the cutting is in progress, the drum is turned until the required piece of graft is excised. The graft is removed immediately from the drum, and the glue on the graft should be wiped off with dry gauze. When using this method the blade should be sharp, the calibration accurate, adhesiveness of the glue strong, and the glue applied evenly. The drum surface should be turned very slowly and should not be inclined. Grafts are easily taken from a flat surface, while in case of depressed parts of the body, such as interspaces between the ribs, physiologic saline should be injected subcutaneously until the depression has been filled. When injecting physiologic saline, the site of entrance of the needle should be at the periphery of the donor area, otherwise physiologie saline may seep out, causing a reduction in the glue's effect.

Thickness of the graft: When skin grafting is performed on the granulation surface, the graft should not be, too thick, otherwise it will not take. A thin split-thickness graft of 0.15 mm–0.2 mm is ideal. When viewing the graft's epidermal surface, the graft is transparent, while on the dermal surface a thin layer of silvery dermis is seen.

Large sheets of graft on the face, hands, and other functional parts ought to be a little thicker; for adults, intermediate split-thickness grafts of 0.3 mm–0.4 mm may be used.

5.2.3.3 Harvesting of Full-Thickness Graft (cf. Chap. XIV)

5.2.4 Harvesting Skin from Unusual Parts of the Body

Repeated harvestings of skin from the scalp play a very important part in the treatment of extensive deep burns.

In 1966, we successfully treated a steel worker with burns to 98% of the BSA, including third degree burns to 90% of the BSA. The only 2% of the BSA not burned was on the scalp and the soles of the feet. Owing to the fact that the scalp is full of hair and the sole is covered by corn, we formerly thought that these areas could not be used as donor sites. How can a burn with such extensiveness be cured with essentially no donor site available at all? However, when we analyzed the histologic constituents of the scalp and the sole, we realized that both scalp and sole have all the common characteristics of skin although they are covered either by hair or by corn, and that they can therefore serve as donor sites. We harvested autografts repeatedly from the scalp and the sole and performed intermingled transplantation of allo- and autografts; in this way we successfully covered the third degree wound surface.

Genuine knowledge originates from practice: after repeated practice through the years, we noted that the scalp as a donor site possesses many advantages, such as resistance to infection and strong healing power due to its thick dermis, deep-seated hair follicles, and excellent blood supply; thus repeated harvestings may be carried out within a short period. Usually, a second thin split-thickness graft can be harvested after an interval of 5–7 days. No scar after healing and no interference with hair growth have been noted. We therefore regard the scalp as the human "natural skin bank." Generally 5–6 harvestings may be carried out at the same site; thus autograft amounting to at least 10% of the BSA may be obtained from 2% of the BSA. In certain patients even as many as 16 harvests have been obtained over a period of 4 years. Nowadays we use the scalp as the principal donor site in managing extensive third degree burns.

The method of harvesting grafts from the scalp is as follows:

1. The head is shaved and cleaned on the morning of the operative day. In the case of repeated harvestings or when the scalp has just healed from burn injury and there is not yet a firm layer of epidermis (speaking scientifically, the dermal-epidermal linkage is still weak), it is only necessary to cut the hair short and to cleanse thoroughly.

2. In order to raise the skin of the scalp and thus facilitate harvesting, 0.25%–0.5% procaine or physiologic saline (in every 100 ml 5–10 drops of

1:1,000 adrenaline may be added to decrease oozing of the donor area) is infiltrated subcutaneously.

3. The skin of the scalp is removed using a Chinese modification of a Humby knife. The thickness of the graft is 0.15 mm–0.2 mm (Figs. III.31–III.33).

4. For the donor site, the semi-exposure method is employed. A single layer of fine mesh gauze is first laid in position and then compressed with a pad soaked in warm saline. The pad is removed when oozing of blood has stopped.

5. To remove the hair from the graft, the following methods may be used:

a) The hair can be scraped off of the dermal surface of the graft using a surgical scalpel.

b) It may be wiped off of the epidermal surface using a piece of Vaseline gauze.

c) It may be washed off by repeated showering of the graft with copious amounts of physiologic saline.

6. When the donor site has healed, the semiexposed gauze should first be softened with liquid paraffin so that new growths of epidermis will not be injured when the gauze is removed.

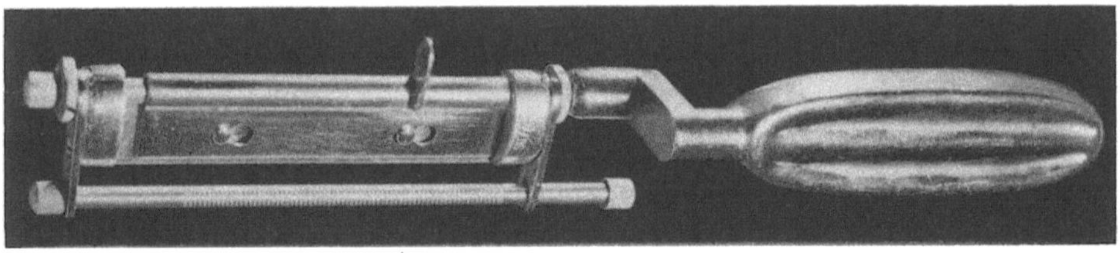

Fig. III.31. Chinese modification of a Humby knife, especially designed for harvesting partial-thickness grafts from the scalp

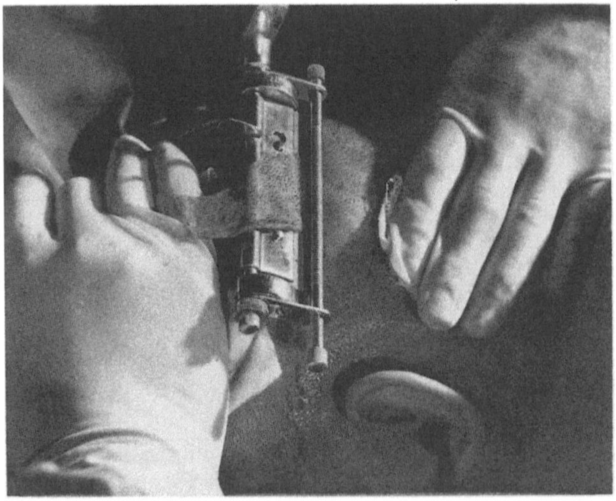

Fig. III.32. Harvesting skin from the scalp

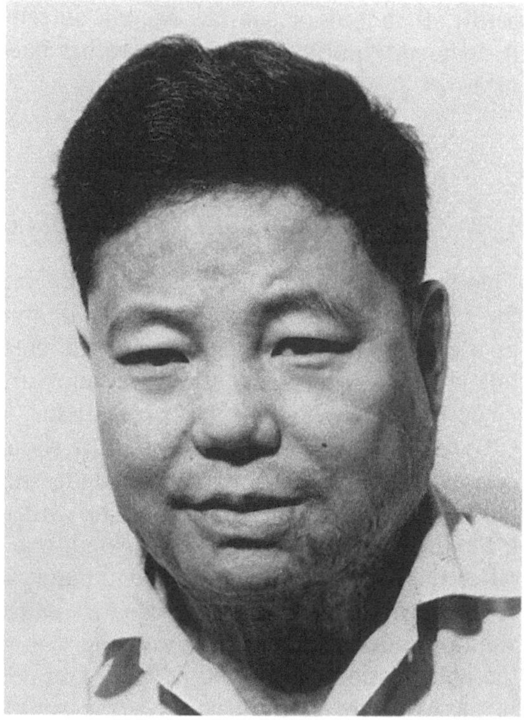

Fig. III.33. In this patient six harvestings were made from the same site on the scalp. The photograph, showing abundant hair growth, was taken 4 years later

The method of harvesting grafts from the sole is as follows:

The sole should be cleansed by washing and the keratinized layer softened by hot compresses and then scraped off. The thickness of the graft taken from the sole must not exceed 0.2 mm because although the keratinized layer is thick, the dermis is thin, and it is quite easy to penetrate too deeply. The donor site of the sole heals slower than that of the scalp: 10 days are needed before another crop of skin can be taken.

Since the keratinized layer of the graft is rather thick, the recipient area should be bandaged with pressure.

We followed up those patients who received skin grafts from the sole and found that after being transplanted the grafts remained hard and there was a good deal of desquamation; therefore one should not graft them on an exposed part of the body.

5.2.5 Care of the Donor Site

After the graft has been harvested, the donor area should be covered with a layer of petrolatum-impregnated gauze or dry gauze and compressed with a gauze pad soaked in warm physiologic saline to stop bleeding. Donor areas on the extremities need to be bandaged with pressure over many layers of gauze. If there is no infection, the dressings may be removed after 2 weeks. If the innermost layer has adhered firmly, it should not be removed by force;

sterilized liquid paraffin may be used to soften it, and it can then be removed gently. If the donor site has become infected, the semiexposure method needs to be used. Antibiotic solution or other bacteriocidal solutions may be applied in drops.

5.2.6 Methods of Grafting

5.2.6.1 Transplantation of Large Sheets of Graft

This method is often used for third degree burns of the functional parts of the body or of the face, and for small third degree burn wounds. After the operation, the function as well as the cosmetic results are fairly promising, but it calls for large and regular donor areas, and the recipient area should be devoid of any remains of necrotic tissue. Meticulous hemostasis in the recipient area should be ensured. The graft should be sutured with fine silk to the periphery of the removed surface under normal (appropriate) tension. If the tension is too great, the grafted sites will tend to contract, while if it is too little, the graft will become corrugated, and linear scar contracture may result. After the graft has been secured on the wound surface, this area should be covered with petrolatum-impregnated gauze or gauze soaked with antibiotic solutions and bandaged evenly. If the wound surface contains depressed areas, these depressions should be padded with cotton before the bandage is applied. If the exposure method is used, the wound should be examined from time to time, and accumulated fluid under the graft aspirated. If the graft is laid

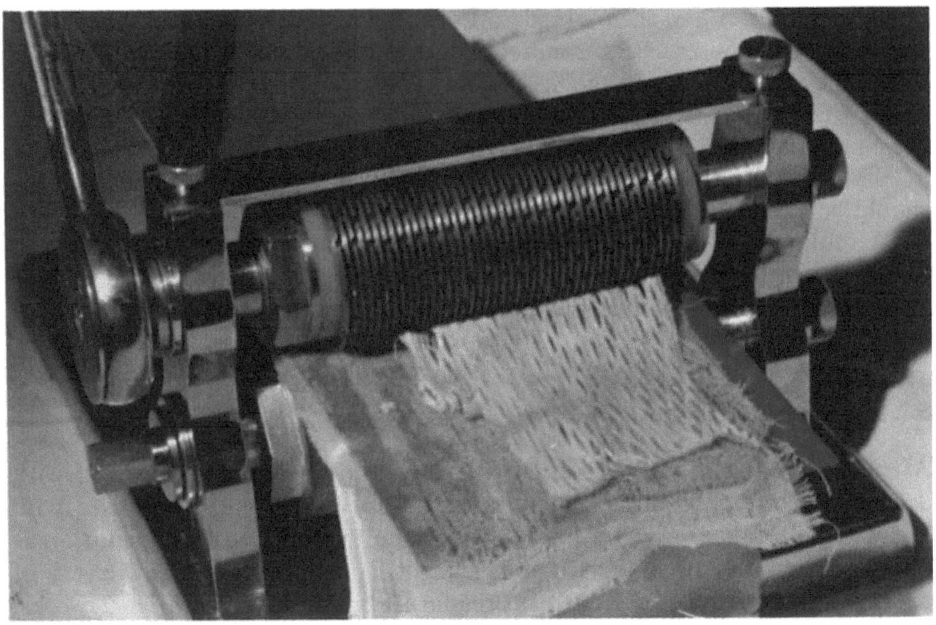

Fig. III.34. The skin mesher

on the functional parts of the joints, immobilization must be efficient in order to avoid displacement of the graft.

5.2.6.2 Transplantation of Mesh Graft

In 1964 Tanner made a sizeable contribution to the method of skin grafting by introducing his "mesher" (the Tanner Vanderput mesh dermatome). Alternative slender incisions are made with distance of 0.05 in. between them. The graft can be expanded by 1.5, 2, or even 3 times the original size. The length of the edges of the graft is increased enormously (according to Tanner, the border surface of 1 $in.^2$ can be increased from 4 in. to 38 in.). The epithelium can creep centrifugally in all directions with an astonishing speed; thus the interspaces of the meshes can be covered within 10 days. The dermal appendages of a mesh graft are evenly distributed to make the healed wound quite resistant against trauma (Fig. II.34).

If the expansion is 1.5 times the original size the functional results will be excellent. For grafting of irregular surfaces such as axilla, chin, and neck, the unexpanded mesh graft gives a better moulding.

For producing meshes, split-thickness graft no less than 0.4 mm thick is employed. The outer border of the graft must be fixed to the wound edge either with sutures or tapes. Fine-mesh Vaseline gauze and bulky pressure bandages are applied.

5.2.6.3 Transplantation of Small Autografts

This method is indicated in extensive burns. For extensive third degree burns, allografts need to be interposed between the small autografts to avoid exposure of the interspaces which would not be covered until weeks later by the extension of the grafted elements. Scar contracture would be inevitable and cosmetic results, poor.

The advantage of transplantation of small grafts is that it is possible to cover extensive third degree wounds with a relatively small amount of autograft. When grafting granulation wounds, it is not necessary to wait for complete dropping off of all the necrotic tissue. Transplantation of small autografts may be performed earlier than that of large sheets.

Procedure: After pasting a large piece of split-thickness skin on to a piece of petrolatum-impregnated gauze or sterilized paper, it is cut into small pieces of 0.3 cm × 0.3 cm to 1 cm × 1 cm (if the thickness is more than 0.2 mm, it is liable to roll up and be difficult to paste). These small autografts are transplanted 1 cm–1.5 cm apart from each other. If small allografts are laid in the interspaces of the autografts, then all exposed areas can be covered, If the granulation surface is large and there is little remaining necrotic tissue, autografting may be performed as follows: Arrange the small autografts on a piece of gauze and then lay it on the recipient surface. After the gauze is removed, the grafts will be evenly distributed with regular interspaces.

After the transplantation, fix the grafts with a layer of petrolatum-impregnated gauze of coarse netting (tulle gras), upon which two or three layers

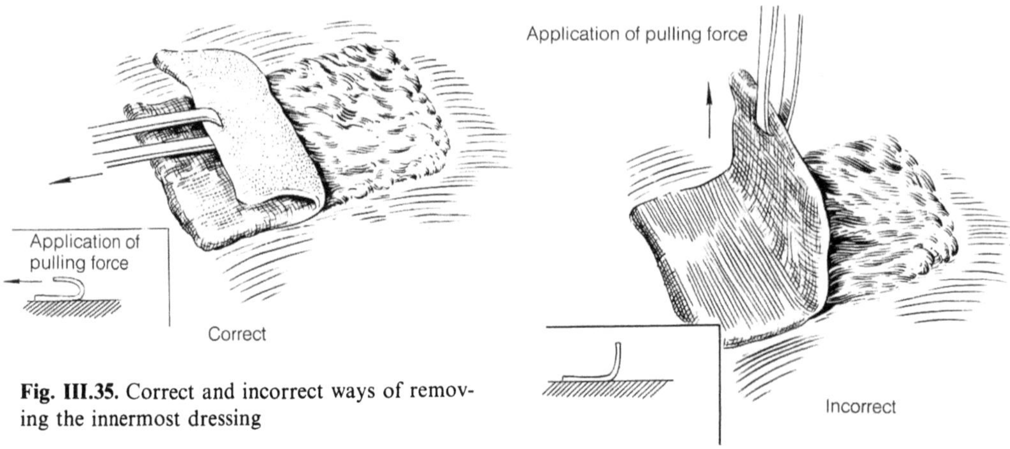

Fig. III.35. Correct and incorrect ways of removing the innermost dressing

of gauze moistened with antibiotic solutions are placed. The wound may be left semiexposed or bandaged under pressure after the addition of a bulky "burn gauze." When bandaging, pressure exerted should be even; the dressings must not be creased or moved to avoid displacement of the grafts. If the pregrafting wound surface was not seriously infected, the dressings may be changed at 1–2 day intervals. If the dressings are changed too early, displacement may occur since the grafts will not have adhered firmly. If the wound surface is seriously infected, at least the outer layers of the dressings ought to be changed 24 h after the operation and the grafts under the tulle gras examined carefully. During the changing of dressings, gentleness is especially important: care must be taken not to displace the grafts. The dressings should be removed with great care along the longitudinal axis (Fig. III.35). If the inner layer is too adherent, it should be moistened with liquid paraffin. If there is little pus on the impregnated gauze, and drainage is good, then only the outer layers of the dressings need to be changed.

If it is evident on changing the dressings for the first time that the grafts have adhered firmly and the epidermis of the grafts is intact, then the grafts have taken. If the grafts turned pink, it means that circulation of blood has been established between the grafts and the recipient surface. Thin split-thickness grafts will turn pink in 3 days, while split-thickness grafts of intermediate thickness will require 5–7 days. Grafts which have taken will, as a rule, begin to expand in all directions 5–7 days after transplantation. If the interspaces between the grafts measure less than 1 cm and there is no evident infection, with the exception of the aged or patients with uncontrolled diabetes, the wound surface should be completely covered about 2 weeks after transplantation.

5.2.6.4 Transplantation of Postage Stamp-Sized Grafts

When autografts are cut square with a surface of 1 cm^2–4 cm^2 they are called postage-stamp grafts. If the third degree burn area is not large and the donor sites are ample, transplantation with postage-stamp grafts will extinguish the wound rapidly. Although the scarring is much less than with small grafts, this method has gradually been replaced by mesh grafts since both the cosmetic and the functional results are better with the latter.

5.2.6.5 Full-Thickness Skin Transplantation (cf. Chap. XIV)

6 Allografts, Xenografts, and Intermingled Transplantation

6.1 Allografts

After the removal of the eschar of extensive burns (either by excision or by natural separation) it is impossible to completely cover the exposed wound with autografts owing to the scarcity of donor sites. If a large surface is exposed and becomes infected, all efforts to retrieve the situation often end in failure. In order to avoid such a calamity, the only effective measure is to cover the wound with allografts.

As soon as the wound has been grafted, the general condition of the patient improves instantaneously. If all the wounds have been sealed temporarily by allografting, the patient can even move about as if nothing has happened. This miraculous effect is, however, soon over. The allografts are bound to be rejected and cast off within 3 weeks after transplantation, and the wound surface will become reinfected. Owing to the remnants of necrotic allodermis left on the wound, the reappearing wounds are not ready to accept further grafting of any kind. Although immense advances have been achieved within the past 10 years in the realm of organ and tissue transplantation, it is acknowledged that the allografts can only serve as a sort of biological dressing. It can protect the body as the autoskin does, but only temporarily. To avoid the aftermath of rejection, the allografts must be torn off before rejoining of the blood vessels takes place, that is, 3–7 days after transplantation. (Three days is more ideal than 7, for there is massive bleeding and oozing when the buds of vessels have already rejoined or grown into the allograft around the 5th postgrafting day.) If there are not enough autografts to cover the whole wound, new sets of allografts are transplanted to cover the still exposed area until sufficient autograft can be harvested to obtain permanent sealing.

If the general condition of the patient does not allow harvesting of a large amount of autograft, allografts may be utilized to win a certain period of breathing space. In some cases, when the ability of the wound surface to receive skin is poor or doubtful, transplantation of allograft may be tried first to ensure that subsequent autografts will survive. After the allografts have survived, they may be torn off and replaced by autografts; alternatively, autografting may be performed to replace the allografts part by part. A 100% take can be achieved by the above-mentioned method.

6.2 Xenografts

The utilization of animal skin as a source of biological dressing had a long enduring history in ancient Chinese medical practice, when the animal used was the cock. Judging by our own clinical observations, it still remains a relatively ideal biological dressing for small granulating wounds. The strange fact is that while xenotransplantation of organs or tissues has been abandoned after successive failures, xenoskin grafts and xenovalvular transplants have won general acceptance. Also strange is the fact that both of the successfully used xenotissues are from the pig. The pig skin – we prefer the term porcine skin – serves as a cheaper biological dressing (in comparison with allografts). Owing to the close resemblance between mammalian epithelial structures, Bromberg and his associates introduced porcine skin as a temporary biological dressing for burns on a scientific basis, hence giving porcine skin to a prominent role in modern surgical practice.

As a biological dressing, porcine skin is applied either on a second degree burn wound or on a wound involving full-thickness injuries. It should be peeled off within 5 days, otherwise adverse effects of xenorejection ensue: the wound is once again exposed and is ill-prepared for grafting, and recovery is further delayed.

If the porcine skin is not peeled off within 2 weeks after transplantation, it becomes well nourished by the human body fluid through osmosis, provided that the porcine skin was applied on a sterile wound after excision. But 2 weeks later, following the ingrowth of the granulation tissue, rejection processes are located around the xenodermal appendages and the epidermis. The reaction is far more intense than in the case of allografts. Nowadays, lyophilized porcine skin is available commercially in Western countries, and glutaldehyde-treated porcine skin is also becoming available, but fresh porcine skin is still preferred in this country for reasons mentioned in the following sections.

6.3 Intermingled Transplantation of Autograft and Allograft

Transplantation of autograft into a larger sheet of allograft (abbreviated as intermingled transplantation hereafter) together with staged excision of the third degree burn eschar constitutes a simple and practical method for the successful management of certain very extensive third degree burns and raises the overall survival rate of patients with extensive deep burns. The intermingled transplanted grafts can be applied either on granulated surfaces or on wounds created by excision of the eschar. As previously mentioned, autografts can expand to a size seven to ten times the original.

After free graft of alloskin, the rejection response begins after revascularization, usually about 6 days after grafting. During these 6 days the epithelial cells are well nourished by osmosis of the body fluid, but the endothelial cells of the allovessels then begin to swell, degenerate, and fragmentate, eventually leading to obliteration. The epithelium then becomes necrotic and gives way to an infected allodermis.

After intermingled transplantation of auto- and allografts, not only does the newly formed granulation tissue grow into the dermis from the grafting bed but also into the interspace between the epidermis and the dermis of the alloskin from both sides of the impregnated autoskins, so as to maintain the integrity of the basal membrane and the basal cell layer, which serve as an efficient barrier against the infiltration of immunocompetent lymphoid cells and even of immunoglobulins. As a result of this process the alloepithelium retains a privileged site; it thus delays rejection and helps the body to win time for the substitution of the alloepithelium by the "creeping" autoepithelium. Under the intact autoepithelium, the allodermis together with the dermal adnexa are rejected in a very slow process which lasts for months. In this way the human body is first protected by the alloepidermis and then by the autoepidermis. The continuous protection by the epidermis and the conservation of the autoskins make possible the survival of patients previously considered hopeless and also leave sufficient autoskins for late reconstructive purposes.

6.3.1 Method of Intermingled Transplantation

Intermingled transplantation usually involves either (a) large sheets of allograft inlaid with autografts for covering third degree wound surfaces after eschar excision or (b) alternating pieces of autograft and allograft to cover the granulation wound after natural separation of third degree burned eschar.

1. Large sheets of allograft with autograft inlays: Slits are made 1 cm apart on a large sheet of allograft which is then grafted onto the surface left after eschar excision. If the allograft appears to have survived after 1–2 days, the slits are transformed into rectangular windows using a pair of thin-blade scissors; the size of these windows must correspond to that of the autografts about to be inlaid. After bleeding from the windows has been checked by pressure, a piece of autograft is inlaid into each window (Fig. III.36) and the wound is bandaged.

At the time of window formation and graft inlaying the following points should be observed: (a) When windows are made in the allograft, care should be taken not to cleave the surrounding allograft, for this would destroy the already established linkage between the allograft and the bed. (b) Bleeding must be checked with meticulous care. There are probably about 500–1,000 small holes in an allograft for one lower extremity. The amount of blood lost may reach as much as 500 ml, even if the blood from each hole is only

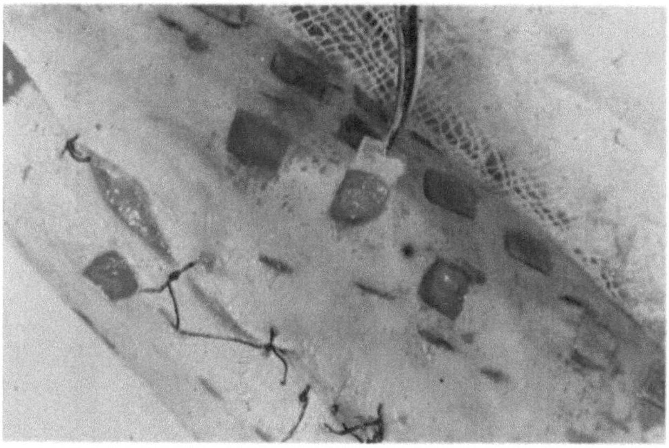

Fig. III.36. Slits are made 1 cm apart on a large sheet of allo- or xenograft and are transformed into rectangular windows into which pieces of autograft will be inlaid

0.5 ml. Blood loss must therefore be fully estimated when the operations for window formation and skin inlaying are in progress.

2. Alternating pieces of autograft and allograft: Cut the allo- and autoskin into small pieces (see Fig. III.18) and then transplant them alternately in a bricklaying pattern on the granulation surface. Semiexpose the wound or bandage it.

6.3.2 Histologic Observations

The thickness of the autografts is approximately 0.2 mm, so that dermal appendages are not involved, while the allografts are 0.5 mm thick, with most of the adnexa intact.

Eight days after transplantation the epithelial cells appear normal. The fact that the dermal vessels have joined with the recipient bed is shown by dilated and congested papillary vessels (Fig. III.37, III.38). At this time, massive lymphoid cells infiltrate the allodermis under the intact epidermis, which indicates

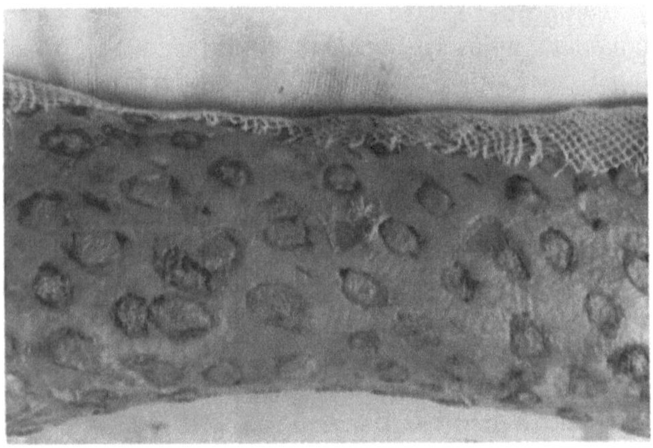

Fig. III.37. Situation 8 days after allografting and 5 days after the insertion of autografts. Two new windows have been "opened", one at the midpoint between two autografts and one adjacent to an autograft. Section of the midpoint specimen is shown in **Fig. III.38**

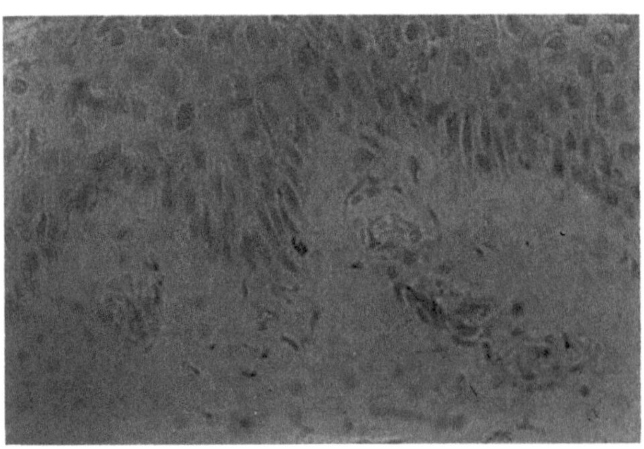

Fig. III.38. Eight days postgrafting. The epithelial cells show a normal appearance. Dilated and congested papillary vessels are seen, indicating joining of the dermal vessels with the recipient bed. H & E, ×580

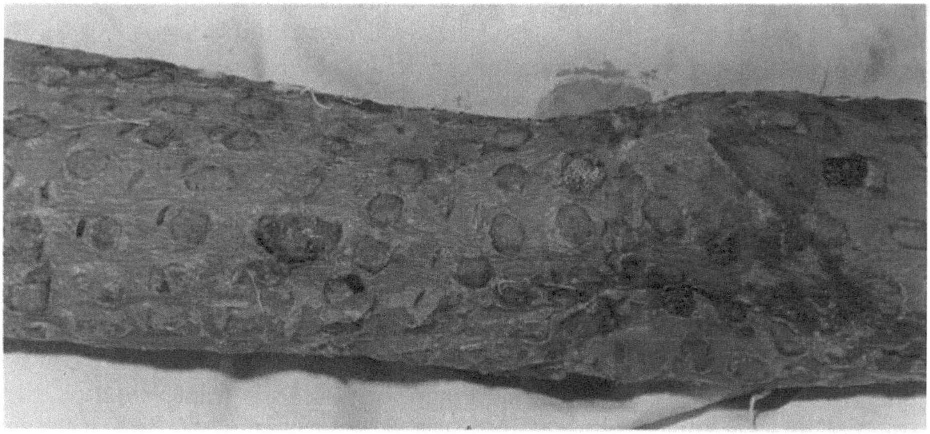

Fig. III.39. Twenty days after intermingled transplantation of allo- and autografts. Repeated desquamation of the alloskin is observed clinically

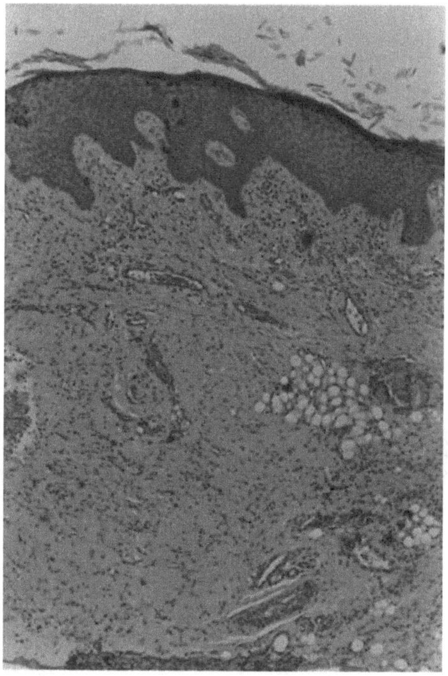

Fig. III.40. Specimen taken from allograft 20 days after intermingled transplantation. The alloepithelium shows acanthosis, and large numbers of lymphocytes are seen infiltrating the allodermis. H & E, ×100

that the rejection process begins as soon as the allografts have communicated with the recipient bed through joined vessels.

In normal skin there are only a few layers of epidermal cells. However, 20 days after grafting the alloepithelium shows acanthosis. A large number of lymphocytes infiltrate beneath the alloepithelium (Figs. III.39, III.40). Under ordinary conditions the onset of acute rejection of allograft from an unrelated donor in a severely burned patient is around 20 days postgrafting, but after intermingled transplantation, a process called the "sandwich phenomenon" will occur after 20 days or more. That is to say, the granulation tissue both from the autotissue and from the autobed will creep and grow between the autoepidermis and the degenerative alloepidermis, and finally substitution of alloepidermis by the autoepithelium will take place. The allodermis will be rejected under an intact autoepidermis (Figs. III.41, III.42). During the process of rejection of the alloepidermis, only scattered areas of dissolution of the basal cells can be observed. Polarizing microscopy reveals degeneration of the allodermal collagen by gradual weakening of its birefringence accompanied by ingrowth of the granulation tissue (Fig. III.43).

Remnants of allodermal adnexa still exist 2 months postgrafting and will disappear 1 month later. The epidermis at that time reveals a normal appearance with H & E stain, but the periodic acid-Schiff (PAS) reaction shows it to contain a large amount of collagen. Eight months after transplantation the structure of skin appears normal under H & E staining, but PAS reaction reveals that the epithelial glycogen is still abundant at the allosites, although it has disappeared at the autosites.

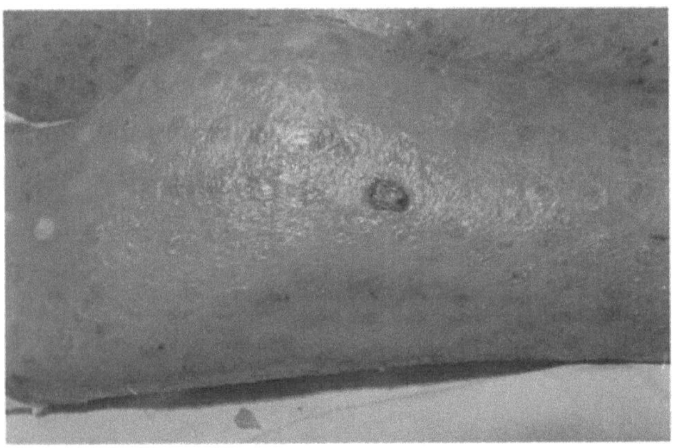

Fig. III.41. Same patient as in **Fig. III.39**, 45 days after intermingled transplantation. The dark spot near the knee joint is the site of biopsy. The microscopic view is shown in **Fig. III.42**

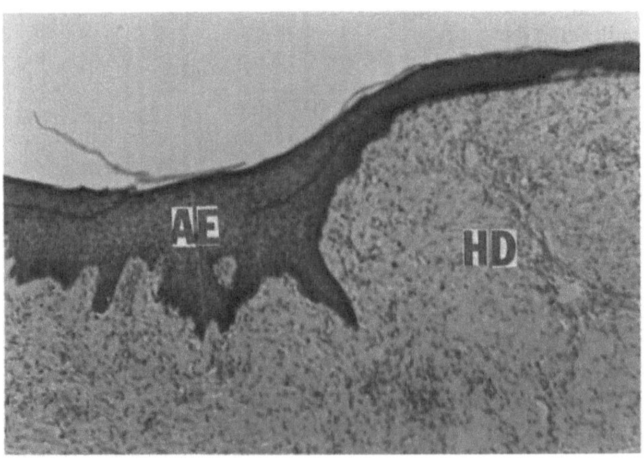

Fig. III.42. Histologic section 45 days after intermingled transplantation. The autoepidermis (*AE*) has crept rightward to "sandwich" the allodermis (*HD*). The allodermis will be rejected insidiously beneath an intact autoepidermis. H & E, ×125

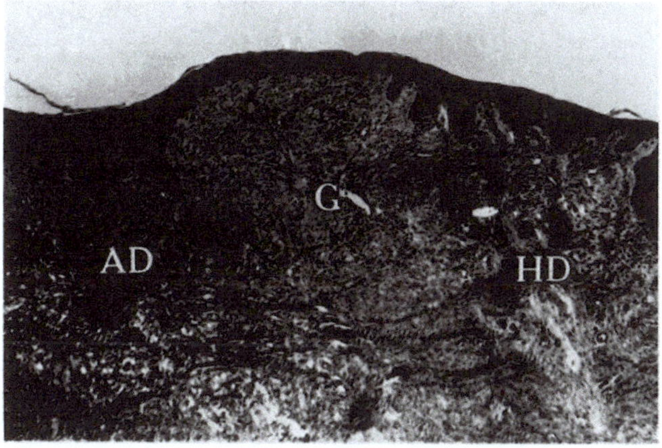

Fig. III.43. Polarizing microscopic view of **Fig. III.42.** *AD*, autodermis; *G*, ingrowth of granulation tissue; *HD*, allodermal collagen showing weakening of its birefringence. × 66

If the inlaid autografts are too small or the distances between them are too great, granulation wounds might appear following the dissolution of the alloepidermis. A few patients showed a "rejection episode" for which the reason is not clear. A "rejection episode" can be defined as acute rejection of the allodermis sandwiched in the autotissue, sometimes together with alloepidermis which has not yet been totally substituted by autoepithelium. During its onset, the grafted site swells with prominent hobnail-like bulging of the autoskins. The episode lasts about 2–3 weeks, during which time there are repeated attacks (Fig. III.44). If acute rejection occurs before 20 days postgrafting, the allograft turns purplish because there is no autotissue under the alloepidermis, and a mesh-like black scab is finally formed. The pathologic sections taken from the scab site show epithelial headings extending above the necrotic allodermis. If the scab is kept uninfected, the autoepidermis from the adjacent autografts

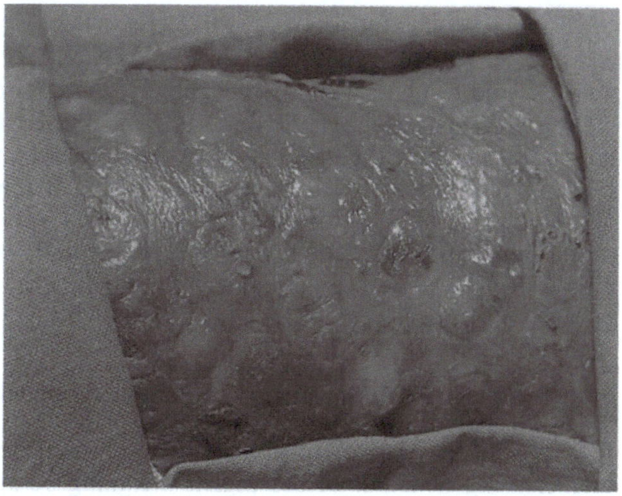

Fig. III.44. "Rejection episode", with hobnail bulging of the autografts and purplish coloration of the allograft

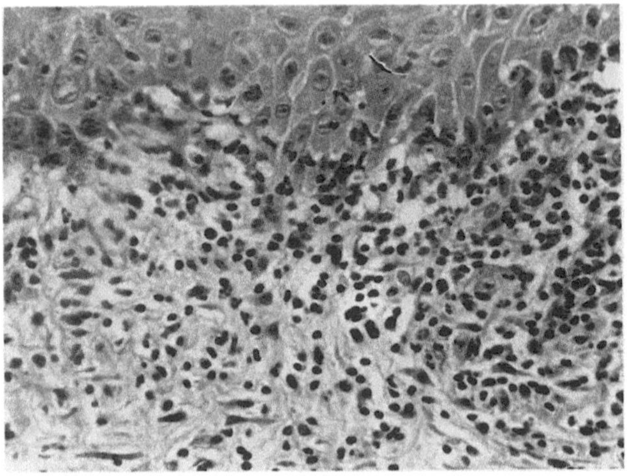

Fig. III.45. Thirty-four days after intermingled transplantation. Rejection episode with destruction of the basal layer of the alloepidermis and patchy infiltration of lymphoid cells. H & E, ×500

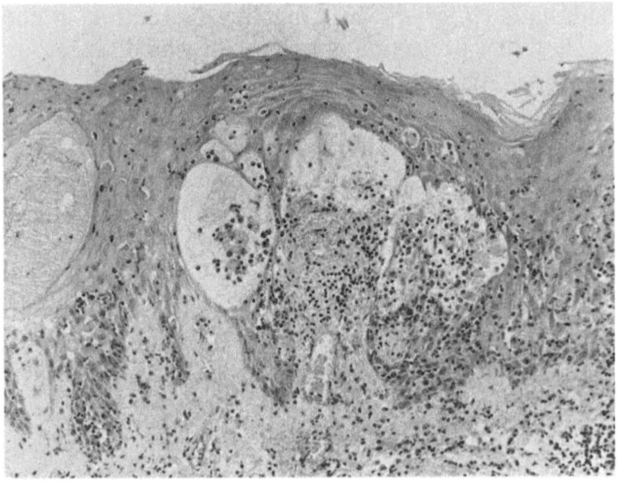

Fig. III.46. Thirty-three days after intermingled transplantation. Rejection episode. Large vesicles containing eosin-stained fluid are seen in a portion of the stratum spinosum; these vesicles may rupture into the dermis. A few layers of epidermal cells are still intact. H & E, ×125

will fuse and result in a subscab healing. If the episode happens 1 or 2 months after grafting, destruction of the basal membrane and patchy infiltration of lymphoid cells into the basal layer of the alloepidermis may be observed (Fig. III.45). There is also lysis of a certain portion of the stratum spinosum. Large vesicles are formed within which there is eosin-stained fluid. These vesicles may rupture into the dermis where the basal layer is destroyed. But, although only a few layers of epidermal cells are left, they still effectively serve the purpose of protection (Fig. III.46).

6.4 Intermingled Transplantation of Porcine Skin and Autograft

It is sometimes possible to use porcine skin in place of allografts, which are in increasing demand. White piglets weighing 10 kg–15 kg are most suitable for use. After killing them by exsanguination and subcutaneous inflation with compression air, the skin is first shaved and then excised together with its subcutaneous tissue in large sheets (preferably as a whole sheet). The skin is placed upside down with the epidermis facing the drum of a Padgett dermatome. A partial-thickness sheet of porcine skin (about 0.4 mm–0.6 mm thick) is thus prepared. Third degree burn eschar is either excised to the deep fascia or tangentially excised down to the healthy tissue. Large sheets of porcine skin are laid on the wound with or without sutures. As with allograft, equidistant slits or windows are made prior to its application. Immediately after the excisional operation or 3 days later, small pieces of autograft (0.2 mm in thickness, and at least 0.25 cm^2 in size) are inserted into the previously prepared windows. No attempt is made to remove the porcine skin by mechanical means, except in patients with autolysis or severe infection of the grafted porcine skin.

The normal porcine epidermis may be divided into layers which resemble the stratum corneum, stratum granulosum, and stratum germinativum, but no

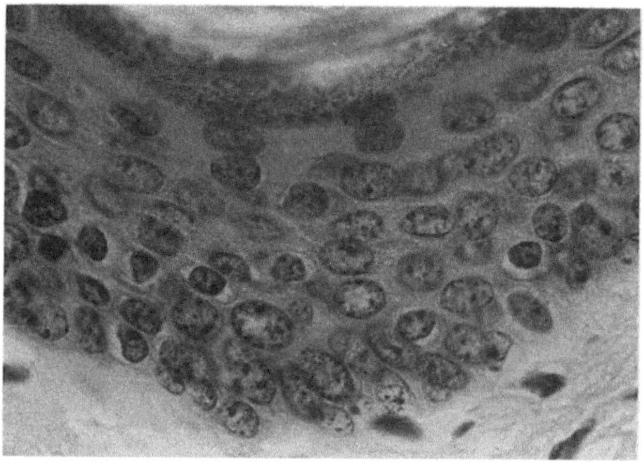

Fig. III.47. Normal porcine epidermis. The stratum corneum, stratum granulosum, and stratum germinativum are shown. No columnar basal cells or melanocytes are to be observed. The chromatin granules are coarse and deeply stained. H&E, ×1,250

distinct columnar basal cells and dendroid melanocytes have been observed. The intercellular bridges of the prickle cells are very coarse and ill-defined in contour. The nuclei are large and consist of coarse and deeply stained chromatin granules (Fig. III.47). The dermal papillae are wide and patent vessels are observed. Hair follicles are large and superficially situated. Only a few deep-seated sebaceous and sweat glands are present. Although no patent vessels were observed following transplantation of the porcine skin, and no lymphoid cells infiltrated the porcine dermal collagen, its epidermal cells were nevertheless integral with normally arranged dermal collagen 9 days after transplantation (Fig. III.48). About 2 weeks after intermingled transplantation a belt of lymphocytic infiltration affected the recipient bed (Fig. III.49). At the same time ingrowth of the granulation tissue into the belt took place except in those areas with large amounts of porcine dermal adnexa; on the other hand, cellular

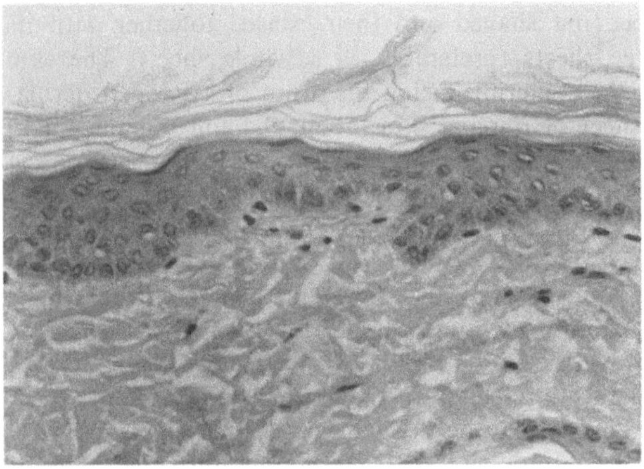

Fig. III.48. Nine days after xenografting. No lymphoid cells have infiltrated the porcine dermal collagen, and the epidermis shows a normal appearance. H & E, × 100

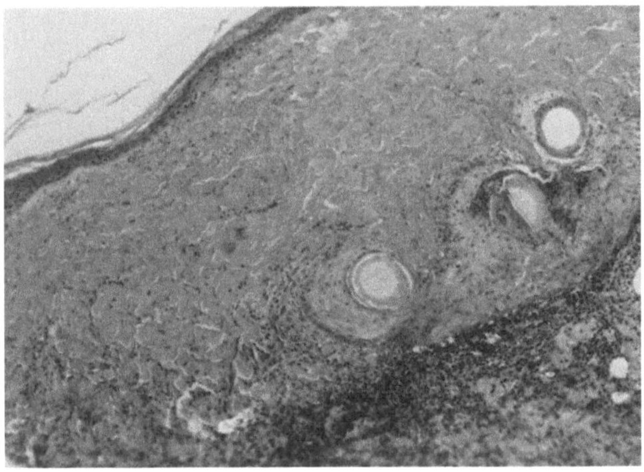

Fig. III.49. Thirteen days after xenografting. Round cells are gathering around the porcine hair follicles. H & E, × 100

infiltration of the porcine dermal collagen was mild, with scattered granulation septa invaded. Three weeks after transplantation the originally xenografted sites were covered with well-differentiated autoepithelium. The dermal papillae vessels reappeared (Fig. III.50). The remnants of the porcine dermal collagen were separated by the ingrowth of the granulation tissue and gradually lost the characteristic birefringence (Fig. III.51).

One month after transplantation; the autoepithelium which grew on the xenografted sites differentiated into distinct layers. Large numbers of dendritic melanocytes were observed. The deposition of melanin could be traced back even earlier, to 2 weeks after transplantation (Fig. III.52) (Fig. III.53).

The following points deserve to be mentioned:

1. The clearance of the bacteria under the porcine skin is not as efficient as with allo- or autografts; transplanting the porcine skin onto granulation

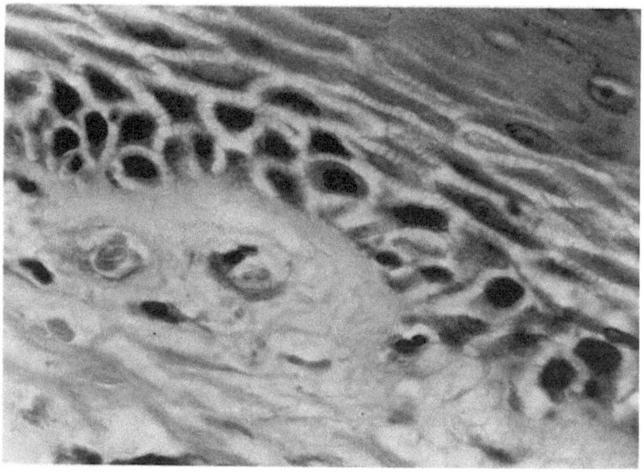

Fig. III.50. Twenty-three days after xenografting; vessels of dermal papillae are seen. H & E, ×1,250

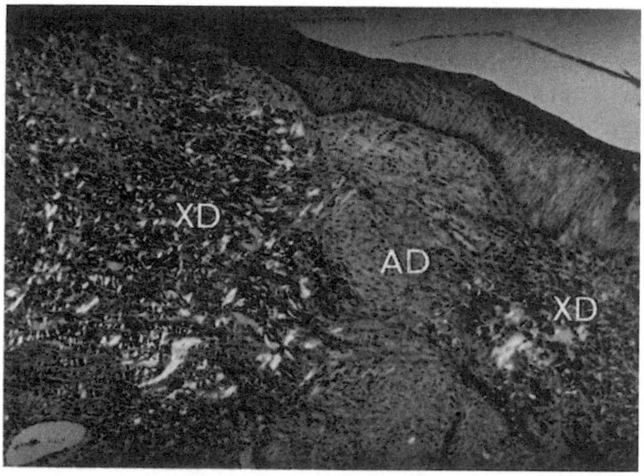

Fig. III.51. Polarizing microscopy. *AD*, autodermis; *XD*, xenodermis. H & E, ×125

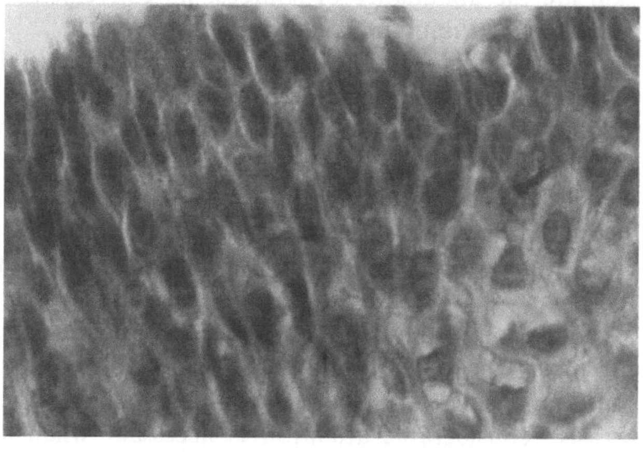

Fig. III.52. Thirteen days after intermingled transplantation of porcine skin and autografts. The autoepidermis "creeps" onto the porcine dermis. A large number of dendritic melanocytes and deposition of melanin are observed. H & E, ×1,250

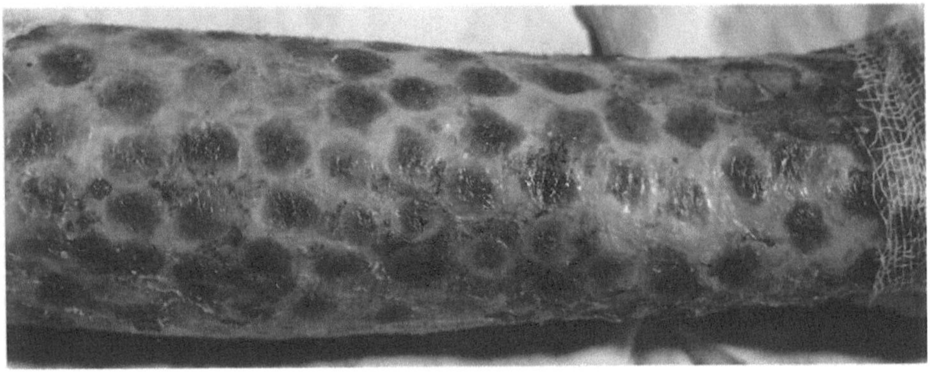

Fig. III.53. Appearance 6 weeks after intermingled transplantation of porcine skin and autografts

tissue usually ends in failure. Therefore porcine skin is mainly used in covering the sterile wounds created by excision of the eschar.

2. Twenty minutes prior to transplantation, the fresh or deep-frozen porcine skin must be dipped into a physiologic saline solution containing 100 mg gentamicin and four thousand units of bacitracin per 100 ml. After the completion of grafting, the same antibiotic solution must be used to irrigate the wound.

3. One must avoid the application of porcine skin to adipose tissue or muscle since it is liable to be infected.

4. If remnants of porcine graft are still present 3 weeks after transplantation, they should be torn off in order to facilitate the early substitution of the xenoepidermis by the autoepidermis.

6.5 Artificial Skin

Artificial skin may be made with synthetic as well as with biologic material. The type we use is double-layered, the outer layer being made of polyurethane film, and the inner layer, of processed cow collagen. The advantages of artifical skin are the abundance of sources, its convenience for use and storage, and the absence of immune reactions.

When artificial skin is used, the wound surface should be fresh and devoid of necrotic tissue. When it is employed on third degree or deep second degree wound surfaces after tangential excision of eschar, the conditions are the same as for allografting, i.e., the bed should be devoid of necrotic and adipose tissue, and hemostasis should be thorough. If artificial skin is used for coverage of wound surfaces with rather large amounts of purulent secretions, then accumulation of pus under that "skin" is inevitable. Therefore, it is necessary to select the wound surface on the basis of strict criteria and with great care. When accumulation of pus is found under the artificial skin, that part of the "skin" must be removed immediately in order to avoid interference with drainage. Since artificial skin is not as pliable as allograft or xenograft and is easily creased, considerable attention is necessary when artificial skin is being laid on the wound surface. It must be laid smoothly and immobilized firmly after application.

The artificial skin is shown to be well pasted on the wound surface if the external appearance of the artificial skin is fairly smooth and a rosy wound surface can be seen through it.

When artificial skin was used as a trial for operation using the intermingled method, we observed that the artificial skin may interfere with the extension of the autograft.

Chapter IV Infection of the Burn

Hsu Wei-shia and Shih Tsi-siang

Translated by Yang Chih-chun and Shih Tsi-siang

At present, infection is still the most frequent cause of death after burns. During the period from 1958 to the end of 1978, 68% of our hospitalized deaths resulted from wound sepsis and septicemia. Many efforts have been made during recent decades to combat infection, yet it still remains a major unsolved problem in the treatment of burns.

Human epidermis has the natural property of being a defensive barrier against bacteria and other microorganisms. After burn, this natural defensive barrier is lost; in addition, the large amount of necrotic tissue resulting from the burn injury serves as an excellent culture medium for microorganisms. Infection of the wound not only causes the conversion of a second degree burn into a third degree wound, but is also the fundamental cause of wound sepsis and septicemia.

It was Teplitz who first defined the concept of "burn wound sepsis" in a scientific way in 1962. Wound sepsis can be said to exist when: "The quantity of the bacteria in the burned necrotic tissue exceeds 10^5 per gram and the subjacent viable tissue has been invaded by the colonized bacteria."

The following experiment was performed by us in 1972. After epilation, the backs of albino rats were scalded with 98 °C water for 10 s, producing a third degree burn to about 20% of the BSA. The burned surface was immediately inoculated with 0.5 ml of a suspension of 2×10^8 of *Pseudomonas aeruginosa* per ml which was isolated from a patient's wound. Ten to fourteen animals were killed 24 h, 4 days, and 6 days postburn, and the bacteria per gram of tissue under the eschar were determined quantitatively. At the same time pathologic section with Giemsa staining was performed. It was found that in animals killed 24 h postburn, the subeschar bacterial count averaged 9.4×10^4 per gram of tissue, but in tissue sections only a few bacterial colonies were seen, these being located around the hair follicles, under the epidermis, and in the superficial layer of the dermis (Figs. IV.1, IV.2). In animals killed 4 days postburn, the amount of bacteria was 2.9×10^7 per gram of tissue. Sections showed large quantities of proliferating bacteria under the epidermis and around the hair follicles, with invasion of the deeper parts of the dermis. The local inflammatory reaction was nil (Fig. IV.3–IV.5). In the 6 days postburn specimens, the quantity of subeschar bacteria per gram of tissue was 1×10^8, and under microscopic examination necrosis and sloughing of the epidermis were seen. Large amounts of bacteria had invaded the deep dermal regions and even the muscular layer. Typical *Pseudomonas* arteritis was observed (Figs.

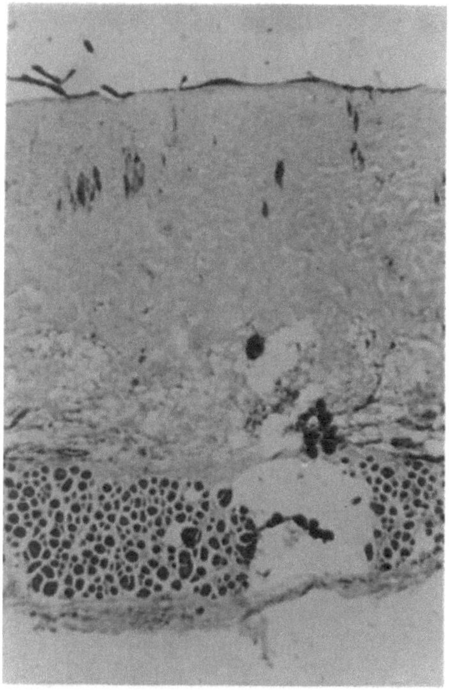

Fig. IV.1. Pathologic section of the burn wound of an albino rat, 24 h postburn. The method of scalding and local innoculation of *P. aeruginosa* are described in the text. A few bacteria are seen under the necrotic epidermis and along the hair follicles. Giemsa, low-power magnification

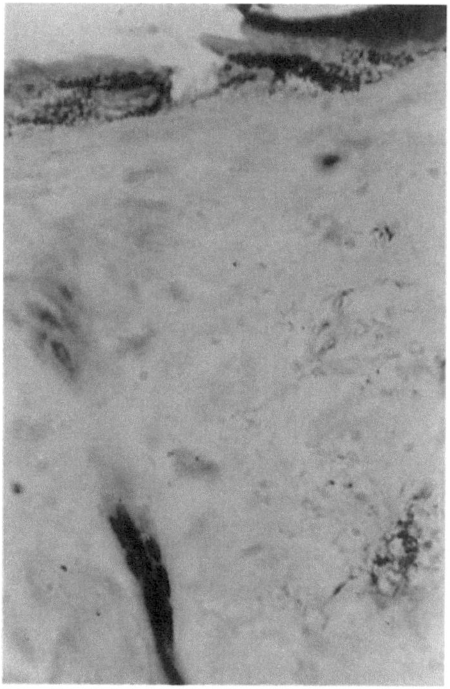

Fig. IV.2. Oil immersion view of a hair follicle from the same rat as in **Fig. IV.1.** Subepidermal bacterial colonies and bacteria along the hair follicle are seen. Giemsa

IV.6, IV.7). These results showed that, with the lapse of time, bacteria entered the subcutaneous lymphatic channels either via the hair follicles or directly from the surface downwards and gradually invaded the deeper layers. Finally they penetrated into the neighboring viable tissue and blood vessels.

In another experimental study we took 98 biopsy specimens from 26 cases of early eschar excision for bacterial quantification. We found that except for 9 sterile specimens the rest invariably showed bacterial growth regardless of the various topical bactericidal agents employed. In 77 specimens the numbers of bacteria per gram of subeschar tissue were 10^3–10^6. These data correlated well with the results of our animal experiments, denoting that after burn, large amounts of bacteria not only proliferate and grow on the burn surface but also invade deeper unburned tissues. If patent blood vessels are involved, positive blood cultures may ensue.

Skin constitutes the largest vital organ of the body. If a huge burn wound is contaminated with proliferating microorganisms it always constitues a great menace to the host. The toxins released by the vast amount of proliferating bacteria are alone already sufficient to kill the patient. Clinically the patient

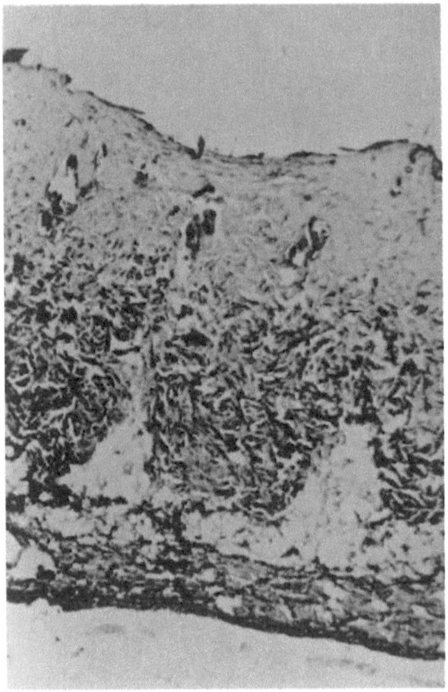

Fig. IV.3

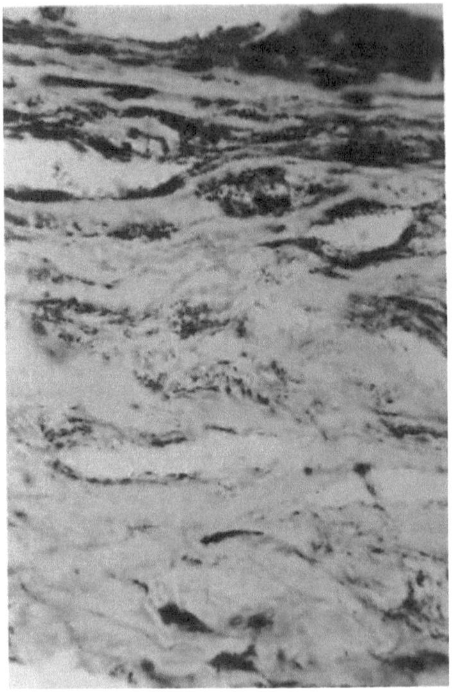

Fig. IV.4

Fig. IV.3. Four days postburn. Bacteria (2.9×10^7/g) are seen proliferating under the necrotic epidermis and around the hair follicle. Giemsa, low-power magnification

Fig. IV.4. High-power view of **Fig.IV. 3.** A large number of bacteria are seen proliferating in the superficial dermal layer. Giemsa

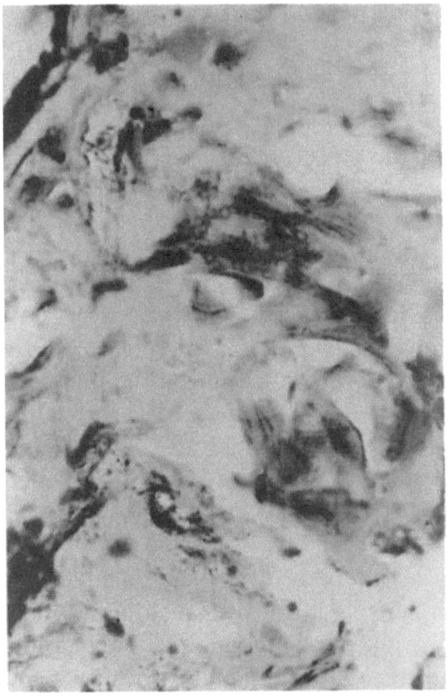

Fig. IV.5. Oil immersion view of **Fig. IV.4.** Pronounced bacterial growth is seen in the deep dermal layer. Inflammatory cells are rarely seen. Giemsa

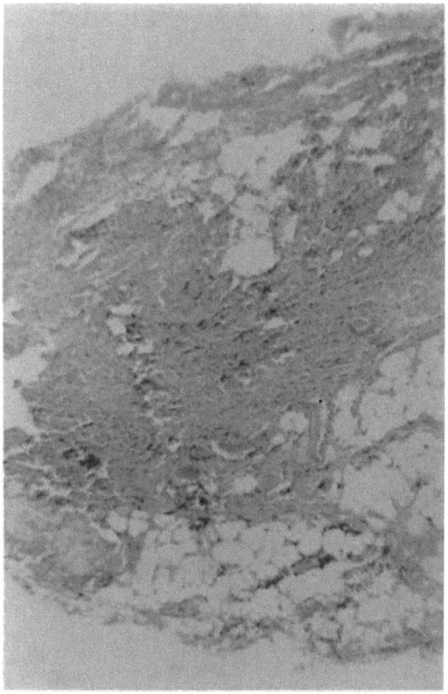

Fig. IV.6. Six days postburn. The epidermis has sloughed off. A large number of bacteria (1×10^8/g) are invading the deep dermal and the muscular layers. H & E, lower-power magnification

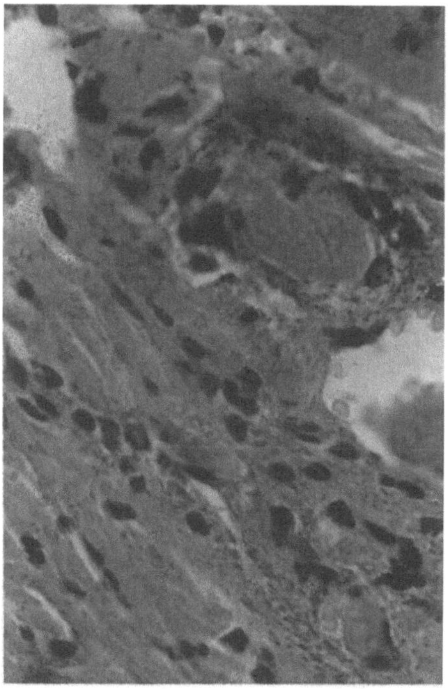

Fig. IV.7. Oil immersion view of **Fig. IV.6.** *Pseudomonas* arteritis and inflammatory cells are observed. H & E

will have all of the most typical symptoms and signs of systemic infection, yet the blood cultures may remain negative provided that the blood vessels are not involved. In this chapter the term "septicemia" is taken to include the concept of "wound sepsis," since although the most frequent cause of septicemia in burns is wound sepsis, foci other than the burn wound, e.g., septic phlebitis and pneumonia, can also lead to invasive systemic infections.

1 The Onset of Septicemia

Before complete closure of the wounds, septicemia may occur at any stage during the entire course of burn treatment. Acute fulminating septicemia may occur within 24 h postburn. Figure IV.8 depicts the incidence and time of onset of septicemias. By understanding the rules concerning its occurrence we can apprehend its onset and prevent it in advance.

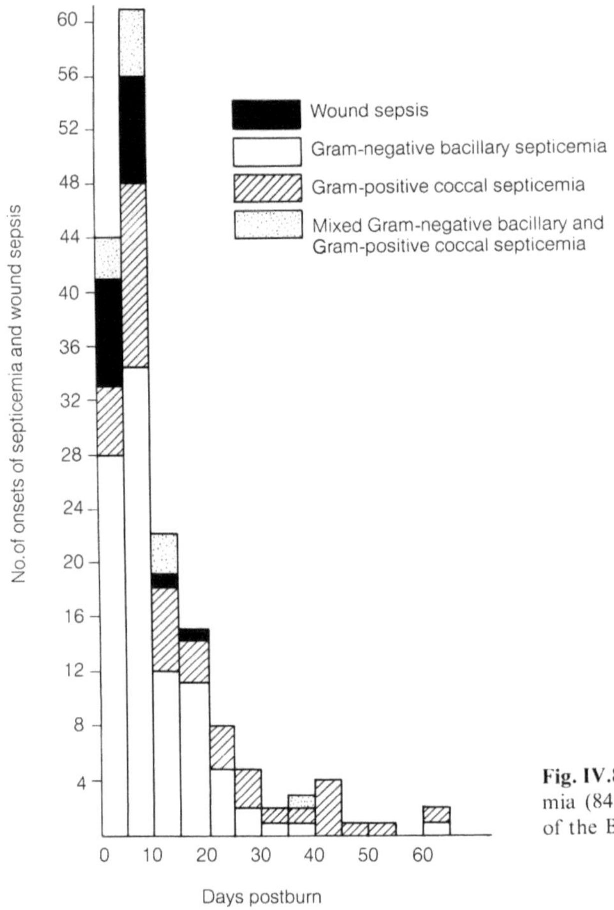

Fig. IV.8. Incidence and time of onset of septicemia (84 patients with burns to more than 80% of the BSA; 168 onsets of septicemia)

1.1 Early Stage (Within 10 Days Postburn)

Figure IV.8 shows clearly that in most patients in whom septicemia occurred, its onset was within 10 days postburn. Sixty-two percent of cases of septicemia occurred at this stage, most of them between 4 and 7 days postburn. During this period, host resistance was lowered due to resorption of the edema fluid, etc. Later on, following the gradual formation of a defensive barrier of granulation tissue underneath the necrotic tissue, the incidence of septicemia decreased significantly.

There is a definite relationship between early stage septicemia and the clinical course of shock. An eventful shock stage will strongly favor the invasion of bacteria into the adjacent viable tissue, as shown by Table IV.1. The majority of the organisms elicited were gram-negative bacilli. Septicemia in the shock stage had a fulminating onset, rapid progress, and poor prognosis. Delay in resuscitation, mishandling of the fluid replacement therapy, or distant transpor-

Table IV.1. The relationship between the nature of shock and early fulminating septicemia

Nature of shock	No. of cases	No. of cases with early fulminating septicemia
Uneventful	35	13
Stormy	47	39
		$P < 0.001$

tation within 72 h postburn may initiate and aggravate fulminating septicemia and should therefore be strictly avoided.

1.2 Stage of Eschar Separation (3–4 Weeks Postburn)

Natural separation of the eschar will invariably be accompanied by subeschar infection. If most of the deep burn eschar has not been removed at the appropriate time, natural separation of large patches of eschar will inevitably ensue, causing exposure of a huge infected wound and leading to a high incidence of septicemia. In patients suffering from malnutrition, granulation tissue is not readily formed, and the probability of development of septicemia is exceedingly high. Staged excisions followed by immediate coverage of the wound are nowadays the most ideal and safest measure in the prevention of septicemia of this stage. For those portions of the eschar which are not suitable for excision, we usually adopt the method of so-called planned natural removal. The parts on which the eschar is temporarily allowed to remain must be kept relatively sterile and free of pressure by proper use of topical antibacterial agents and by timely turning of the patient. Chinese herb medicine is applied topically to hasten the separation of those areas of the eschar planned for removal. The extent of application is limited each time to about 10% of the BSA in very extensive burns and 20% of the BSA in extensive burns in order to avoid separation of the eschar all at once.

If subeschar healing cannot be achieved, lysis of an infected deep second degree eschar usually occurs 2 weeks postburn. At this time the wound surface usually has not yet been epithelialized and it must be protected by topical antibacterial agents.

1.3 Late Stage

Septicemia developing later than 1 month postburn is usually due to further lowering of host resistance in patients with a wound which has been uncovered for a prolonged period. Septicemia developing at this stage closely correlates with the extensiveness of the exposed wound. In high-risk, protractedly debilitated patients an infected wound of 10% of the BSA may lead to septicemia.

The presence of foci other than the burn wound should not be overlooked as a potential source of development of septicemia at this stage.

2 Symptoms of Septicemia

2.1 Systemic Symptoms

1. *Body temperature:* The temperature of patients who have sustained extensive burns usually fluctuates above the normal range during the whole course of treatment. After change of dressing the temperature rises more significantly, with a short period of shivery sensation. If the body temperature suddenly rises to above 40 °C with shivering or there is a precipitous drop to below 36 °C, septicemia is to be strongly suspected. Hypothermia is a grave sign of systemic invasion by gram-negative bacilli. If the patient has a sustained or remittent fever of over 39 °C, the possibility of septicemia should be considered.

2. *Heart rate:* Sinus tachycardia below 120/min is regarded as normal manifestation of extensive burns. If heart rate exceeds 140/min (in children, even higher), it may be regarded as another symptom of invasive infection. In the case of hypothermia, the temperature and pulse curves dissociate. The use of *Digitalis* cannot lower the heart rate. In the event of complicated myocardial damage, gallop rhythm or arrhythmias may occur.

Upon impending death, sometimes only monosyllabic heart sound can be heard, and heart rate drops to below 60 per minute.

3. *Respiration:* The change in the pattern of the patient's respiration is more diagnostic than either temperature or pulse rate. The first noted change is fast, shallow breathing, which then gives way to prolongation and increasing effort of expiration. Cheyne-Stokes respiration is a still later symptom. In terminal wound sepsis, respiratory failure usually precedes cardiac arrest.

When tachypnea and dyspnea cannot be attributed to primary obstruction of the respiratory tract or to electrolyte and acid-base disturbances, the possibility of septicemia should always be considered.

4. *Mental disturbances:* The majority of the patients affected by septicemia first show excitation. The chief manifestations are irritability, delirium, hallucination, and restlessness. Later, excitation turns to depression, which is evidenced by disorientation, lethargy, cloudy sensorium, indifference, and even coma.

5. *Abdominal distention:* This is an important symptom. At first the abdomen is slightly distended. Both the pitch and the frequency of peristalsis are decreased upon auscultation. In late cases the abdomen is distended like a drum owing to paralytic ileus (Fig. IV.9). Acute dilatation of the stomach may further aggravate this condition. Brownish gastric contents with sloughing necrotic mucosa can be aspirated through a nasogastric tube. Intractable abdominal distention is a reliable diagnostic symptom.

6. *Diarrhea:* Odorless watery diarrhea characterizes disturbances of the normal intestinal flora. Whether diarrhea is the cause or the sequel of septicemia remains to be established.

7. *Edema:* In the early stage retention of sodium and water will be demonstrated clinically by the reappearance of the subsided burn edema. In the majority of cases, location of the edema in the vicinity of the wound only denotes heavy infection of the wound.

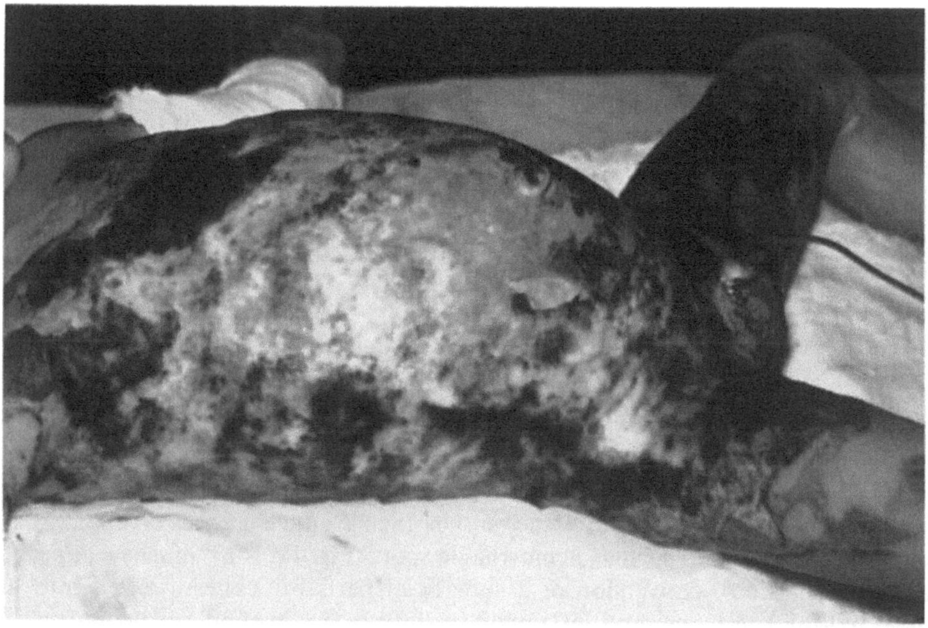

Fig. IV.9. Fulminating gram-negative rod wound sepsis. Black necrotic patches are seen, and the abdomen is distended

8. Tremor of the tongue and limbs, hemorrhagic tendency, and jaundice signify that the condition is very serious.

2.2 Changes in the Appearance of the Wound

The appearance of the wound sensitively mirrors the systemic changes. Sometimes a change in the wound's appearance occurs earlier than the systemic manifestations of invasive infections; therefore the wound should be placed under close observation. The pathogenesis which causes the change of the wound are the invasion of bacteria into the viable subjacent tissue and the lowering

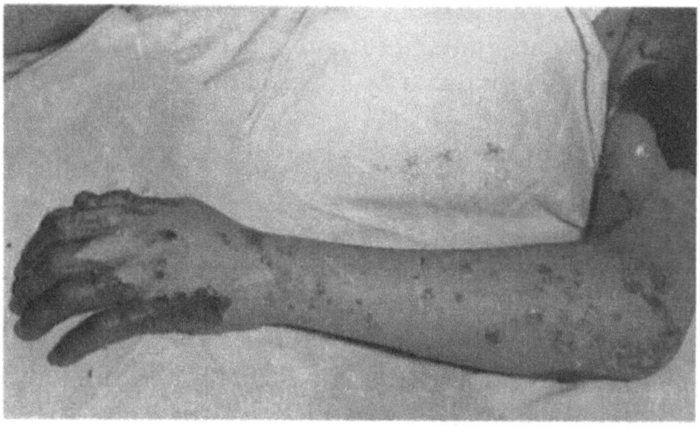

Fig. IV.10. Hemorrhagic spots on the burn wound

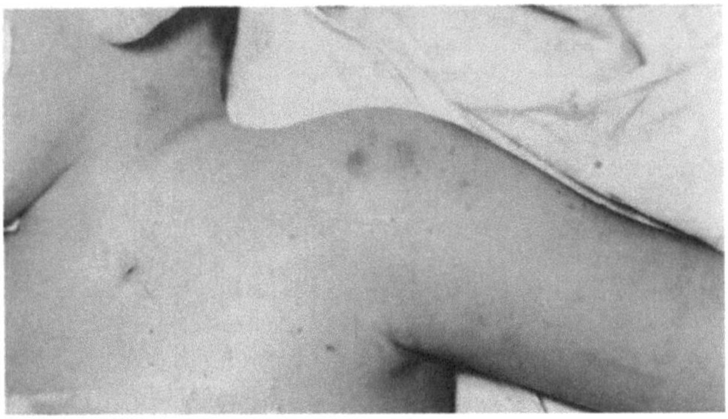

Fig. IV.11. Purplish-black hemorrhagic necrotic spots (erythema gangrenosa) on the previously normal skin

of the host resistance. Local inflammatory swelling, thrombosis of the vessels involved, and progressive necrosis of the tissue on the one hand and deterioration of the general defense mechanism, impairment of local cellular reaction, and destruction of the granulation tissue on the other produce a series of observable changes of the wound such as hemorrhagic spots (Fig. IV.10), "mushy" appearance (maceration), conversion of a superficial partial-thickness wound into a deep full-thickness one, and inflammatory infiltration around the wound with hyperemia and edema. In very severe cases, the wound turns dark and dry with no pus formation, the wound edge becomes sunken, the epithelial growth ceases, and purplish-black hemorrhagic necrotic patches (erythema gangrenosa) may appear over the wound or even over the normal skin (Fig. IV.11). These patches have a broad base and are hard to the touch. They may penetrate deep into the subcutaneous tissue, muscle, or even reach the bone and are a sign of impending death. The most frequent causal microorganism is *Pseudomonas aeruginosa*, while *B. anitratum, Klebsiella pneumoniae,* and proteus are sometimes the causal bacteria. Various fungi may also be isolated.

2.3 Changes in the Appearance of the Tongue

The tongue turns dark red or even purplish with a scorched yellow or blackish coating; sometimes it may be "bare" (uncoated, with papillae flattened or atrophied), fissured, and dry. The patient cannot extrude his tongue or can do so only with extreme difficulty and tremor. Tongue changes are very early signs of systemic infections, but in children and in patients with systemic mycotic infections the tongue may appear normal at first. Most patients suffering from invasive infections have a dry tongue (Fig. IV.12).

2.4 Laboratory Findings

1. *Blood picture:* In extensive burns the white cell count is generally above 10,000/mm^3, the exception being the period of resorption of edema of shock stage. There is a slight leftward shift of the Schilling's count, and few toxic granules may be seen within the granulocytes. During the edema resorption period the white cell count may fall to below 10,000/mm^3 before rising again

quickly. This ebb and flow does not necessarily correlate with infection, but during the remaining course of the trauma, decrease of the white cell count to below $10{,}000/mm^3$ or a sudden rise to above $20{,}000/mm^3$ with a marked leftward shift of the Schilling's count is highly indicative of septicemia. The fall in the leukocyte count to below $5{,}000/mm^3$ usually denotes a fulminating invasive infection of gram-negative bacilli. Therefore the kinetic changes of the white cell count must be kept under daily review. No changes of the red blood cell count or the hemoglobin value are to be observed. In very rare cases septicemia may be followed by anemia which is not easy to correct.

2. *Electrolytes:* Hypernatremia and hypokalemia may develop in some patients.

3. *Verdoglobinuria:* Under long wave ultraviolet light and sometimes under natural light in severe cases, the urine has a green color. This is a specific sign of septicemia due to *P. aeruginosa* (Fig. IV.13)

2.5 Summary

The above-mentioned symptoms and signs may not all exist in any one case of septicemia. For instance (a) abdominal distension is a frequently observed symptom, but some patients never suffer from it; (b) some patients remain alert even just prior to their death; and (c) although subnormal temperature and leukopenia are of diagnostic significance in gram-negative bacillary septicemia, high fever and immense leukocytosis are not infrequent. Therefore in the diagnosis of septicemia, one must observe and analyze all aspects; one

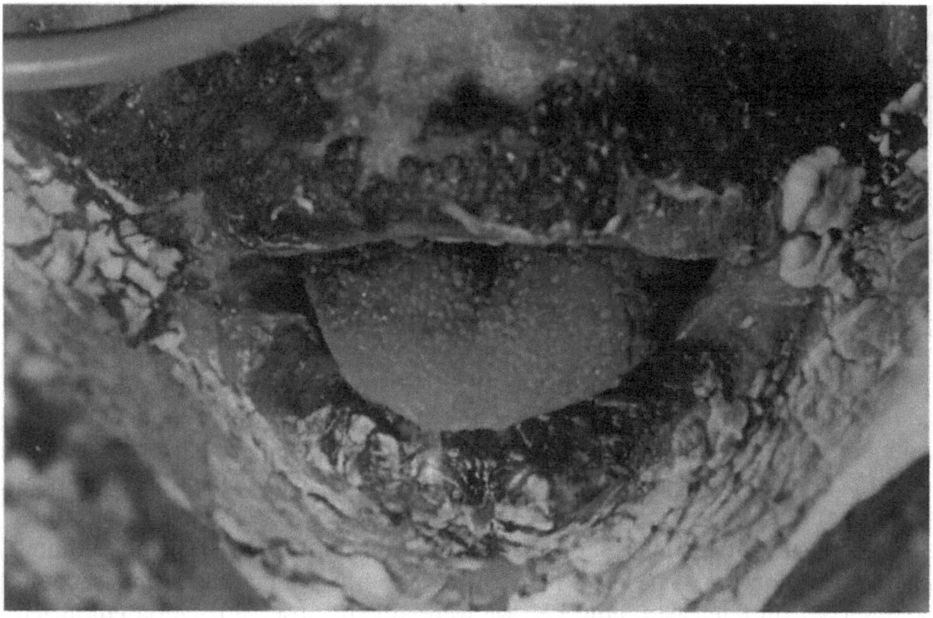

Fig. IV.12. Dark red, "bare", fissured, and moistless tongue, typical for septicemia

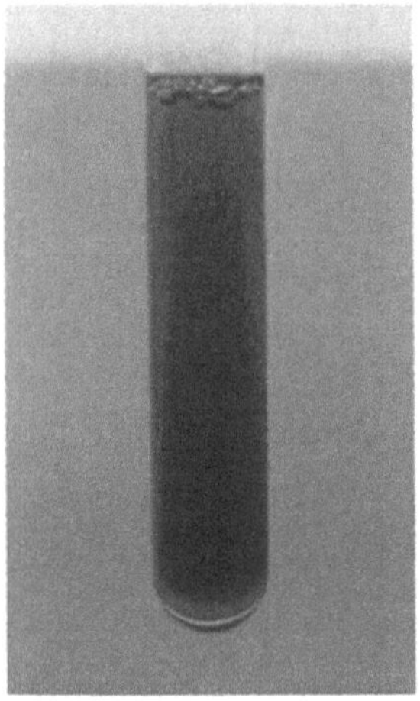

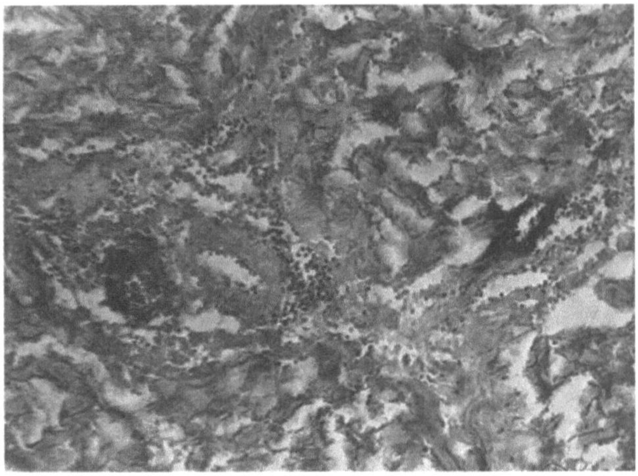

Fig. IV.13. Verdoglobinuria. Under long-wave ultraviolet light the urine appears green

Fig. IV.14. Section through a necrotic patch. The small dark-blue rings represent sites of arteritis and periarteritis caused by gram-negative bacilli. Giemsa, low-power magnification

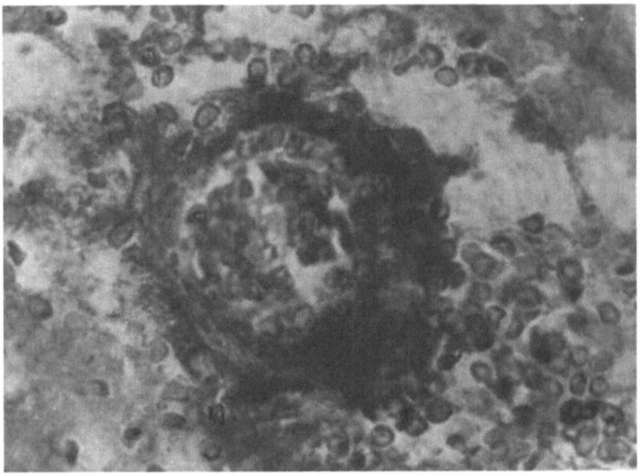

Fig. IV.15. Oil immersion view ▷ of the perivascular cuffing (dark-blue rings) shown in **Fig. IV.14.** The intima, media, and adventitia have been destroyed and replaced by gram-negative rods. Giemsa

must not fail to diagnose septicemia and thus cause a delay in treatment just because certain signs and symptoms are absent.

2.6 Erythema Gangrenosa

From January 1966 to December 1973, we treated 53 cases of fulminating gram-negative septicemia with necrotic patches (erythema gangrenosa) on their wounds; only nine of these patients survived. The etiologic bacteria isolated were *P. aeruginosa*, *Klebsiella pneumoniae*, *Proteus*, *B. anitratum*, and fungi. Bacterial quantification per gram of tissue varied between 10^6 and 10^8. Sections through the necrotic patches showed necrosis and hemorrhage. Only mild inflammatory reaction was revealed. In early cases only punctating necrosis could be observed; in late cases, however, we were able to observe bacteria colonized along the adventitia and media of the blood vessels. Under Giemsa staining and low-power magnification, the arteritis and periarteritis caused by gram-negative bacilli gave an appearance of small dark-blue rings (Fig. IV.14). Under oil immersion, gram-negative bacteria could be identified, but rarely in the lumina of affected vessels, except in very late cases (Fig. IV.15).

In patients with erythema gangrenosa, new necrotic patches may appear after septicemia has been controlled, even though the general condition is improved. This indicates that the vascular lesions far exceed the extent of necrosis observed by the naked eye. Consequently one should apply topical antibacterial agents over all wound surfaces and keep the agent in close contact with those surfaces.

Prior to the deterioration of the wound there is a certain period during which the patient is extremely irritable, while other clinical symptoms, such as hypothermia or leukopenia, may not be apparent. The use of large doses of sedatives is rarely effective. In children, irritability and restlessness are usually accompanied by itching of the wound. This should not be misinterpreted as itching caused by healing of superficial burns.

Careful observation and comprehensive analysis facilitate early diagnosis. If diagnosis and treatment are delayed, gram-negative bacillary septicemia will inevitably lead to fatal septic shock.

3 Early Diagnosis of Septicemia

Early diagnosis is especially important in gram-negative bacillary septicemia, because its development is rapid and septic shock will occur within a few hours. By the time symptoms and signs of sepsis manifest, effective treatment may already be difficult to achieve.

In regard to early diagnosis, two questions are require attention: First, is septicemia present? Second, what is the causative organism?

The key to early diagnosis is full understanding and keen observation of the early symptoms and signs of septicemia. Blood cultures drawn from patients suffering from wound sepsis may remain negative throughout the whole course; besides, even if a positive report is received, the installation of treatment is usually too late by that time. In some cases the nature of the invading microorganisms may have changed.

A characteristic feature of infection in burns is that the bacteria colonized on the wound will invade and grow into the deep layer of unburned tissue. Sometimes the bacteria on the burn surface are not identical with the bacteria cultured from the subeschar tissues. Therefore subeschar bacterial culture with quantitative investigations will give more reliable information for the diagnosis of wound sepsis.

Examinations were made of 97 specimens taken from different sites after early eschar excision in 28 patients in whom evidence of wound sepsis had not been observed. Quantification of subeschar bacteria revealed counts of above 10^5/g in only 21 sites (21.6%), the maximum being 10^6/g (Table IV.2).

On the other hand, in 18 biopsies taken from five patients with wound sepsis, 15 sites (89%) had a bacterial count exceeding 10^5, the highest being

Table IV.2. Subeschar bacterial counts in 97 specimens taken after early eschar excision from 28 patients without wound sepsis

Bacteria/gram tissue	No. of specimens
0	9
10^1	4
10^2	7
10^3	33
10^4	23
10^5	15
10^6	6

Table IV.3. Subeschar bacterial count of 18 specimens procured from five patients who had erythema gangrenosa or died of sepsis

Bacteria/gram tissue	No. of specimens
10^3	1
10^4	1
10^5	1
10^6	7
10^7	2
10^8	5
10^9	1

10^9 (Table IV.3). In albino rats, bacteria are seen in histologic sections under oil immersion when the subeschar bacterial count exceeds 10^5/g tissue. By using a cryostat, analysis of sections can be performed immediately after biopsy; if bacteria are observed, it denotes that the number of bacteria per gram tissue exceeds 10^5, and even if the blood culture is sterile, the presence of wound sepsis should be strongly suspected and treated accordingly.

Biopsies are taken by means of a corneal trephine 6 mm in diameter; 0.02 g tissue is removed each time for bacterial quantitation (cf. Appendix). The amount of tissue obtained by this method is small, and specimens can be taken from various areas, making it possible to achieve a better understanding of the subeschar condition. Biopsies can be taken at any time and can be of value in the early diagnosis of wound sepsis, in the selection of topical and systemic antibacterial agents, and in the selection of the areas for eschar excision. Nevertheless, for early diagnosis, close dynamic observation of burn wounds still remains the most important procedure. The possibility of septicemia or wound sepsis should always be considered in patients who develop hyper- or hypothermia, marked shivering, shallow and rapid breathing, continued irritability, systemic edema, abdominal distention, intractable diarrhea, extremely dry and dark red tongue, leukopenia, markedly leftward shift of Schilling's count, low red blood cell count and hemoglobin value (for which no other cause can be found), hypernatremia, hypokalemia, verdoglobinuria, etc. For early diagnosis of oncoming fulminating sepsis during the shock stage, the following symp-

Table IV.4. Clinical characteristics which differentiate gram-positive coccal wound sepsis from gram-negative bacillary wound sepsis

	Gram-positive cocci infection	Gram-negative bacilli infection
Wound	Lysis of granulation tissue	Focal black or violaceous discoloration, deepening of the wound, erythema gangrenosa
Clinical course	Insidious	Fulminating
Disturbance of consciousness	Severe	Slight or none
Body temperature	Hyperthermia	Hypothermia
White cell count	Usually increased	Sometimes decreased

toms and signs are of diagnostic value: oliguria, labile blood pressure (with adequate fluid replacement), restlessness, and wounds retaining a "mushy" appearance, without formation of dry eschar.

Hypothermia, leukopenia, prolonged expiration, paralytic ileus, and wound turning dark with sunken edges and necrotic patches are late signs of very severe septicemia.

It is very difficult to differentiate clinically a gram-negative bacillary septicemia from a gram-positive coccal septicemia. Some points for reference are given in Table IV.4.

4 The Prevention and Treatment of Septicemia

There are four cardinal measures in the prevention and treatment of sepsis: raising host resistance, proper management of the burn wound, appropriate usage of antibiotics, and reasonable handling of isolation measures.

4.1 Ameliorate the Host Resistance

Feasible measures for raising the general resistance of the patient are beneficial nutrition, oral Chinese herb medicine, and immunotherapy. Nutrition and oral Chinese herb medicine are discussed in Chaps. XII and V respectively; therefore only immunotherapy is dealt with below.

4.1.1 Anti-*Pseudomonas* Hyperimmune Globulin

Serum agglutination tests on 73 strains of *P. aeruginosa* isolated from burn patients of Rui Jin Hospital revealed the majority to be of types I and IV.

Table IV.5. Prophylactic effect of anti-Pseudomonas hyperimmune globulin in albino mice[a]

Group	Prophylactic dosage administered before the attack	Concentration of attacking micro-organisms[b] (10^8/ml)	Dosage of attacking micro-organisms[b] (ml)	No. of mice	Result (dead/survived)		
					1st day	2nd day	3rd day
Control		20	0.5	5	5/0	–	–
		10	0.5	5	4/1	5/0	–
		5	0.5	5	4/1	4/1	4/1
		2.5	0.5	5	2/3	4/1	5/0
		1.25	0.5	5	0/5	0/5	0/5
Treatment	0.25	20	0.5	5	0/5	0/5	0/5
	0.25	10	0.5	5	0/5	0/5	0/5
	0.25	5	0.5	5	0/5	0/5	0/5
	0.25	2.5	0.5	5	0/5	0/5	0/5
	0.25	1.25	0.5	5	0/5	0/5	0/5

[a] Data from the Shanghai Biological Product Institute
[b] *P. aeruginosa*

Table IV.6. Relationship between the time of prophylactic treatment and the prophylactic effect of anti-*Pseudomonas* hyperimmune globulin in mice[a]

Groups	Prophylactic group[b]	Early-treated group[c]	Late-treated group[d]	Control
No. of experimental animals	6	10	15	6
No. of deaths within 7 days	0	1	8	6
P	<0.01	< 0.01	> 0.01 <0.05	

[a] Data from the Shanghai Biological Product Institute; concentration of attacking microorganisms, 10^8/ml; dose of attacking microorganisms, 0.5 ml
[b] Anti-*Pseudomonas* hyperimmune globulin injected 24 h prior to attack
[c] Anti-*Pseudomonas* hyperimmune globulin injected on day of attack
[d] Anti-*Pseudomonas* hyperimmune globulin injected 24 h after attack

Table IV.7. Comparison between the prophylactic effects of anti-*Pseudomonas* hyperimmune globulin and human serum γ-globulin[a]

Group	Prophylactic dose (ml)	Concentration of attacking micro-organisms[b] (10^8/ml)	Dosage of attacking micro-organisms[b] (ml)	No. of animals	Result (dead/survived)		
					1st day	2nd day	3rd day
Control			0.5	10	10/0	–	–
		40	0.5	10	10/0	–	–
		20	0.5	10	7/3	9/1	9/1
		10	0.5	10	5/5	9/1	9/1
Anti-*Pseudomonas*	0.25	40	0.5	10	5/5	9/1	9/1
hyperimmune	0.25	20	0.5	10	0/10	6/4	7/3
globulin	0.25	10	0.5	10	0/10	1/9	2/8
Human serum	0.25	40	0.5	10	10/0	–	–
γ-globulin	0.25	20	0.5	10	7/3	10/0	–
	0.25	10	0.5	10	6/4	9/1	9/1

[a] Data from the Shanghai Biological Product Institute
[b] *P. aerugionosa*

Therefore hyperimmune globulin was procured from horses immunized with type I and IV strains of *P. aeruginosa*. This hyperimmune globulin effectively protected mice inoculated with a lethal dose of *P. aeruginosa* (Table IV.5), although its prophylactic effect proved to be much greater than its therapeutic effect (Table IV.6). No protection could be provided by nonspecific human serum γ-globulin (Table IV.7). These results show that in clinical practice anti-*Pseudomonas* hyperimmune globulin is useful only for prophylactic purposes; a therapeutic effect against invasive *Pseudomonas* infection has rarely been proved.

Patients with a negative skin test to tetanus antitoxin may receive anti-*Pseudomonas* globulin: 5 ml must be given intramuscularly on the day of injury

Table IV.8. The relationship between the extent of third degree burn and the incidence of septicemia and wound sepsis; an analysis of 133 cases with burns to 80% of the BSA

Group	No. of cases	Average BSA burned (%)	Average BSA with third degree burns (%)
Septicemia and/or wound sepsis	84	90.9	58.2
No septicemia and/or wound sepsis	49	87.7	26.1

and then every other day. The protective effect of each injection lasts for only 48 h. Immunoglobulin should be administered until there is no longer any danger of systemic *Pseudomonas* infection. If the injection has been discontinued for more than a week, hypersensitivity will develop and it should not be used again.

4.1.2 Convalescent Blood or Plasma

Blood or plasma withdrawn from patients with extensive or medium burns 2 months to 1 year postburn is termed convalescent blood or plasma. The antibody titers of convalescent plasma against the commonly isolated bacterial flora are high, especially those from extensive third degree burns. Therefore repeated infusions of 200–400 ml convalescent blood or plasma may be beneficial.

4.2 Proper Management of the Wound

Proper management of the wound is another key to the prevention and treatment of septicemia. If the wound is managed properly, infection will be slight, repair will be quicker, coverage will occur earlier, and the incidence of septicemia will be markedly reduced. The incidence of septicemia is much more closely related to the extensiveness of the third degree burns than the patient's total BSA burned, so it is evident that the management of third degree burn wound is of prime importance. The stress on the importance of the third degree wounds does not mean that one can neglect the care of the second degree wounds. If the second degree burn wound is not treated properly, septicemia is also liable to develop, especially among the children. Even if the patient is already afflicted with septicemia, management of the wound still remains the key link in the chain of treatment.

Wound treatments are mostly dealt with in Chap. III. At this point, we are concerned only with the principle and application of various topical agents and the surgical removal of infected foci. Since local vascular obliteration is one of the characteristic histologic changes of wound sepsis, once sepsis is established antibiotics administered systemically are rarely able to reach the burn wound in concentrations sufficient to control the rapid proliferation of the wound flora. After the pathophysiologic changes of burn wound sepsis had been clarified in the early 1960s, the use of topical antimicrobial agents became a standard practice.

4.2.1 10% Sulfamylon Cream

Dr. John Moncrief first introduced Sulfamylon for the treatment of burns in 1964. It can penetrate deep into the subeschar tissue and can reach an effective bactericidal concentration. It has a broad antimicrobial spectrum. Most of the gram-negative and gram-positive bacteria, and *B. clostridia* are sensitive. It is especially effective against *P. aeruginosa*.

Though it has many untoward side effects, its toxicity is low. In vivo, Sulfamylon is disintegrated by aminoxidase into *p*-carboxyl benzyl sulfonamide, which is highly soluble and will never tend to crystalize out in urine. *p*-Carboxyl benzyl-sulfonamide is a strong carbonic anhydrase inhibitor. When it is assimilated in large quantities, it may inhibit the clearance of the hydrogen ions as well as the reabsorption of the bicarbonate ions by the renal tubules. It is acidic in nature, so it will further increase the hydrogen ion load of the patient. After topical application, Sulfamylon is readily absorbed and disintegrated rapidly, thus causing acute metabolic acidosis soon after its use. The human body compensates by increasing the amplitude and frequency of respiration (to as many as 40–50 times per minute). When Sulfamylon is applied to most of the BSA in extensively burned patients, a concomitant quantity of sodium bicarbonate must be infused (see Chap. VI) since the patient is rarely able to bear such a vast amount of hydrogen ion load. Sulfamylon is contraindicated in patients with ARDS, pneumonia, or any other respiratory disturbances. In children the respiratory compensatory mechanism is not yet well developed, so application of Sulfamylon to a large area is again inappropriate.

Sulfamylon acetate is prepared in the form of 10% water miscible cream and is painted on the wound in sufficient thickness. A single layer gauze or bandage is applied to ensure retention of the cream. When the dressing is changed the previously applied "cream" must be washed off with physiologic saline solution. The medicament can penetrate the deep tissue layers within 3 h after application, and there is rarely any Sulfamylon left in the base 6 h after application. Therefore dressings should be changed twice a day. If the infection is severe, the number of applications may be suitably increased.

Side effects such as pain, allergic dermatitis (which can be effectively combated by a large dose of phenergan), superimposed fungi infection, acid-base disturbances and delay in separation of the necrotic tissue must be kept in mind.

4.2.2 Silver Sulfadiazine Cream

Silver sulfadiazine was compounded in 1968 and popularized thereafter by Prof. Charles Fox Jr. It is extremely insoluble in water and has a very strong bactericidal effect. Its antimicrobial spectrum is broad, and it exhibits a strong inhibitory effect against *P. aeruginosa*. Pus, necrotic tissue, and para-aminobenzoic acid do not reduce its action. In tissue, silver sulfadiazine is disintegrated by nucleic acid, liberating sulfadiazine and silver ions. Sulfadiazine has its own bactericidal actions, while silver ions probably conjugate with deoxyribonucleic acid of the *Pseudomonas* bacilli and inhibits its replication. Silver sulfadiazine has the less ability to penetrate through the eschar. Its advantages over Sulfamylon are that it does not cause pain, elicite allergic reactions, or disturb the acid-base balance. Its main drawback is that it delays separation of necrotic tissue and induces superimposed fungi infection. The method of application is essentially the same as for Sulfamylon cream.

4.2.3 Gentamicin Cream

In 1966 Stone introduced the use of gentamicin cream; 0.1% was the concentration employed. However, after a certain period of application, resistant strains would be formed, which greatly restricted its usage.

4.2.4 Combinations of Drugs

Owing to the fact that separation of the necrotic tissue is inevitably delayed after the application of Sulfamylon or silver sulfadiazine cream, ultimate wound closure can not be achieved and the course of treatment is protracted. Therefore we have been using Sulfamylon or silver sulfadiazine with a slight modification: We mix equal volumes of Sulfamylon or silver sulfadiazine cream with Burn and Scald Ointment and double the strength of the former. This combination not only controls the local infection, but also promotes separation of the necrotic tissue. In addition, healthy granulation tissue is readily formed.

Case Illustration. Male, aged 2.5 years. The patient had second degree burns to 40% of the BSA. The shock stage was stormy, and after it was over, the patient seemed irritable with a high fever of 40 °C and weak and thready pulse of dorsalis pedes. On the 8th day postburn, gentamicin was administered intravenously and the wound was bandaged with 10% Sulfamylon wet dressings. During that night, the patient became extremely restless with hyperpnea. Next morning necrotic patches were observed on the wound, and the white blood cell count dropped to $9{,}300/mm^3$, with marked leftward shift of the Schilling's count. The diagnosis of wound sepsis with *Pseudomonas* erythema gangrenosa was established. Topical antimicrobial agent was changed to silver sulfadiazine. Polymyxin B, convalescent blood, γ-globulin, and corticosterone were given for 3 days. Although the number of necrotic patches increased, with invasion of the unburned skin, an improvement in the patient's general condition was nevertheless observed. The patient's mental condition became clear, and he was willing to answer questions and to take food. On the 4th day the local application was changed to a mixture of silver sulfadiazine and Burn and Scald Ointment. The dressings were changed every 4 h. During the following days, necrotic patches continuously dropped off and numerous undermined pus pockets were found. After skin grafting, the patient recovered.

4.2.5 Surgical Removal or Drainage of Infective Foci

Possible insidious foci must be looked for, and particular attention should be paid to establishing whether septic thrombophlebitis or infected necrotic muscles are present.

Case Illustration. Female, age 23 years. The patient had burns to 60% of the BSA, including third degree burns to 24.5%; the cause of burn was a blast. On the 8th postburn day patient's condition suddenly deteriorated. Polypnea of 36/min and dyspnea appeared, and generalized edema flared up. Marked inflammatory infiltration of the wound edge on the right leg was observed. Blisters were seen on normal skin of the distal portion of the involved leg. On the wound, a round necrotic patch with a very hard and broad base was found at the lower inner aspect of the right leg. The patient's general condition soon deteriorated further. She was in respiratory distress, and her tongue became extremely dry and could barely be extruded. Emergency operation was performed under combined intravenous anesthesia. After excision of the third degree eschar of the lower left extremity, thrombosis of the femoral vein at the midthigh level, causing wet gangrene of the right leg, was found. After midthigh amputation and allografting of the stump, the patient's respiratory distress ameliorated. She had an uneventful recovery.

In fulminating gram-negative bacillary wound sepsis an astonishing number of bacteria colonize on the wound, and the patient might go into septic shock within a few hours. If it is possible to excise the wound in a single stage, emergency excision might be carried out in order to reduce the number of bacteria to a level which the human body can tolerate.

Case Illustration. Male, aged 27. The patient had second degree burns to both lower extremities, the perineum, and the buttocks – a total of 41% of the BSA. Fifteen days postburn patient revealed wound sepsis with necrotic patches and positive blood culture of *P. aeruginosa*. The patient's blood pressure suddenly dropped to zero, and even with large doses of vasopressors, systolic pressure could hardly be maintained above 70 mmHg. He became unconscious with Cheyne-Stokes respiration. Assistance of respiration through intubation was mandatory. An emergency operation was performed 3 h after septic shock. Excision was performed down to the deep fascia, and in addition several necrotic patches on the nonburned area were removed. A tremendous amount of exudation was found under the eschar. The area excised was 40% of the BSA and the wound was covered with large sheets of fresh porcine skin. The excised tissue weighed 1,600 g and contained $2–5 \times 10^6$ bacteria per gram of tissue removed. Organisms were found to be *P. aeruginosa* and *Klebsiella pneumoniae*. No more than 60 ml ether was needed to perform such a major operation. It required 10,600 ml colloids (8,000 ml blood and 2,600 ml plasma) to maintain blood pressure at a level of 90–100/60–70 mmHg. After the operation the patient's condition improved and he recovered consciousness. His blood pressure stabilized, and vasopressors were withdrawn 12 h after the operation.

On the next day numerous new necrotic patches appeared on the remaining wound. Seven of them were excised under local anesthesia. Quantitative determination of bacteria of the excised necrotic patches showed counts of $3 \times 10^6–4 \times 10^8$. The organisms identified were *P. aeruginosa* and *Bacterium anitratum*. The rest of the necrotic patches were treated by topical application of Sulfamylon cream.

The patient's condition was complicated by bilateral bronchopneumonia with disseminated foci confirmed by X-ray. Sputum culture showed growth of *P. aeruginosa* and *K. pneumoniae,* which suggested that the pneumonia was hematogenous in origin. Systemic polymyxin B, gentamicin, and carbenicillin were employed, and the bronchopneumonia was finally controlled. The porcine skins were replaced by large sheets of allograft intermingled with small pieces of autoskins, and the patient recovered.

Septic thrombophlebitis: In extensively burned patients the incidence of septicemia after central venous catheterization is exceedingly high. The phlebotomy sites are likely to be sites of entrance for bacteria. Therefore, except during the shock stage, we now rarely thread any catheter into the central veins of an extensively burned patient. The peripheral veins, and especially the scalp veins, are used instead (see Chap. XII). In using peripheral veins one must be aware of possible septic thrombophlebitis which develops insidiously and causes undue prolongation of treatment. *Staphylococcus aureus* is often found to be the pathogenic bacterium in the venous foci. In most instances it is necessary only to ligate the proximal end of the venous cutdown. If pus is found at the proximal end, that entire section of the vein should be dissected out and excised by making an incision along its course. In patients with clinical symptoms and signs of septicemia, the venous route as the site of entry must be strongly suspected if a venous catheter has been placed. If septicemia is suspected, we usually remove the venous catheter and culture its tip for microorganisms.

4.3 Reasonable Use of Antibiotics

Since wound sepsis is the major cause of septicemia, the causal bacteria of burn septicemia are usually the same as those isolated from the wounds.

Table IV.9 gives the breakdown of 5,499 strains of bacteria isolated from the burn wounds of 481 patients either with a total burn exceeding 50% of the BSA or with third degree burns to more than 20% of the BSA. Of the 5,499 strains found, gram-negative bacilli formed 65.4% and gram-positive cocci formed 34.6%. With respect to species, *P. aeruginosa* (27.9%) and *Staphylococcus aureus* (25.6%) were the most frequent (Table IV.9).

Sulfamylon and silver sulfadiazine have been extensively used in our burn unit since 1973, and since that time bacteria from the wound have shown some distinct changes. *Pseudomonas* decreased from 34.8% to 21.4%, while *K. pneumonia* increased significantly. Prior to the use of these two topical sulfa drugs, *Klebsiella* was isolated in only a very few cases, but from 1973 to 1978 the positive wound culture of this organism increased to 10.9%. It also occupies 15% of all the positive blood cultures, second only to *Staphylococcus* and *Pseudomonas*. Sometimes we can obtain positive growth of *K. pneumoniae* from the cultures of necrotic patches or the viscera of patients who have died as a result of their burns.

During the same period (1973–1978) and among the same group of patients, in 134 positive blood cultures, gram-negative bacilli dominated (70.1%). With

Table IV.9. Nature of 5,499 strains of bacteria isolated in 481 patients with burns exceeding 50% of the BSA or

Years	Bacteria						
	Staphylococcus aureus	*Pseudomonas aeruginosa*	*Escherichia coli*	*Paracolobacterium*[a]	*Bacterium anitratum*	*Streptococcus pyogenes*	*Streptococcus faecalis*
1966–1972	24.1	34.8	2.3	5.8	3.7	4.4	4.1
1973–1978	26.6	24.1	2.7	5.6	7.7	0.6	8.6
1966–1978	25.6	27.9	2.6	5.7	5.9	2.4	6.5

[a] Before 1973, *Slomonella arizonae*, *Citrobacter*, *Providencia*, and late-lactose-fermenting *Escherichia coli* were reported as *Paracolobacterium*

[b] Before 1973 *Klebsiella* were not differentiated

regard to species. *P. aeruginosa* took first place (38.1%), *S. staphylococcus* second (14.2%), and *Streptococcus faecalis* third (12.7%). In cases of wound sepsis with repeated negative blood cultures, most of the subeschar cultures revealed gram-negative bacilli. Twenty-eight out of 30 strains found in the subeschar unburned tissues of five patients who died after onset of wound sepsis were gram-negative bacilli (Table IV.10); among them *P. aeruginosa* formed 56.6% and again occupied first place. *K. pneumoniae* formed 22.2%, which coincides with the increase of incidence of this particular microorganism on the burn wound surface.

4.3.1 Indications for Systemic Administration of Antibiotics in Burns

1. In the presence of early clinical symptoms and signs of septicemia, antibiotics selected on the basis of the results of cultures from the wound should be given without hesitation. It is not necessary to wait for the report on the blood culture or subeschar bacterial quantification – to do so will always render action too late.

2. Antibiotics are used as a protective measure during and after eschar excision over a large area and debridement, or during the period of spontaneous separation of extensive eschars.

3. During occurrence of various serious complications, when the defensive mechanism of the body is lowered (e.g., massive gastrointestinal bleedings, uncontrolled stress diabetes).

4. In the presence of bronchopneumonia or other infective foci.

Systemic antibiotics are not indicated in hyperthermia, leukocytosis, and noninvasive wound infections.

4.3.2 Plan for the Systemic Administration of Antibiotics

1. Benzyl penicillin is still the routine antibiotic employed for the first 2–3 days postburn, although there is no clinical evidence of early streptococcal infection in our cases.

with third degree burns exceeding 20% of the BSA

Proteus	*Aerobacter aerogenes*	*Bacillus alcaligenes*	*Klebsiella pneumoniae*[b]	Total no. of strains
11.2	4.9	4.0	–	1,598
12.5	1.3	1.9	10.8	2,901
12	3.0	2.9	5.8	5,499

Table IV.10. Bacteria (or fungi) cultured from 18 sites of subeschar nonburned tissue in five patients whose condition was complicated by wound sepsis with erythema gangrenosa or who died as a result of sepsis

Bacteria (or fungi)	No. of strains
Pseudomonas aeruginosa	17
Klebsiella pneumoniae	8
Bacterium anitratum	1
Aerobacter aerogenes	1
Paracolobactrum[a]	1
Staphyloccus aureus	1
Monilia albicans	1
Total	30

[a] Before 1973, *Arizona, Citrobacter, Providencia*, and late-lactose-fermenting *E. coli* were reported as *Paracolobactrum*

2. In very extensive burns, combinations of polymyxin B and gentamicin, polymyxin B and Chloromycetin, or tobramycin, Chloromycetin and amikacin is employed from the 3rd or 4th postburn day through the period of resorption of edema. These antibiotics should be discontinued after a few days if there are no clinical signs or symptoms of septicemia. Among 36 occurrences of septicemia within 5 days postburn, cocci were found only 5 times, gram-negative bacilli 28 times, and mixed infection 3 times. Therefore the above-mentioned antibiotics are mainly directed at *Pseudomonas* and other gram-negative bacilli.

3. In the presence of signs or symptoms of septicemia, two or three antibiotics should be given intravenously in large doses; they should be selected on the basis of the results of wound surface cultures and their sensitivity tests. As soon as the condition becomes stable, antibiotics should be withdrawn.

4. Benzyl penicillin remains the first choice antibiotic against *Streptococcus pyogenes*. If this organism is found on the granulation wound, large doses of benzyl penicillin should be given before and after the grafting operation.

Table IV.11. The sensitivity of *P. aeruginosa* isolated from burn wounds to polymyxin B

Year	No. of strains	No. of sensitive strains (%)	Year	No. of strains	No. of sensitive strains (%)
1964	362	332 (99.4)	1972	99	88 (89)
1965	151	141 (99.3)	1973	54	49 (89)
1966	35	33 (94.3)	1974	102	102 (100)
1967	29	29 (100)	1975	111	91 (82)
1968	47	45 (95.7)	1976	39	34 (87.2)
1969	39	39 (100)	1977	122	113 (92.6)
1970	99	96 (97)	1978	80	79 (98.8)
1971	59	54 (91.5)			

If the patient is hypersensitive to penicillin, the second choice is erythromycin or cephalothin.

5. In late-stage septicemia (1 month postburn) the principal pathogens found are gram-positive cocci, mostly *Staphylococcus aureus*. Figure IV.8 shows that in 13 times of septicemia occurring after more than 1 month postburn, gram-positive cocci were found nine times (*S. aureus* 7), gram-negative bacilli three-times, and mixed infection once. Therefore, if symptoms of septicemia appear 1 month or more after injury, antibiotics effective against *S. aureus* should be chosen, oxacillin being the first choice. However, the possibility of infection by gram-negative bacilli must not be overlooked. In the case of *Streptococcus faecalis* infection, vancomycin may be considered the first choice. The antibiotics may be readjusted later according to the results of sensitivity tests.

6. In the case of gram-negative bacillary septicemia, the possibility of *Proteus* infection should be considered if the symptoms cannot be controlled by polymyxin B or Chloromycetin. Gentamicin, tobramycin, or amikacin may be used, and subsequent readjustment should be made on the basis of the results of sensitivity tests. Sometimes *Proteus* is sensitive to carbenicillin or sulfocillin.

7. In septicemia caused by undetermined pathogens or mixed infection, the two effective combinations are (a) polymyxin B, gentamicin, and oxacillin and (b) polymyxin B, Chloromycetin, and erythromycin.

8. When broad spectrum antibiotics are used, oral nystatin 500,000–1,000,000 units should be given.

When the wound is infected by *P. aeruginosa,* it appears green and there is an unusual foul odor. When infected by coliform bacteria, the purulent exudate is thin with a fecal odor. When infected by *Streptococcus pyogenes*, the purulent exudate is milky in color, with evidence of invasion of the wound periphery and the appearance of scarlatinoid dermatitis. When infected by *Streptococcus faecalis*, the wound edge shows marked inflammatory edematous infiltration, and mental disturbances are evident. The knowledge of these symptoms may be useful for reference in choosing antibiotics when reports on cultures are not yet available.

4.3.3 Choice of Antibiotics in the Light of Past Experience

1. *Benzyl penicillin: Streptococcus pyogenes* infection is the main cause of failure of skin grafting. To combat it the antibiotic of first choice is benzyl penicillin, which is sometimes administered routinely as a preventive measure. Booster dose intravenous dripping may be effective in the case of *Streptococcus faecalis* infection.

2. *Oxacillin:* Oxacillin, together with cloxacillin and dicloxacillin, belongs to the group of semisynthetic isoxazolyl penicillins. They have cross resistance. When oxacillin was first used, 100% of penicillin-resistant *Staphylococcus aureus* strains were susceptible to it, but at present this figure is only 40%. Oxacillin is usually resisted by *Streptococcus faecalis*.

3. *Carbenicillin and sulbenicillin:* These are the carboxyl and sulfo-derivatives of benzyl penicillin. They are effective against *Proteus* and against *Pseudomonas* in high serum level (50–100 γ/ml). They have a synergistic action with gentamicin,

but should not be mixed together in one injection. They are prescribed clinically for *Pseudomonas* and indole-positive *Proteus* infections, especially in patients with impaired renal function.

Out of 218 strains of *Klebsiella pneumoniae* isolated from the burn wound, only 19 were susceptible to carbenicillin.

4. *Cephalothin:* Of the *Staphylococcus aureus* strains isolated from burn wounds, 80% are sensitive to cephalothin, 59% being highly sensitive. However, only 7 out of 17 strains of isoxazolyl penicillin-resistant *Staphylococcus aureus* are susceptible to cephalothin, which denotes that there is some, at least, partial cross-resistance between cephalothin and β-amidase-resistant penicillins. *Streptococcus faecalis* is resistant to cephalothin. As for gram-negative bacilli, most strains of *Pseudomonas*, indole-positive *Proteus*, *Serratia*, coliform bacteria, and *Klebsiella* are usually resistant.

5. *Erythromycin:* This is a good antibiotic against gram-positive cocci infection. In burn infections, 54.4% of *Staphylococcus aureus*, 50% of *Streptococcus faecalis*, and 80% of *Streptococcus pyogenes* are susceptible to erythromycin. Therefore a combination of erythromycin and Chloromycetin is quite effective in *Streptococcus faecalis* infection.

6. *Clindamycin:* The antimicrobial spectrum of clindamycin is similar to that of erythromycin. Most strains of *Staphylococcus aureus* isolated from burn wounds are resistant to clindamycin. Therefore it is only indicated for the proven susceptible strains, although the anaerobes, with the exception of *Clostridium*, are sensistive to it. Therefore in the case of gas gangrene we prefer to prescribe benzyl penicillin in preference to clindamycin.

7. *Novobiocin:* Owing to its adverse side effects, novobiocin is rarely used as a first line drug. In isoxazolyl penicillin-resistant and erythromycin-resistant staphylococcal infection, novobiocin may sometimes give promising results. Whenever novobiocin is employed, it should not be prescribed over a long period because side effects always appear after long-term administration.

8. *Vancomycin:* It exerts strong bactericidal effect upon the majority of the gram-positive cocci. *Staphylococcus aureus*, *Streptococcus faecalis*, and *Streptococcus pyogenes* isolated from burn wounds are highly susceptible to Vancomycin. Drug-resistant strains are rarely seen. It has no cross-resistance with other antibiotics. Vancomycin is the drug of choice in *Streptococcus faecalis* infection, and we usually prescribe Vancomycin, with satisfactory results, in *Staphylococcus aureus* infection when other antibiotics have failed to have an effect. Using Vancomycin, we have treated several cases of *Staphylococcus aureus* enterocolitis with miraculous results.

9. *Chloromycetin:* It is not easy for *Staphylococcus* to become resistant to Chloromycetin. Despite extensive use of Chloromycetin in our burn unit for more than 20 years, 68.9% of *Staphylococcus aureus* strains isolated are still sensitive to it. The sensitivity of *Streptococcus faecalis* is about 56.3%, and that of *Streptococcus pyogenes,* about 80–90%. Although it is not effective against *Pseudomonas* and *B. anitratum*, 60% of the isolated *Proteus* strains, and 40% of *Klebsiella* are susceptible to it. Therefore despite its toxicity we frequently combine its use with polymyxin B or gentamicin.

Table IV.12. The result of serologic typing of 73 strains of *P. aeruginosa*

Type	I	III	IV	VI	VIII	IX	Unclassifiable
Strains	48	1	17	3	1	1	2
%	65.7	1.4	23.3	4.1	1.4	1.4	2.7

Table IV.13. Antibiotic sensitivity tests of 36 strains of *P. aeruginosa*

Serologic types	No. of strains	No. of strains resistant to various antibiotics				
		Streptomycin	Chloromycetin	Neomycin	Polymyxin B	Gentamicin
I	22	20	18	18	0	14
III	1	1	1	1	0	1
IV	8	8	7	4	0	0
VI	1	1	1	1	0	0
VIII	1	0	0	0	0	0
IX	1	1	1	1	0	0
Unclassifiable	2	2	2	2	0	0
Total	36	33	30	27	0	15
Antibiotic-resistant strains (%)		91.7	83.3	75	0	41.7

Besides exfoliative dermatitis, the most severe side effect of Chloromycetin is the suppression of bone marrow; therefore a daily blood picture examination should be made. Bone marrow is also suppressed in severe gram-negative bacillary infection of burn patients, and there are manifestations of leukopenia and thrombocytopenia. Such a case must be differentiated from one resulting from the toxic effect of Chloromycetin. Chloromycetin is not contraindicated when leukopenia is caused by gram-negative bacillary infection; on the contrary, if infection is controlled by the administration of Chloromycetin, the white blood cell count may be raised.

10. *Polymyxin B:* Most of the gram-negative bacilli, e.g. *Pseudomonas*, coliform bacteria, *Aerobacter*, *Alcaligenes*, *B. anitratum*, and *Klebsiella* are sensitive to polymyxin B. It is resisted by *Proteus* and gram-positive cocci. From 1964 to 1978 the susceptibility of *Pseudomonas* to polymyxin B remained more than 90%, which was much higher than its susceptibility to gentamicin and carbenicillin. Therefore during the past 2 decades polymyxin B has continuously played a leading role in treating gram-negative bacillary infection in burns dealt with by our unit.

From Tables IV.12 and IV.13 we can see that the drug resistance of *Pseudomonas* of different serologic types against streptomycin, Chloromycetin, neomycin, gentamicin is empirically very similar. No strain is resistant to polymyxin B. More than half (63.6%) of the type I strains are resistant to gentamicin, one strain of type III is also resistant, and the rest are sensitive. Regardless of their serologic types, all the *Pseudomonas* cultured are resistant to streptomycin, Chloromycetin, and neomycin.

Pseudomonas septicemia in extensively burned patients was in many cases controlled by polymyxin B. Therefore in gram-negative bacillary infections combinations of polymyxin B and gentamicin or polymyxin B and Chloromycetin are used.

The nephrotoxicity of polymyxin B is manifested by albuminuria, granular casts, azotemia, and salt-losing nephritis. However, these consequences are reversible, and after cessation of administration of polymyxin B the kidney will soon recover. The course of administration is not necessarily to be restricted. In 14 survivors of very extensive third degree burns, within the 1st month of hospitalization polymyxin B was prescribed for an average of 20 days. During continuous usage of this antibiotic, urinary excretion of sodium and potassium was greatly increased. The daily urine output rose to 5,000 ml–6,000 ml, with the loss of 20 g each of sodium and potassium. Therefore, if polymyxin B is employed continuously for more than 1 week, water and electrolyte disturbances must be watched for. The daily urinary volume and urinary output of sodium and potassium must be precisely recorded and suitably replenished. The rate of intravenous dripping of polymyxin B must be kept slow. If the blood concentration reaches 30 μg per milliliter, it will cause respiratory arrest, and respiratory assistance is mandatory. Respiration can be restored after cessation of polymyxin B administration. The other side effects, such as paresthesia of the mouth, will disappear after discontinuation of therapy.

11. *Kanamycin:* The use of kanamycin is gradually being replaced by gentamicin. Kanamycin is indicated in only two instances: (a) for patients who have preexisting tuberculous foci and (b) for *Shigella* carriers, especially carriers

Table IV.14. The sensitivity of polymyxin B and gentamicin to eight common gram-negative rods isolated from burn wounds

Bacteria	Polymyxin B sensitivity %[a]	Gentamicin sensitivity %[b]
Pseudomonas aeruginosa	94.8	64.3
Escherichia coli	86.9	76.7
Paracolobacterium[c]	88	56.8
Bacterium anitratum	95	42.3
Proteus	35.6	70.5
Aerobacter aerogenes	90	73.1
Bacillus alcaligenes	91	53.6
Klebsiella pneumoniae[d]	92.5	53.3

[a] Data from 1966 to 1978
[b] Data from 1969 to 1978
[c] Before 1973 *Salmonella arizone*, *Citrobacter*, *Providencia*, and late-lactose-fermenting *E. coli* were reported as *Paracolobacterium*
[d] Data from 1973 to 1976

Table IV.15. Year-by-year comparison of the sensitivity of *P. aeruginosa* to gentamicin

Year	No. of strains	Drug-resistant strains (%)	Year	No. of strains	Drug-resistant strains (%)
1969	14	2 (14.3)	1974	70	21 (30.0)
1970	98	4 (4.1)	1975	114	31 (27.1)
1971	57	9 (15.9)	1976	36	19 (52.8)
1972	97	49 (50.5)	1977	119	49 (41.2)
1973	53	22 (41.5)	1978	87	33 (37.9)

of *Shigella flexneri*, because after extensive burns the previously quenched dysentery will usually flare up; in such cases administration of kanamycin may be adopted as a preventive measure.

12. *Gentamicin:* *Proteus* is highly sensitive to gentamicin, more so than to kanamycin: of 286 strains isolated from burn wounds, 211 are susceptible to gentamicin. Other gram-negative bacilli are less sensitive, and of *Klebsiella pneumoniae*, *Bacterium anitratum*, and *Bacterium alcaligenes* strains, only ca. 50% are susceptible (Table IV.14).

Staphylococcus aureus strains are sometimes susceptible to gentamicin, and all ten strains of *Streptococcus faecalis* isolated are sensitive; however, *Streptococcus pyogenes* strains are usually resistant.

The drug resistance of *Pseudomonas* to gentamicin develops readily: its susceptibility has decreased from 85%–95% to ca. 50% (Table IV.15).

As Pseudomonas develops resistance to gentamicin readily, therefore gentamicin is rarely used as a first-line drug for *Pseudomonas* infection, with the exception of infection caused by proven sensitive *Pseudomonas* strains. In practice gentamicin is used in combination with polymyxin B to compensate the defect of the latter, which is resisted by *Proteus*, *Staphylococcus aureus*, and *Streptococcus faecalis*. The combination of the above-mentioned antibiotics possesses the widest antibacterial spectrum. If there is definite coexisting staphylococcal infection, oxacillin may be added. In the case of coexisting *Streptococcus faecalis* infection, erythromycin and Chloromycetin are the supplementary drugs of choice.

The nephrotoxicity of gentamicin is similar but milder than that of polymyxin B. It may also cause damage to the vestibular nerve. Gentamicin occasionally causes hematuria, which is alleged to be a sort of hypersensitiveness not related to the dosage administered.

13. *Tobramycin:* Our laboratory data show that 70%–80% of indole-positive and indole-negative *Proteus*, coliform bacteria, *Aerobacter* and *B. alcaligenes* strains are sensitive to tobramycin, which is slightly greater than their sensitivity to gentamicin. As to *Citrobacter* and *A.c. lwoffi*, their susceptibility to gentamicin is somewhat inferior, reaching only 30%. Only 60% of *Pseudomonas* strains are sensitive to tobramycin, but 6 out of 17 strains resistant to gentamicin are sensitive to tobramycin. Therefore the latter may be administered if strains proven to be sensitive are found. Only a few *Staphylococcus aureus* strains are sensitive to tobramycin and it has no effect on gentamicin resistant gram-negative bacilli other than *Pseudomonas*.

14. *Amikacin:* Though it belongs to the aminoglycoside group and possesses a similar pharmacodynamic action to kanamycin A, amikacin is usually effective against most of the kanamycin- or gentamicin-resistant bacteria, especially *Pseudomonas*. Of the *Pseudomonas* strains isolated from burn wounds, 73% are sensitive to amikacin. This figure is lower than the sensitivity of *Pseudomonas* strains to polymyxin B, but greater than that to tobramycin and gentamicin. Ten out of 17 gentamicin-resistant strains and 6 out of 12 tobramycin-resistant strains of *P. aeruginosa* are sensitive to amikacin. The sensitivity of indole-positive and indole-negative *Proteus*, *Klebsiella pneumoniae*, *Aerobactar aerogenes*, and *Citrobacter* strains is between 70% and 80%. Fifty percent of coliform bacteria and *B. anitratum* and 90% of *A.c. lwoffi* strains are sensitive to amikacin.

Except in the case of *Proteus*, polymyxin B is always more effective than amikacin in gram-negative bacillary infection, yet amikacin is always more effective than gentamicin and tobramycin. Therefore amikacin remains an important weapon against gram-negative bacillary infection.

The sensitivity of *Staphylococcus aureus* strains to amikacin is around 50%. Amikacin is essentially ineffective in *Streptococcus faecalis* infection.

The above-mentioned findings and conclusions are only the sum of our past experience; continuous improvement in treatment and the emergence of various newly found or newly synthesized antibiotics and new drug-resistant strains will necessitate their modification. Therefore they can only be regarded as a point of reference.

5 Fungal Infection

Early in the 1950s clinicians were aware that fungal infection was tending to increase and in the 1960s the massive amount of literature on the subject confirmed the increasing incidence of fungal infection in debilitated patients whose host defence has been altered. Contributing factors include:

1. Greater frequency of acute or chronic debilitating conditions, such as leukemia, malignant disease, diabetes mellitus, and severe burns;
2. The use of corticosteroids;
3. The extensive use of broad-spectrum antibiotics;
4. Immunosuppressive therapy;
5. Radiation therapy;
6. The use of total parenteral nutrition;
7. Increased life expectancy and other immunosuppressed conditions.

In severely burned patients, especially those with extensive third degree burns, prolonged systemic antibiotic therapy is often necessary for the treatment of infection because of the extensive uncovered wound and their compromised host defences. It is well known that the use of broad-spectrum antibiotics may result in the development of resistant strains and fungal superinfection. Many microorganisms, including fungi, formerly considered to be nonpathogenic have assumed a new importance as lethal pathogens, and carry a high risk of mortality. It is obvious that the topical antibacterial agents used may further interfere with the host microbial ecology and permit the emergence of drug-resistant fungi from a polymicrobial wound in a severely burned patient.

From 1970 through 1979, 25 patients with severe burns developed confirmed invasive fungal infection. There were 18 deaths (mortality, 72%) in this group, either due to disseminated fungal sepsis or to associated bacterial sepsis. The breakdown of pathogenic organisms was: *Candida*, 17; *Aspergillus*, 4; Phycomycetes group, 2; *Cephalosporium*, 1; and *Nocardia*, 1. The average extent of burns was 77% ± 10% of the BSA, and the average area affected by third degree burns was 54.3% ± 26.6%. The average survival period for the 18 patients who died was 38 days. All of the patients in this group had concurrent bacterial infections or wound sepsis and both systemic antibiotics and topical antimicrobial agents were repeatedly used during treatment.

Fungal infection in these burned patients could conveniently be classified into three categories:

1. Those involving the burn wound;
2. Those involving mucous membranes (oral, esophageal, gastrointestinal, tracheal, bronchial, urinary);
3. Disseminated (septicemia, pneumonia, encephalitis, endo-peri- and myocarditis, pyelonephritis, etc.).

5.1 Fungal Infection of Burn Wounds

The majority of fungi found in burn patients are ubiquitous microorganisms which are commonly encountered in the hospital environment (Fig. IV.16). The fungi grown on burn wounds are not necessarily invasive; they are considered

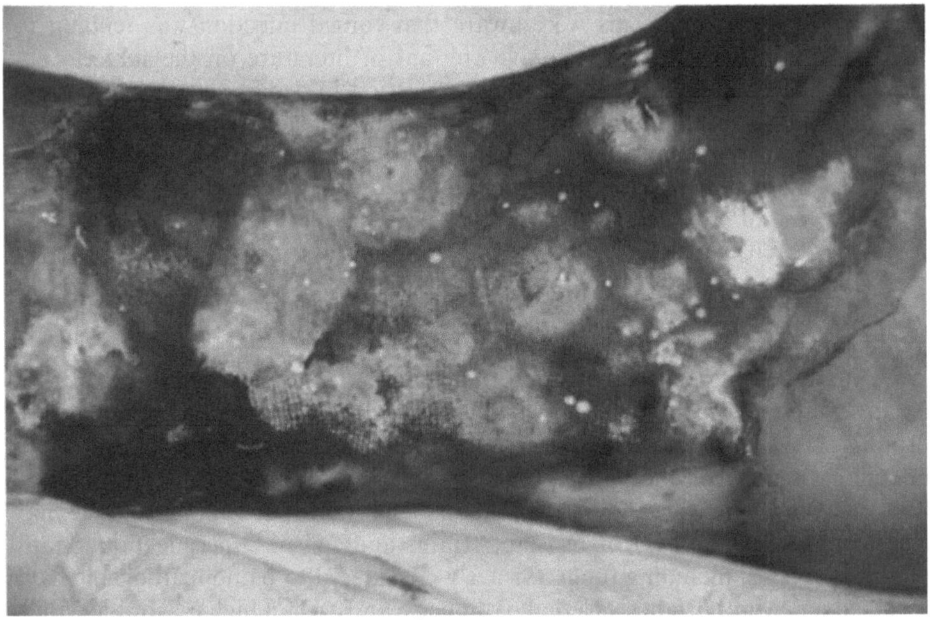

Fig. IV.16. Superficial fungal growths on the burn wound, which are not necessarily invasive

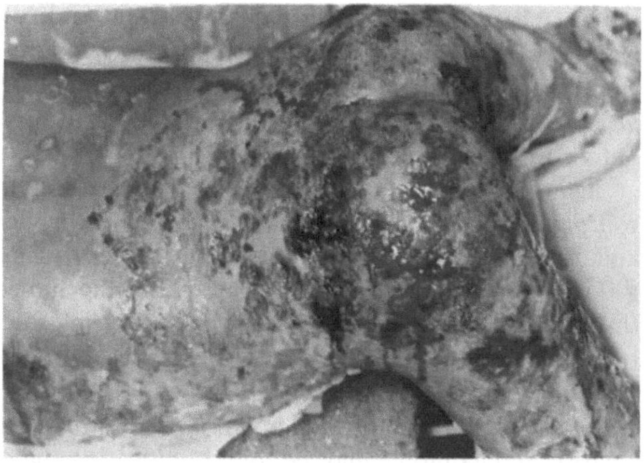

Fig. IV.17. Invasive *Candida albicans* infection, with necrotic patches on the wound

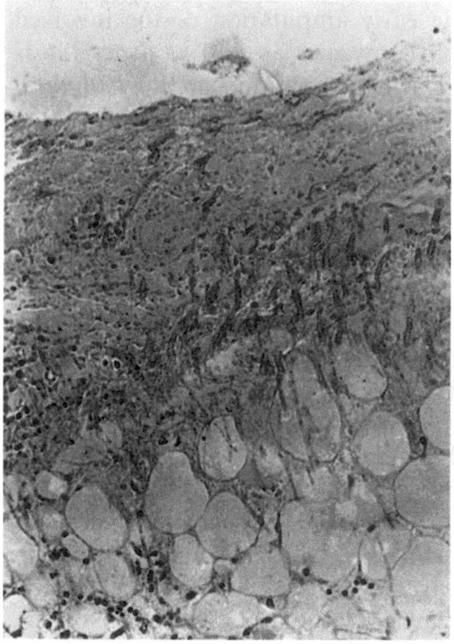

Fig. IV.18. Pathologic section of a fungal necrotic patch, showing subeschar hyphae which invade the viable subcutaneous fat. PAS

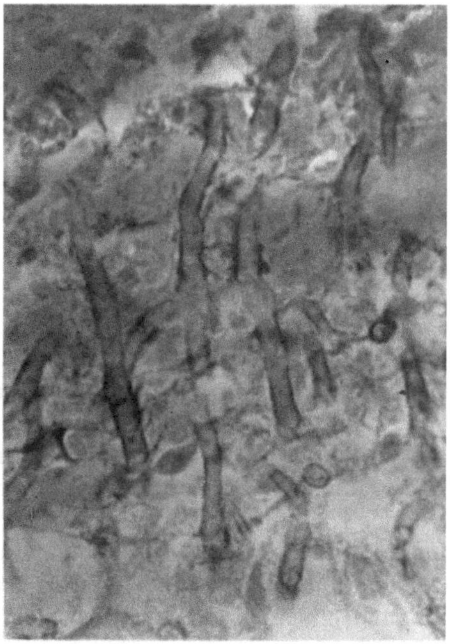

Fig. IV.19. Oil immersion view of the specimen shown in **Fig. IV.18.** PAS

invasive only when they penetrate beyond the depth of the original necrosis and invade the adjacent viable tissue. Using this criterion, only seven cases of invasive fungal infection of the burn wounds were diagnosed during a 10-year period. All of these cases were confirmed histologically. Six of them were associated with bacterial wound sepsis. All except one of these patients died of bacterial wound sepsis (Figs. IV.17–IV.19). The pathogenic organisms were *P. aeruginosa* and species of Enterobacteriaceae. The concomitant fungal invasion of burn wounds in these cases may be merely a result of the terminative state of the wound and the use of systemic and topical antimicrobial agents. Only a few cases of invasive *Candida* infection of burn wounds result in disseminated spread. On the other hand wound sepsis involving true fungi, e.g., *Aspergillus* spp. and the Phycomycetes group, may lead not only to serious morbidity but also to death.

The Phycomycetes group includes members of the genera *Mucor*, *Absidia*, *Rhizopus*, and *Mortierelle*; they appear in tissue as branching nonseptate hyphae and have a special affinity for blood vessels. The organisms may penetrate the vascular walls of arteries, grow within the lumen, and cause septic fungal thrombosis. Later, the fungi may invade veins and lymphatics as well. The presence of these invasive organisms in the burn wounds may produce rapid arterial thrombosis and deepen the wound, which may become ischemic and necrotic. Soon after the initial invasion, widespread proximal and distal muscular necrosis and gangrene may be found, indicating the invasion of relatively larger vessels of the involved muscle. If the wound is located on the face they may also invade the eyes and cause meningitis. Phycomycosis thus carries a high risk of mortality. Several authors advocate early amputation of the involved limbs as a life-saving measure. Invasive phycomycosis as well as aspergillosis are difficult to diagnose and are lethal. The cutaneous morphology of both aspergillosis and phycomycosis is not sufficiently distinctive in the early stage to make a clinical diagnosis. We feel that the only way to make a definite early diagnosis is to rely on wound biopsy. The treatment consists of wound excision and the use of topical and parenteral antifungal agents to control the infection.

Case Illustration. Male, aged 19. The patient sustained an extensive burn involving 75% of the BSA, including third degree burns to 33%. Initial treatment was quite satisfactory. He had been treated in a local hospital for nearly 4 weeks and was transferred to our hospital 26 days postburn. On the 8th day postburn the third degree eschar over the limbs had been excised and immediately covered with xenografts. On the 10th day infection occurred in the excised and grafted wound. The nonviable transplanted xenograft became black and ischemic, and there was widespread necrosis underneath the base of the wound. Histologic examination of the wound revealed *Phycomycetes mucor* which had penetrated into the lumen of the vessels. After biopsy, microscopic examination of the infected wound tissue revealed mucoraceous invasion with necrosis, sloughing, and ulceration. There was vascular thrombosis caused by invasion by the fungus of the walls and lumens of blood vessels of the muscles. The involved muscles were ischemic and necrotic. Associated bacterial infection occurred owing to the patient's debilitated state. We decided to treat the patient conservatively with topical 1% clotrimazole in propylene glycol combined with intravenous amphotericin B. The result was astonishingly good. Surgical excision was carried out 2 days later, after which toxemia and high fever were brought under control. On the 41st day the wounds were sufficiently replaced and closed with autografts, and the patient was discharged from hospital 76 days after the injury.

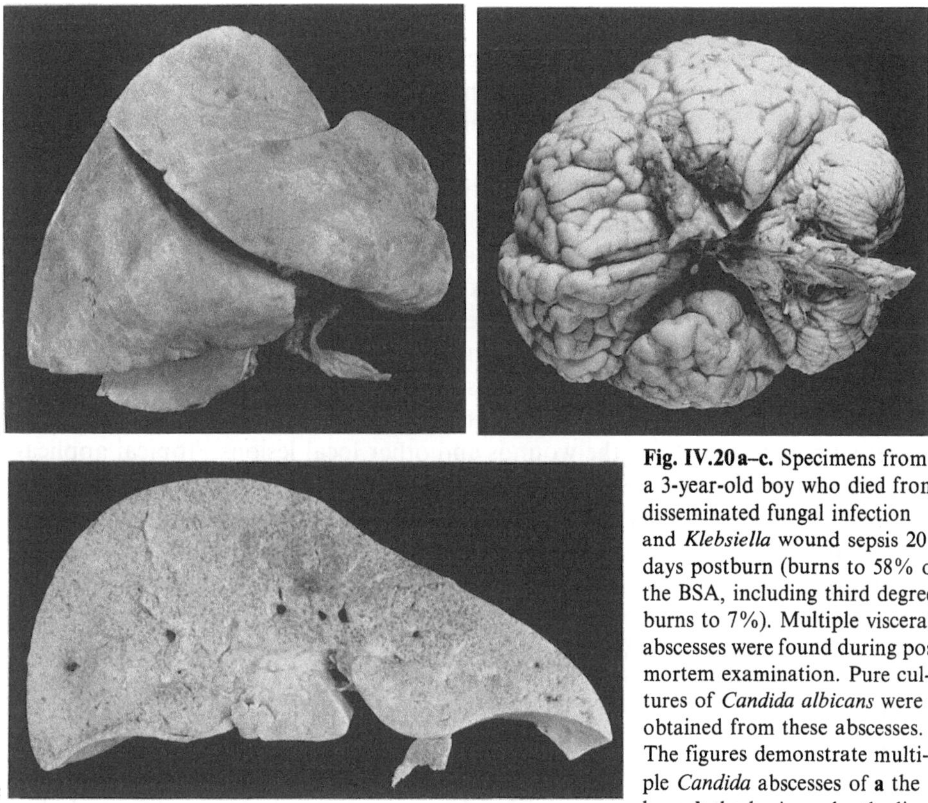

Fig. IV.20 a–c. Specimens from a 3-year-old boy who died from disseminated fungal infection and *Klebsiella* wound sepsis 20 days postburn (burns to 58% of the BSA, including third degree burns to 7%). Multiple visceral abscesses were found during post-mortem examination. Pure cultures of *Candida albicans* were obtained from these abscesses. The figures demonstrate multiple *Candida* abscesses of **a** the lung, **b** the brain and **c** the liver

5.2 Invasive Fungal Infection of the Mucous Membranes and Disseminated Fungal Infection

Candida albicans may be cultured from the mouth, throat, urine (urinary tract), sputum (trachea and bronchi), and feces (gastrointestinal tract). Foci of infection may also be found in the kidneys, heart, lungs, central nervous system, spleen, and other organs (Fig. IV.20). Fungal infection is considered to be localized when the infection is within the confines of the mucous membrane of hollow organs. The normal subject with intact defense mechanisms is able to resist fungal invasion even when the organisms are present in large numbers, whereas patients with altered defense mechanisms cannot. The evolution of fungal invasion in a burn patient is dependent on the number of invading organisms and the defence mechanisms of the host.

The developement of fungal septicemia with metastatic visceral lesions usually begins in the orpharynx, esophagus, or gastrointestinal tract; it spreads directly from the alimentary tract or indirectly from the respiratory organs. The disseminated form of fungal infection carries a high risk of mortality: only two out of six patients with disseminated fungal infection survived, and one of the survivors never regained consciousness after brain involvement and died a year later.

5.3 Treatment

In the prevention and treatment of fungal infections, strict control of the use of antibiotics in the course of treatment of burns should be combined with intensive efforts to raise the host defence. The environment as well as the burn wounds should be kept dry. Oral prophylactic therapy with nystatin should be used during the treatment with antibiotics for bacterial sepsis to reduce the incidence of fungal superinfection. When topical antimicrobial agents are used and if fungi appear on the wound surface, 1% clotrimazole cream should be added. For the prevention of invasion of fungi via other portals of entry, indwelling bladder and intravenous catheters should be removed whenever fungi infection is suspected. Cultures of wounds, sputum, urine, and feces should be taken at least once a week, and biopsy is indicated in any suspicious wound infection. The essential means of preventing wound sepsis and fungal infections is energetic management of the wounds and other local lesions. Topical application of antimicrobial agents such as clotrimazole and nystatin may be effective, but the ultimate method is the surgical excision of the nonviable tissue.

The results of current therapy in invasive mycoses are still discouraging. Amphotericin B and 5-fluorocytosine remain the most useful agents, and of the newer drugs, miconazole seems promising for clinical use in systemic mycoses. Miconazole is a newer broad-spectrum antimycotic imidazole derivative and can be administered both orally and intravenously. Drug-induced resistance is rare and it is remarkably free from toxic effects.

Amphotericin B: Amphotericin B is currently the agent of choice for the treatment of systemic fungal infection. This polyene, which is not well absorbed from the gastrointestinal tract, must be given intravenously to provide a reliable systemic therapeutic effect. However, its use has been associated with significant toxic effects including headache, fever, chills, phlebitis, anemia, hypokalemia, and azotemia as well as nephrotoxicity. It is customary to begin administration with a small test dose, 1 mg administered over 30 min. The dose should generally be increased gradually, but rapidly if the patient tolerates it well.

All of the patients in our series were given pretreatment with salicylates. Subsequent doses were raised in 5-mg increments daily up to about 0.5–1 mg/kg per day in order to obtain an effective serum level in a relatively short period. We added 25 mg–50 mg Hydrocortisone succinate into the infusion bottle for patients who tolerated such doses poorly. The total dose given was less than 3 g in all cases. Dosage schedules for the drug should be governed by frequently repeated measurement of creatinine clearance in patients with impaired renal function.

5-Fluorocytosine: This fluorinated pyrimidine is a competitive inhibitor of cytosine. It is well absorbed from the intestines after oral administration. No metabolism of the drug occurs in human beings and up to about 80% is excreted in the urine. The spectrum of inhibition is rather narrow; it includes only *Cryptococci*, *Candida*, and some strains of *Aspergillus*. The toxicity of 5-fluorocytosine is rather low; very few adverse effects have been observed, only diarrhea and leukopenia being occasionally noted. The white blood cell (WBC) count has sometimes continued to decrease even after the drug had been stopped for some days. We have met with three cases in which the WBC dropped to 4,900, 2,900, and 6,200/mm^3 after total dosages of 88.5 g, 44 g, and 4.5 g respectively. All three patients had leukocytosis before the treatment with 5-fluorocytosine was started. Recovery to the former count took 15, 11, and 6 days respectively. In the treatment of *Candida* infections confined to the gastro-intestinal tract, tracheobronchus, urinary tract and other mucous membrane sites, 5-fluorocytosine is usually the agent of choice, for it can control the early phase of fungal invasion. Nevertheless, drug resistance arising during therapy has been a major cause of therapeutic failure. Encouraging results have been observed in patients with urinary tract infection: fungi disappeared in all patients with urinary tract candidiasis.

In the treatment of serious mycoses, a combination of amphotericin B and 5-fluorocytosine is usually used. The combination has been said to be additive or synergistic. Amphotericin B acts by impairing the selective permeability of the fungal cell membrane to cause damage and lysis of the fungus, whereas 5-fluorocytosine can penetrate into the cell and exerts its effect by deamination to 5-fluorouracil, a known metabolic antagonist. Furthermore, it was hoped that the combination therapy might be equally effective when using low and relatively non-toxic doses of Amphotericin B. Based on this assumption, Amphotericin B was given in 0.3–0.6 mg/kg body weight in one of our cases, and proved to be effective. The currently recommended dose of 5-fluorocytosine is 150 mg/kg per day, which gives serum levels of 44–78 μg/ml. 5-Fluorocytosine can penetrate across the blood-brain barrier: cerebrospinal fluid levels are 60%–75% of the serum levels.

Clotrimazole is an imidazole derivative and has definitive action against a variety of pathogenic fungi in vitro. Despite initially enthusiastic reports that this drug was effective in the treatment of systemic mycosis, it has subsequently been proved to be of little value as a systemic agent. However, we found that the drug, either in the form of water miscible cream or propylene glycol solution, is of value as a topical agent in the treatment of mycotic infections of the burn wounds.

Chapter V Traditional Chinese Treatment of Burns *

Hsu Wei-shia

Translated by Ling Li-li

In China, methods for the treatment of burns were documented as early as the Tsin Dynasty (265–420 A.D.) in *Zhou Hou Fang (Prescriptions for Emergencies)*. The methods mentioned therein are as follows: "use aged lime alone or mix with oil as a dressing" and "fry the white cortex of willow in lard to make ointment for external application." In traditional Chinese medical literature of the past centuries, the majority of the voluminous prescriptions for burns dealt with external applications to the wound surface. However, while in minor burns of a small surface area it is sufficient to treat with external application only, in burns of a large surface area the damage may involve Qi, Xue, and Zang-fu[1,2,3] and causes various kinds of internal dysfunctions; therefore both the internal and the external condition of the patient should be considered in treatment in order to achieve satisfactory results. Cheng Shi Duo of the Ching Dynasty (1644–1911 A.D.) pointed out: "An effective medical treatment will rescue the viscera from being damaged by the malicious agent."[4] In the management of massive burns with integrated treatment involving both traditional Chinese and Western medicine, the traditional Chinese medical treatment is an important component. Therefore, it is our aim to investigate and compile the rich experiences of traditional Chinese medicine.

This chapter begins with a discussion of clinical practice, and we then sum up our experiences with traditional Chinese medicine, which has resulted in continuous improvement of our cure rate. On this basis we attempt to establish the rules governing successful use of Chinese medical treatment and thus to provide a guide for future clinical practice. Comments will be made on the

---

* It should be noted that the terminology used in this chapter is somewhat unusual. Those terms which will be unfamiliar to the reader are explained at first usage by way of footnotes

1 *Qi:* From the point of view of physiology, the meaning is twofold: a) Fine, small, and nutritional substances flowing in the body. b) Functional state of the internal organs

2 *Xue:* "blood" from the physiological point of view

3 *Zang-fu* consists of two parts: five "organs" and six "viscera." The former are the heart, liver, spleen, lung, and kidney. These terms basically represent the same organs as in modern medicine, but they do have different features. For instance, "heart" embraces both the physiologic functions of the heart proper and the circulatory system and also the activities of the central nervous system (such as mental activity and thinking). The six "viscera" are hollow organs in the peritoneal cavities: gallbladder, stomach, large intestine, small intestine, bladder, and "three Chiao" (functional unit for digestion, assimilation, and excretion). Again their functions are not exactly the same as those of organs with the same names in modern medicine

4 *Malicious agent* is a general term for various kinds of pathogenic factors and factors which cause pathologic damage

following three items: (a) treatment following discrimination of symptoms and signs in burns, (b) the principles of treatment and medication, and (c) the diagnostic significance of the "pulse picture"[5] and "tongue picture"[6].

1 Treatment Following Discrimination of Symptoms and Signs in Burns

In the ancient literature, classical works all considered burns as "heat poisoning"[7]: Such works are *Qian Jin Fang (A Thousand Gold Remedies)*, written in 652 A.D. of the Tang Dynasty (618–907 A.D.): *Wai Ke Zheng Zong (The Classics of Surgery)*, written in 1617 A.D. during the Ming Dynasty (1368–1644 A.D.); *Wai Ke Da Cheng (Encyclopedia of Surgery)*, written in 1665 A.D.; and *Yi Zong Jin Jian (The Golden Mirror of Medicine)*, written in 1739 A.D. during the Ching Dynasty. For instance, in *Wai Ke Zheng Zong* it was mentioned that "the intense heat of hot water and fire compels the poison to attack the interior." *Wai Ke Da Cheng* pointed out: "In the splashing of hot water and fire burn, the disaster comes from the outside; if the heat is extremely intense, the fire poison will attack the interior"[8]. *Yi Zong Jin Jian* stated: "Although the disease is caused by an external factor, the conditions must be classified as mild or severe. The mild cases can be promptly cured with treatment, while in the severe cases it is important to prevent the fire poison and hot gas from attacking the interior and causing fretfulness, vomiting, constipation, and even coma and suffocation." On the basis of the theory cited above, the medication used at that time for treating burns caused by hot water or fire was concerned mainly with the dispersal of heat and detoxication. Frequently used decoctions of medicinal herbs were: compound decoction of flos *Lonicerae* and radix *Glycyrrhizae* (composed of flos *Lonicerae* and radix *Glycyrrhizae*); compound decoction of rhizoma *Coptidis* for detoxication (composed of rhizoma *Coptidis*, cortex *Phellodendri*, radix *Scutellariae*, and radix *Pittospuri*); and Si Shuen Ching Liang Ying ("Four Soothing Cold Drinks," composed of radix *Sileris*, fructus *Forsythiae*, radix *Glycyrrhizae*, radix *Angelicae sinensis*, radix *Paeoniae rubra*, rhizoma et radix *Notopterygii*, radix et rhizoma *Rhei*, and medulla *Junci*).

In burns, the body is suddenly attacked by a thermal force causing damage to the skin, muscles, and "channels"[9] and leading to "stagnation of vital

---

5 *Pulse picture* denotes the sensation of pulsation felt by the fingers and comprises the frequency, rhythm, degree of fullness, state of patency and range of flow

6 *Tongue picture* denotes the morphology, color, sap, and other conditions concerning the tongue and its coating

7 *Fire poison (heat poison)*: Infection in burns

8 *Attack of the interior by fire poison*: Invasive infection in burns

9 *Channels*: From the point of view of modern medicine, "channels" might be considered to include the structure and certain functions of the nerves, blood vessels, and endocrine glands. This cannot, however, fully account for the "channel theory" as a whole; further investigation is required

energy and blood stasis"[10]. The local manifestations of burns by water and fire, such as thrombosis of the arborescent vessels and formation of eschar in third degree burns and pain in the wound, are all considered to be the manifestations of "stasis"[11] according to traditional Chinese medical theory. The large amount of necrotic tissue caused by the burn will unavoidably lead to "stasis and obstruction" of the vital energy and blood. Blood stasis will produce "heat," and the mechanism of such phenomena as high fever, thirst, bitterness in the mouth, fretfulness, red and dry tongue, and rapid pulse in the early postburn stage should be considered as "stasis" and not as "heat poison." We believe that wound healing can be accelerated once symptoms and signs of blood stasis have been discriminated and the blood circulation improved.

On the basis of our clinical observations and our understanding of the pathology of burns from modern medicine, we are of the opinion that the fundamental mechanism of burns[12] is injury and not heat poison, and injury will cause stasis. The necrotic tissue formed after a burn and the formation of wound surface are manifestations of blood stasis, and in treatment more emphasis should be placed on the administration of drugs that will disperse the stasis. Systemic infection in extensively burned patients is closely related to the condition of the wound surface and differs from the ordinary "fevers." According to traditional medical theory, the wound sepsis or septicemia which appears during the course of disease is considered to be the result of "attack on the interior by the malicious poisons"; it corresponds to the "deep going"[13] of "pyogenic poisons"[14] in traditional Chinese surgery and belongs to the category of "deep going complications."

As to treatment, both the internal and the external condition of the patient should be considered. The treatment of the former aims mainly at strengthening the bodily vital energy and "lifting" the poison to the outside; to this end the method of "internal support"[15] is employed. Internal support involves the use of drugs that will nourish the body and increase the vital energy and blood (i.e., increase the resistance of the body) and "drive" the poison outwards.

---

10 *Stagnation of vital energy and blood stasis:* Stagnation of vital energy is a pathologic concept. The chief clinical feature is local distention or pain, and prolonged stagnation of vital energy will cause blood stasis with aggravation of pain and resultant formation of a mass or maceration of the muscles

11 *Stasis* is a kind of pathologic concept which is much broader than the concept of blood stasis in modern medicine. It can be considered to include circulatory disturbances (especially disturbances of the microcirculation), the metabolic and nutritional imbalance due to circulatory disturbances, spasm of the internal organs and the striated muscles, impairment of blood supply or abnormal excitation of the afferent nerves due to spasm, and also changes in the tissues, such as proliferation or atrophy. Injury by external forces, swelling and pain due to inflammation, and surgical infection are all considered to be related to stasis

12 The *mechanism of disease* consists of the causation and site of disease and the mechanism of the changes in the disease process

13 *Deep going:* Invasive infection

14 *Pyogenic poison:* The infection in deep-lying tissues

15 *Internal support* (strengthening the vital energy and "lifting" the poison): This is a method of treatment which, by the use of medicine, helps in strengthening body resistance or the power of defense and regeneration in order to prevent invasive infection

This will prevent the malicious poison from transmitting to the interior and is therefore a very important method of treatment. The traditional Chinese work on surgery, *Wai Ke Jin Yao (The Essence of Surgery)*, which was written in 1263 A.D. during the Sung Dynasty (which lasted from 960 to 1280 A.D.), pointed out: "A surgeon dealing with pyogenic conditions cannot even for one day get good results without the method of internal support." *Wai Ke Jin Yi (The Essential Principles of Surgery)*, written in 1335 A.D. during the Yuan Dynasty (1280–1368 A.D.), stated "if the pus has not yet been formed, one should hasten its early formation; if the wound has already ruptured and pus has escaped to the outside, one should hasten the early growth of new flesh; if both vital energy and blood are deficient, then one should nourish them through internal support; if there is disharmony between "Yin" and "Yang"[16], one should regulate it by internal support." According to traditional Chinese medical theory, prevention of the complication of pyogenic infection by septicemia is based upon the balance between the external causative factor and bodily resistance; the method of lifting the poison or giving nourishment and support will accelerate suppuration of the local pyogenic infection and drainage of the pus and increase the local defensive power. The same principle should be followed in the prevention and in the treatment of systemic infection in burns. Cheng Shi Duo of the Ching Dynasty made remarks to this effect in his famous work *Shi Shi Mi Lu (Secret Records in a Stone Room)* (1686 A.D.) on the treatment of burn with *Tso Huo Tang (Remedy for Expelling Fire)*, which is composed of radix *Astragali*, radix *Angelicae sinensis*, radix et rhizoma *Rhei*, radix *Scutellariae*, rhizoma *Coptidis*, herba *Schizonepetae*, radix *Sileris*, *Poria cocos*, and radix *Glycyrrhizae*. In addition, Cheng made the following comments: The nicety of this prescription lies especially in the introduction of radix et rhizoma *Rhei* in addition to radix *Astragali* and radix *Angelicae*; this will not only nourish the vital energy and blood but also expel the malicious fire. It is even more important to use herba *Schizonepetae* and radix *Sileris* for inducing radix *Astragali* and radix *Angelicae* to nourish the vital energy and blood, to give birth to the new, and to expel the old. The highlight of this prescription lies in the use of 90 g *Poria cocos* to flush the fire gas[17] through the bladder once for all, thus relieving the pain of the skin. Radix *Glycyrrhizae* and radix *Scutellariae* are used simply for modulation and cooling."

---

16 *Yin* and *Yang*: According to ancient Chinese philosophy, everything is related to the opposition and unification, increase and decrease, and transformation of Yin and Yang. The concept of Yin Yang is a very broad one, and it embraces many aspects in the field of medicine. Yin denotes substance and Yang denotes function. Thus disharmony between Yin and Yang is a imbalance of substance and function

17 *Fire gas* is the pathologic manifestation of hyperfunction in the human body. The clinical manifestations include high fever, thirst, fretfulness, mania, and insomnia. The tongue is red with a yellow, rough coating. The pulse is rapid and forcible

2 Methods of Treatment and Medication

The principles of treatment are chiefly as follows: strengthening of vital energy and lifting the poison, easing the Yin and improving the blood circulation[18], and nourishing the Yin and dispersing heat[19]. The following prescription is recommended:

Prescription:	Radix *Astragali*, raw	30 g
	Angelica sinensis, whole plant	15 or 30 g
	Radix *Paeoniae rubra*, fried	9 g
	Radix *Salviae*, purple	12 g
	Flos *Carthami*	9 g
	Semen *Persicae*, mashed	9 g
	Flos *Lonicerae*	30 g
	Fructus *Forsythiae*, pure	15 g
	Radix *Rehmanniae*, fresh	30 g
	Cauli *Dendrobii*, fresh	30 g
	Radix *Glycyrrhizae*, raw	9 g

Since methods of both traditional Chinese and Western medicine are used in the treatment of burns, and antibiotics are always used in cases complicated by infection, medication for dispersal of "heat" (which corresponds to the antibiotics used) is of secondary importance.

In the prescription mentioned above, the raw radix *Astragali* helps to strengthen vital energy and lift the poison, while radix *Angelicae* helps to improve blood circulation and alleviate pain. When acceleration of pus formation and resolution of poison are indicated, radix *Angelicae* is generally the drug of choice. In prescriptions for internal support in surgery, radix *Astragali* and radix *Angelicae* are usually used in combination, being important drugs in lifting the poison. With regard to drugs for improving blood circulation, semen *Persicae*, flos *Carthami* and radix *Salviae* (all stasis-resolving drugs) are chosen. For dispersal of heat, drugs such as flos *Lonicerae* and fructus *Forsythiae* are the drugs of choice. In clinical practice, other drugs may be added to or deducted from these prescriptions according to the stage of the burn process and the various symptoms appearing during its course.

During the shock stage, hypovolemic shock may occur as a result of an increase in capillary permeability and loss of plasmalike fluids. According to traditional Chinese medical theory, burn first causes stagnation of vital energy and blood and then leads to deficiency of vital energy and blood, followed by great exhaustion and loss of corporeal secretions. In the basic prescription, drugs for dispersal of heat, such as flos *Lonicerae* and fructus *Forsythiae*, may

18 *Easing of Yin* and *improvement of blood circulation* is a kind of treatment for blood stasis

19 *Nourishment of Yin and dispersal of heat:* In infectious diseases, the body fluids and nutritional substances are exhausted due to persistent fever. The patient is feverish and thirsty with a red tongue and dry lips. Radix *Rhemanniae*, radix *Ophiopognis*, radix *Scrophylariae*, and caulis *Dendrobii* should be used. Any traditional Chinese medicament for nourishing body fluids is antipyretic and will promote secretions

be omitted, and radix ginseng, radix *Ophipogonis*, fructus *Schisandrae*, and semen *Zizyphi jujubae* may be added.

In elderly patients or those with very extensive burns, the following symptoms of involvement of Yang, following damage to Yin or symptoms of deficiency of "Yang vital energy," may appear immediately after injury: hypothermia, thready pulse, weariness, loss of vitality, drowsiness, cold extremities, etc. Under these conditions, medicinal herbs with a warming effects may be used. Compound decoction of radix ginseng and radix *Aconiti carmichaeli* praeparata may be used as the basic prescription with modifications according to the patient's condition.

During the shock stage, rhizoma *Imperatae* and herba *Plantaginis* (or similar drugs) may be used for the dispersal of heat and for diuresis in order to protect the kidneys and to increase urinary output. They can be stewed and made into a drink as a substitute for tea, and the dosage should be large: as much as 120 g–150 g rhizoma *Imperatae* and 30 g herba *Plantaginis*. It is much better to use fresh plants.

When the shock stage is over, the edema subsides, but the patient often has a high fever and psychic symptoms of varying degrees of severity. One may use Calculus Bovis Balls (one to three balls per day according to the severity of symptoms), "Surgical Secretio Bufonis Balls" (eight balls per dose, three times a day), or "Plum-blossom Tongue Stippling Balls" (two balls per dose, twice a day)[20].

When the wound is infected, the skin is macerated, and it is possible for the external poison to attack the interior. Emphasis should then be placed on preventing the malicious poison from attacking the interior. Shen Xiao Tuo Li San ("Miraculous Internal Support Powder," composed of radix *Astragali*, radix *Angelicae sinensis*, flos *Lonicerae*, and radix *Glycyrrhizae*) and Hui Du Ying Hua San ("Resorption of Poison and flos Lonicerae Powder," composed of radix *Astragali* and flos *Lonicerae*) may be used. Besides the external treatment for the extraction of pus and removal of macerated tissue, internal treatment for the improvement of blood circulation and dispersal of stasis should be employed. For the latter purpose, semen *Persicae*, flos *Carthami*, radix *Salviae*, and the like may be used for accelerating regeneration of the tissue of the wound surface. Our basic prescription listed on p. 144 is formulated according to this principle. During this stage of the disease, the basic prescription may be used and slight modifications made according to the clinical symptoms.

Once the malicious poison has attacked the interior, there will be wound sepsis or septicemia. Clinically, the most frequent symptoms are as follows: high fever, thirst, fretfulness, coma and delirium, papular rash, tendency to bleed, deep red and dry tongue with either a yellow, little, or no coating, and wiry rapid or thready rapid pulse. According to the classification of symptoms and signs in "fevers"[21], these symptoms belong to the category of "burn-

---

20 All three prescriptions are given in the form of ready-made pills

21 *Fevers* correspond to infectious diseases in modern medicine. According to traditional Chinese medical theory, the complicated manifestations of infectious diseases can be divided into four stages, namely, "Wei," "Qi," "Ying," and "Xue"

ing" of both vital energy and blood[22]. Medicinal herbs for internal support and improving blood circulation and dispelling stasis should be used in combination. Radix *Scrophylariae*, fried cortex *Paeoniae*, rhizoma *Coptidis*, radix *Astragali*, and fructus *Gardeniae* may be added to the basic prescription listed on p. 144. By this time, the patient often has a high fever and different kinds of mental symptoms, such as delirium, visual hallucination, insomnia, and even mania. Aromatic medicinal herbs for "opening the orifices" may be used selectively, such as Calculus Bovis Balls, Zhi Xue Dan ("Voilet Snow Powder"), and Zi Bao Dan ("Most Precious Powder")[23]. Calculus Bovis Balls should be used for severe mental symptoms, Zhi Xue Dan for high fever with convulsions, and Zi Bao Dan for coma.

If damage to the vital energy of Yang occurs there may be such symptoms as hypothermia, loss of vitality and deficient vital energy, sluggishness in response, loss of mental control, drowsiness, weakness, coldness of fingertips, tremor of extremities and tongue, and a feeble and thready pulse. Regaining of Yang and "resuscitate of backset"[24] are urgently demanded. To the basic prescription for strengthening vital energy, lifting poison, cooling blood, and dispersing heat, 15 g radix ginseng and radix *Aconiti carmichaeli* praeparata may be added.

During the stage of internal attack by the malicious poison, various kinds of complications frequently occur:

Pulmonary Symptoms. There may be shortness of breath and asthmatoid attacks. These symptoms may be due to bronchopneumonia or wound sepsis and may also be seen in the early stage of burn with resorption of edema.

Prescription:	Rhizoma *Phragnitis*, fresh, with removal of knots	60 g
	Cortex *Mori radicis*	9 g
	Semen *Banincasae*	30 g
	Bulbus *Fritillariae cirrhosae*	9 g
	Radix *Platycodi*	9 g
	Rhizoma *Pinelliae* treated with succus *Bambosae*	9 g
	Os Madreporariae	12 g
	Concha Meritricis	12 g
	Herba *Houttuyniae*	30 g
	Rhizoma *Fagopyri cymosi*	30 g
	Oleum succus *Bambosae*, diluted	60 g

22 *Burning of both vital energy and blood* denotes the syndrome composed of the stages Qi and Xue in infectious diseases. The chief symptoms are high fever, thirst, fretfulness, coma, convulsions, papular rash, and various kinds of hemorrhage, such as hemoptysis, bleeding from the nose, and melena. The tongue is red with a rough coating

23 Again, both Zhi Xue Dan and Zi Bao Dan are given in the form of ready-made pills

24 *Regaining of Yang and resuscitation of backset* is the method of treatment for loss of Yang, which is manifestated as incessant perspiration, cold sweat, coldness of the body and extremities, proclivity for hot drinks despite lack of thirst, feebleness of breath (sluggish reaction, shallow respiration), and extremely feeble and almost absent pulse. This kind of condition is usually seen in patients who are in shock

Gastrointestinal Symptoms. Abdominal distension, diarrhea, thin black stools, nausea and vomiting, and anorexia are often manifestations of wound sepsis. The following medicinal herbs may be chosen according to the symptoms:

1. For abdominal distension: lignum *Aquillariae resinatum*, radix *Aucklandiae*, fructus *Aurantii*, pericarpium *Arecae*, radix *Linderae*, etc.

2. For diarrhea: If the symptoms are those of deficiency and cold[25], Li Zhong Tang (compound decoction composed of radix ginseng, rhizoma *Zingiberis*, rhizoma *Atractylodis*, and radix *Glycyrrhizae*) may be used. If the cold is extreme, radix *Aconiti carmichaeli* praeparata may be used. If the symptoms are those of excess and heat[26], we can use the compound decoction of radix *Puerariae*–radix *Scutellariae*–rhizoma *Coptidis*; alternatively Xiang Lian Wan (composed of radix *Aucklandiae* and rhizoma Coptidis) can be used with modifications.

3. For nausea and vomiting: Er Chen Tang (compound decoction composed of rhizoma *Pinelliae*, *Poria cocos*, pericarpium *Citri reticulatae*, and radix *Glycyrrhizae*) or Zuo Jin Wang (balls made of rhizoma *Coptidis* and fructus *Evodiae*).

4. For anorexia: radix *Codonopsitis*, *Anas domestica*, burned fermented almond compound, pericarpium *Citri reticulatae*, lignum *Aquillariae resinatum*, radix *Aucklandiae*, fructus *Hordei germinatus* etc. or Xiang Sha Liu Jun Zhi Wan.

Symptoms of Deficiency of Vital Energy. The manifestations are fatigue and weakness, edema, dyspnea, tremor of the tongue and extremities, pinkish and puffy tongue, and deficient and thready pulse.

Ginseng, which has a sweet taste and nourishes the bodily vital energy efficiently, should be the drug of first choice. One may stew 3–9 g red ginseng to make a drink which acts as a substitute for tea. This prescription improves the patient's mental condition and appetite.

During the course of extensive burns, symptoms of polyuria are not infrequent. They may be caused by the development of postburn stress diabetes or by salt-losing nephritis due to prolonged use of antibiotics which are toxic to the kidneys. The mechanism of disease consists of deterioration of the Yang of the kidney[27], impotence, and deficiency and failure of absorption of the vital energy in the lower part of the body. The principles of treatment are warming of the kidney[28], strengthening of vital energy, and consolidation of absorption[29]. Remedies such as Su Quan Wan or ootheca *Mantidis* powder may be used with modifications.

---

25 *Symptoms of diarrhea* due to hypofunction of the digestive system. They consist of loss of appetite, loss of taste, undigested food in the stools, pale tongue, and small and feeble pulse

26 Diarrhea due to bacterial infection

27 *Deterioration of the Yang of the kidney:* Decline of the energy metabolism in the human body

28 *Warming of the kidney* is the method of treating deficiency of the Yang of kidney, the chief manifestations of which are a sensation of coldness, loss of vitality, lumbar soreness, loss of control of discharge, impotence, frequent urination, and clear and profuse urine

29 *Consolidation of absorption* is the method of treating deficiency of the kidney with frequent urination

Prescription:	Radix *Codonopsitis pilosulae*	9 g
	Radix *Astragali*	30 g
	Rhizoma *Dioscoreae*	30 g
	Radix *Trichosanthis*	30 g
	Fructus *Rosae laevigatae*	15 g
	Ootheca *Mantidis*	15 g

In thrombophlebitis of the lower extremities the following prescription may be used.

Prescription:	Rhizoma *Sparganii*	9 g
	Rhizoma *Curcumae zedoariae*	9 g
	Semen *Persicae* (mashed)	5 g
	Flos *Carthami*	9 g
	Radix *Angelicae sinensis* (tail)	9 g
	Radix *Salviae*	12 g
	Paeonia Rubra	9 g
	Radix *Achyranthis bidentatae*	9 g
	Myrrh	9 g
	Frankincense	9 g

For external application, *Allium sativum* and *Mirabilitum depuratum* (minced together) may be applied for 2 h, and then, as a substitute, *Rhei* paste (made with vinegar) is applied for 8 h. It must be noted that *Allium sativum* and *Mirabilitum depuratum* are strongly irritative to the skin. During their application, tincture of benzoic acid should be applied locally at the same time, and the skin should be covered with two layers of vaseline gauze for protection.

3 Diagnostic Significance of "Pulse Picture" and "Tongue Picture"

Most burn patients have a wiry pulse and nearly every patient has a rapid pulse. When infection occurs, the pulse is frequently full and rapid. If the bodily vital energy is deficient, the pulse will become feeble and rapid. A thready and feeble pulse signifies the decline of the real "Yang".

Assessment of the tongue picture was a characteristic diagnostic measure in traditional Chinese medicine. The tongue is closely related to the viscera: diseases of the viscera and channels will be revealed by the tongue, and changes in the tongue picture indicate a change in the state of the disease. The tongue picture in burn patients is of some value in assessing the severity of infection and in prognosis. Changes in the tongue picture sometimes appear in the early stage of wound sepsis or septicemia.

The tongue picture in patients with wound sepsis (or septicemia) usually has the following features: a crimson or purplish tongue proper, a small amount of secretion and even dryness and cracks, prominent papillae, and a dry yellow or dry black coating or absence of coating. These changes in tongue picture may occur before the appearance of other clinical symptoms of wound sepsis (or septicemia) and are therefore of value in early diagnosis; they also aid prediction of the outcome. Changes in the tongue proper are more important than those of the coating, and changes in the sap of the tongue proper are more significant than changes in coloration, especially in the early diagnosis of wound sepsis (or septicemia). If the tongue proper is sapful, the secretions are abundant; if, however, it is sapless, there is secretory deficiency. Sometimes the variations in the degree of moisture of the tongue may precede the color changes of the tongue proper; therefore the degree of moisture of the tongue should be observed. The great majority of patients have a dry, sapless tongue when wound sepsis (or septicemia) is present. Clinically, if there are no other explanations for the lack of secretions or dryness (no secretions on palpation) of the tongue proper, it is very important to keep a close watch for the possibility of wound sepsis (or septicemia). Improvement of the patient's condition is indicated when the dry and sapless tongue proper becomes sapful.

When performing diagnosis by examination of the tongue picture, we found that some of the patients had a dry and sapless tongue due to long-term use of large doses of broad spectrum antibiotics. This possibility should be considered if the wound sepsis (or septicemia) has been controlled and other symptoms have been ameliorated, but the tongue picture shows no corresponding improvement, with persistent deficiency or absence of secretions.

To avoid gaining a false impression from the appearance of the tongue, it should be palpated to assess secretory activity.

Case Illustration. Female, aged 28. The patient sustained flame burns to 98% of the BSA, including third degree burns to 81%. On the 9th day postburn, pulmonary infection occurred. Moist rales could be heard over the anterior aspects of both lungs, and chest films showed bilateral bronchopneumonia. The following prescription was first tried:

Radix *Phellodendri*	9 g
Nelumbo nucifera	3 g
Radix *Angelicae sinensis*	15 g
Gypsum fibrosum	60 g
Bulbus *Fritillariae thunbergii*	9 g
Radix *Atractylodis*	9 g
Talcum (packed)	30 g
Radix *Glycyrrhizae*	9 g

The clinical condition was not improved after two successive doses, possibly owing to accumulation of sputum heat in the lungs. The principles of treatment were altered to flushing of the lungs, dispersal of heat, and resolution of the sputum. The modified prescription was as follows:

Rhizoma *Phragmitis* (fresh)	60 g
Semen *Benincasae*	15 g
Semen *Coicis*	15 g
Succus *Bambusae* (diluted)	90 g

Rhizoma *Pinelliae* treated with succus *Bambusae*	9 g
Concha *Meritricis*	30 g
Os Madreporariae	12 g
Cortex *Mori radicis*	9 g
Bulbus *Fritillariae thunbergii*	9 g
Radix *Platycodi*	3 g
Gypsum fibrosum	60 g
Rhizoma *Anemarrhenae*	9 g
Radix *Glycyrrhizae*	9 g

Three doses of this decoction were taken successively. Pulmonary infection gradually subsided, the body temperature fell, and the rales markedly decreased, those on the left lung field disappearing. The pulmonary infection was controlled after another two doses, and the patient survived.

Case Illustration. Male, aged 44. The patient sustained flame burns to 80% of the BSA, including third degree burns to 50%. On the 4th day after this extensive burn, the patient had diarrhea, especially after feeling coldness of the abdomen. The diarrhea was not accompanied by abdominal pain or gurgling intestinal sounds, and there was no burning sensation in the anus. The patient was thirsty and enjoyed hot drinks, and there were also mental symptoms. The tongue had a thin white coating. These were the symptoms of the inward attack of the malicious poison. The condition was diagnosed as "deficiency cold" with diarrhea. The treatment was Li Zhong Tang with some additions:

Radix *Codonopsitis pilosulae*	9 g
Rhizoma *Atractylodis*	9 g
Rhizoma *Zingiberis* (carbonized)	3 g
Cortex *Magnoliae officinalis*	3 g
Poria cocos	9 g
Radix *Glycyrrhizae*	9 g

The diarrhea was controlled after two successive doses, but the symptoms of inward attack of the malicious poison became more marked, including fretfulness, tremor of the whole body, and slight abdominal distension. Blood culture showed growth of *Aerobacters*. The following medication was given to strengthen the vital energy and "lift" the poison, to ease "Ying" and to disperse heat:

Radix *Astragali*	60 g
Radix *Angelicae sinensis*	30 g
Radix *Paeoniae rubra*	9 g
Radix *Salviae*	12 g
Flos *Lonicerae*	30 g
Fructus *Forsythiae*	15 g
Radix *Glycyrrhizae*	9 g

The clinical condition had improved greatly after two doses, and the patient survived.

Chapter VI Water-Electrolyte and Acid-Base Balances

YANG CHIH-CHUN

Translated by NYI PAO-CHUN

In the treatment of extensive burns it is vital that full consideration is given to the water-electrolyte and acid-base balances, which are subject to disturbance for the following reasons:

1. During the shock stage, large amounts of fluid and electrolytes escape from the burned surface and "sequester" into the interstitial spaces. Even when blood volume has been well replenished, peripheral perfusion will not yet be restored. This causes incomplete degradation of carbohydrates, fats, and proteins, and, in addition, there is an increase of antidiuretic hormone and aldosterone secretion.

2. An enormous amount of water is lost from the burn wound surfaces by evaporation and from the granulation surfaces by exudation. At the same time, water is also lost through solute diuresis owing to significantly increased catabolism and by salt-losing nephritis caused by long-term administration of aminoglycosides or polymyxin. Hence water must be properly supplemented to avoid disturbances of the aforementioned balances.

1 Water-Electrolyte Balance

1.1 Introduction

1.1.1 Calculating Units

For the expression of the concentration of various constituents of the body fluids, comparable units should be chosen. Interaction of the substances in the extracellular fluid takes the form of molecules or ions. Therefore, it is suitable that gram-molecule or milligram-molecule and gram-equivalent or milliequivalent are used.

1. *Gram-mole (mol) and Milligram-mole (mmol):* One mole of a certain substance is the molecular weight of that substance in terms of grams. It reflects under certain defined physical conditions the number of particles contained in a certain unit volume. In any given gasified substance, at a temperature of 0 °C and an atmospheric pressure of 760 mmHg, the number of particles contained in a definite volume is the same.

For example, the atomic weight of sodium is 23; chloride, 35.5; and potassium, 39.1. One mole of NaCl is $23+35.5=58.5$ g.

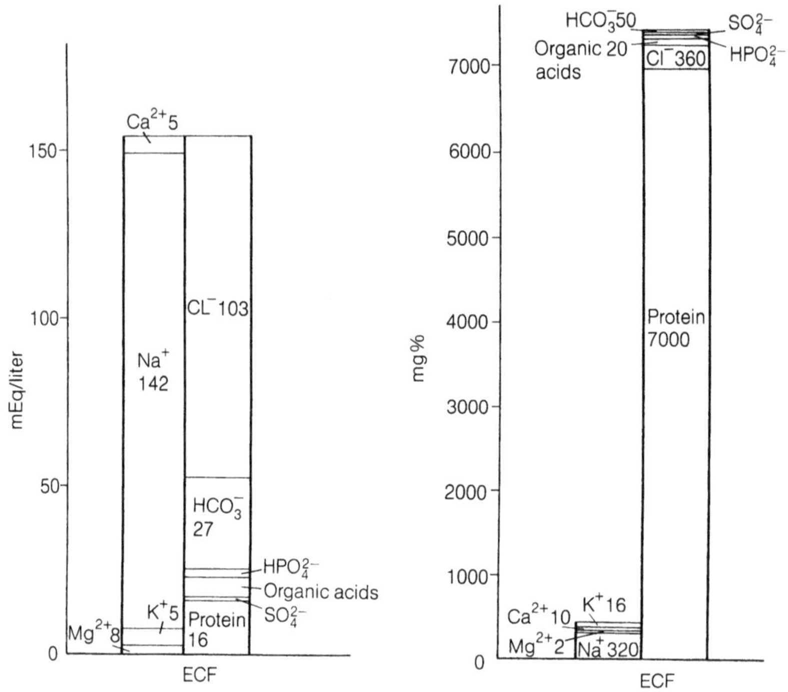

Fig. VI.1. The concentrations of various constituents of the extracellular fluid (*ECF*) expressed in milliequivalents per liter and milligrams percent

Taking ions: 1 mol $K^+ = 39.1$ g; 1 mol $Na^+ = 23$ g; 1 mol $Cl^- = 35.5$ g; and 1 mol $HCO_3^- = 1 + 12 + 3(16) = 61$ g.

If one desires to change grams or milligrams into millimoles, the method of calculation is as follows:

1 g = 1,000 ÷ molecular weight = x mmol. For example, 1 g NaCl = 1,000 ÷ 58.5 = 17.1 mmol.

2. *Equivalent (Eq) and Milliequivalent (mEq)*: For electrolytes, equivalents and milliequivalents are generally used; they reflect the number of electric charges carried by the particles contained in a certain unit volume.

One milliequivalent is the milliatomic weight of the ion divided by the atomic valence.

The number of millimoles of monovalent ions is similar to the numerical value of mEq. Under a certain physical condition, in a certain unit volume, the number of electric charges carried by the particles in a bivalent ion is twice the number of millimoles. One millimole of a bivalent ion is equal to 2 mEq. For instance, a Ca^{2+} ion carries two positive electric charges; therefore the number of milliequivalents of the particles is twice the number of millimoles. Therefore 1 mmol $Ca^{2+} = 2$ mEq Ca^{2+}. It can interact with 2 mEq Cl^- to form $CaCl_2$.

In the body fluids, the numbers of positive electric charges and negative charges are the same. Therefore when the water-electrolyte balance is concerned, milliequivalents are used as the calculating unit (Fig. VI.1).

1.1.2 Method of Unit Transformation

Although we use milliequivalents as the calculating unit for the water-electrolyte balance, we often use grams as the unit when electrolytes are supplemented intravenously or orally, e.g., oral administration of 6 g sodium chloride per day, intravenous infusion of 9 g potassium chloride. One might then ask, how many milliequivalents are 6 g sodium chloride or 9 g potassium chloride equal to. In a compound formed by two monovalent atoms, we may use the following values for the transformation of units:

One gram of any substance = 1,000 ÷ molecular weight of that substance = mEq. Therefore:

1 g $NaCl$ = 1,000 ÷ 58.5 = 17.1 mEq Na^+
1 g KCl = 13.4 mEq K^+
1 g $NaHCO_3$ = 12 mEq Na^+
1 g sodium lactate = 9 mEq Na^+
1 g $CaCl_2$ = 18 mEq Ca^{2+}
1 g calcium gluconate = 5 mEq Ca^{2+}
6 g $NaCl$ taken orally = 102.6 mEq Na^+ and 102.6 mEq Cl^-
9 g KCl injected intravenously = 120.6 mEq K^+ and 120.6 mEq Cl^-.

We can transform milligrams percent into milliequivalents per liter by the following formula: $\frac{\text{mg\%} \times 10 \times \text{atomic valence}}{\text{atomic weight}} = \text{mEq/liter}$

In order to simplify the procedure, we make use of $\frac{10 \times \text{atomic valence}}{\text{atomic weight}}$ to calculate a transfer factor; it is only necessary to multiply the mg% value by the transfer factor to obtain the number of milliequivalents per liter (Table VI.1). For example, to transform a given value of Na^+ serum electrolyte of 326 mg% into milliequivalents, multiply by 0.435, i.e., $326 \times 0.435 = 141.8$ mEq/liter.

Some other laboratories report in milliequivalents, which can be converted into grams if desired. For example, a certain patient excretes 250 mEq K^+; how many grams of KCl would that be? The answer is $250 \times 74.5 = 18{,}600$ mg KCl, i.e., 18.6 g (74.5 is the molecular weight of KCl).

Table VI.2 shows the normal values of serum and urinary electrolytes (data from Rui Jin Hospital, Shanghai Second Medical College).

Table VI.1. Conversion factors of various electrolytes

Electrolytes	Conversion factors
Na^+	0.435
K^+	0.256
Cl^-	0.282
HCO_3^-	0.446
Ca^{2+}	0.5

Table VI.2. Normal values of serum and urine electrolytes (Rui Jin Hospital)

Electrolytes	Serum concentration (mEq/liter)	Urine concentration (mEq/liter)
Na^+	130–140	40–90
K^+	4–5.6	20–60
Cl^-	95–105	40–120
HCO_3^-	24–27	
Ca^{2+}	5	

1.2 Sodium Balance

1.2.1 Hypernatremia

Hypernatremia may be defined as the presence of a serum sodium concentration of more than 145 mEq/liter. It occurs frequently in burn patients, but is rarely caused by excessive intake of NaCl; rather it is usually the result of a greater water loss in relation to sodium loss. In fact the total exchangeable sodium value may still be within normal limits or even lower than normal. The vast amount of water loss is, as previously mentioned, caused by either evaporation from the wound surfaces or solute diuresis in combination with failure to give supplement at the appropriate time. The clinical manifestations of hypernatremia are thirst, restlessness, disorientation, confusion, delirium, and even coma.

There are three groups of substances which cause solute diuresis, namely:

a) Substances only partially reabsorbed by the renal tubules, such as glucose, urea, sodium chloride, ketones, and organic acids

b) Substances mostly not reabsorbed by the renal tubules, such as sulphates

c) Substances not reabsorbed by the renal tubules, such as mannitol and sorbitol

When the quantity of the above-mentioned substances is too large or they are not reabsorbed, they will accumulate in the collecting tubules; this causes very high osmotic pressure in the urine in the collecting tubules, effecting a large reduction in water reabsorption by the renal medulla. Therefore large amounts of water are excreted along with the solutes; hence the term "solute diuresis."

Before the solutes (with the exception of solute diuresis caused by sodium chloride) reach the collecting tubules, the major portion of Na^+ has already been reabsorbed by the renal tubules. Therefore during solute diuresis the ratio between water and Na^+ (H_2O/Na^+) is correspondingly increased, that is to say, more water than sodium is excreted. Consequently, even when body fluids are isotonic, insufficient supplement of water may cause them to become hypertonic, resulting in dehydration hypernatremia. Hypernatremia caused by solute diuresis in burned patients often occurs after prolonged nasal feeding of hypertonic liquid diet without sufficient water intake or when complicated stress diabetes has not been controlled in time.

1.2.1.1 Tube-Feeding Syndrome

All burn patients require high caloric and protein diet, but dehydration hypernatremia is very likely to result if only caloric value or protein quality is emphasized and supplement of water is neglected. When urea nitrogen (breakdown of lean body mass) is excreted as solute, it will carry a large amount of water, and hypertonic dehydration will ensue.

Fig. VI.2. Tube-feeding syndrome in a patient with burns to 66% of the BSA, including third degree burns to 40%. Changes in **a** the levels of serum sodium, serum potassium, and serum chloride and **b** the water balance are shown ▷

Case Illustration. Female, aged 46. The patient had burns to 66% of the BSA, including third degree burns to 40%. She passed the shock stage uneventfully. During the shock stage nutrition was increased gradually every day. Up to the 7th day after injury, the patient was receiving 3,500–4,000 cal and about 150 g protein each day. On the 8th postburn day she became irritable, and on the 10th day she became semiconscious and did not respond when addressed. Her respiration rate increased and body temperature rose. On the 11th postburn day her response was sluggish, and she was in a confused state of mind. Her respiration became rapid and was complicated by gastrointestinal hemorrhage and bronchopneumonia. The hemoglobin level was 19 g%; serum sodium increased from 140 mEq/liter immediately after burn to 167 mEq/liter on the 10th day after injury; urinary sodium decreased from 300 mEq/liter to 55.5 mEq/liter; nonprotein nitrogen increased from 35.5 mg% to 98 mg%; and urea nitrogen rose from 15 mg% to 53 mg%. Urinary nitrogen excretion increased day by day from 26 g/day to 41 g/day. Although water intake was up to 4,000 ml, 3,500 ml urine was excreted per day, showing a negative balance.

Beginning from the 9th day postburn, her caloric intake was limited to 1,400–3,000 cal per day. On the 10th, 11th, 12th, and 13th days, daily water intake was 7,000, 9,800, 9,300, and 7,000 ml respectively. By the use of these measures, serum sodium, nonprotein nitrogen, and urea nitrogen gradually dropped to normal levels. The patient's general condition improved; she became mentally clear, gastrointestinal hemorrhage stopped, and pneumonia was controlled (Fig. VI.2). The patient survived.

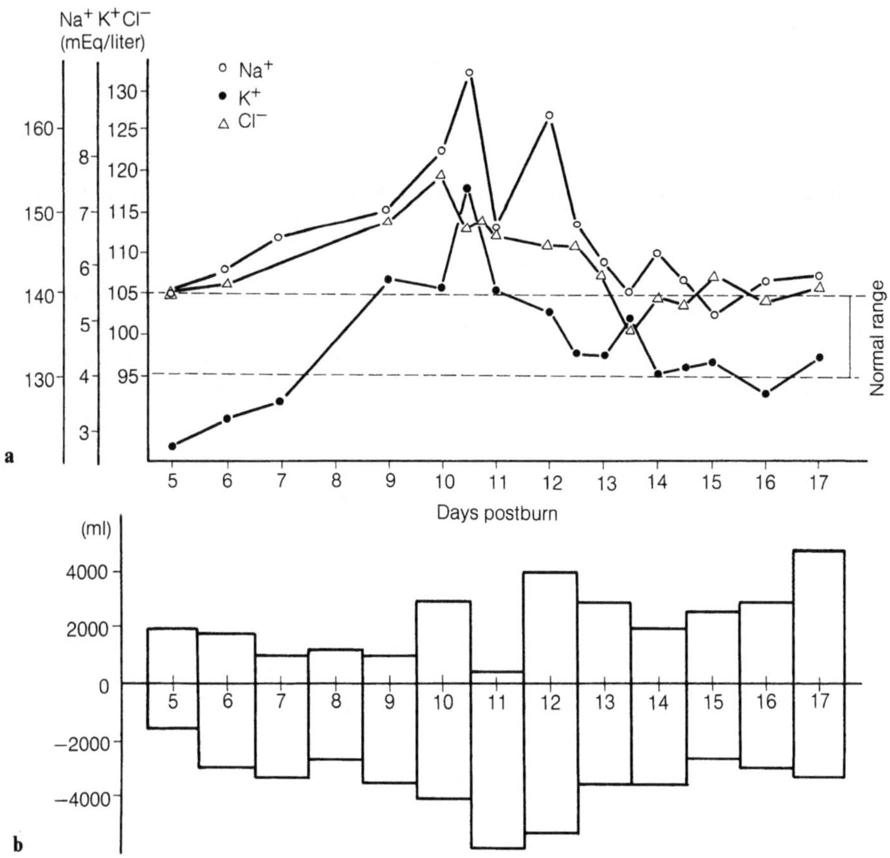

1.2.1.2 Hypernatremia Induced by Uncontrolled Diabetes

Ordinarily the increased concentration of glucose in extracellular fluid draws water out of cells and dilutes the extracellular compartment, causing hyponatremia, but in cases of long-term uncontrolled stress diabetes, especially in those patients with insulin resistance, glucose together with intermediate metabolites of fat and protein will cause a prolonged solute diuresis, resulting in dehydration hypernatremia.

Case Illustration. Male, aged 23. The patient had burns to 95% of the BSA, including third degree burns to 85%. After the patient passed through the shock stage uneventfully, he took large quantities of food. He became very thirsty, drank a lot of water, and passed large amount of urine frequently. The intake of water was about 7,000 ml per day with a urinary output of around 4,000 ml, and sugar in the urine was +++ to ++++. On the 8th postburn day second eschar excision was performed. The patient was at first irritable and later became indifferent. The rate of his respiration increased. Serum sodium then increased, reaching 155 mEq/liter on the 11th day after injury; at this time the blood sugar level was 410 mg%, and urea nitrogen, 60 mg%. Urinary sodium dropped from 72 mEq/liter (24-h total, 215 mEq) to 38 mEq/liter (24-h total, 172 mEq); 24-h urinary excretion of potassium rose from 190 mEq to 273 mEq; and 24-h urinary excretion of nitrogen increased from 23 g to 38 g.

Beginning from the 11th day postburn, the patient was treated with insulin, and urinary output decreased significantly. After a daily supplement of 7,000 ml–8,000 ml water and 60–120 mEq potassium, dehydration hypernatremia was corrected (Fig. VI.3).

Under normal conditions, the ratio (mEq:g) of potassium to nitrogen in urine is 2.7:1, but as long as diabetes has not been rectified, large quantities of protein, fat, and glycogen are broken down. Fat and glycogen do not contain nitrogen, but they do contain potassium. In the above patient, on the 11th day after injury the ratio of potassium to nitrogen in the urine was as high as 7:1. In patients with an extensive burn surface area complicated by diabetes, water loss is often greater than loss of potassium, and potassium loss is in turn greater than sodium loss. Therefore the level of serum potassium is sometimes normal and sometimes subnormal, while the serum sodium level is often higher than normal, manifesting clinically as serious hypertonic body fluid syndrome.

1.2.2 Hyponatremia

Hyponatremia may be defined as a serum sodium level of lower than 130 mEq/liter. In the presence of hyponatremia, nausea, vomiting, somnolence, lack of facial expression, loss of emotion, muscular twitching, acute gastric dilatation, increase of body weight, pitting edema, weakened or loss of tendon reflex, and even convulsion and coma may appear clinically.

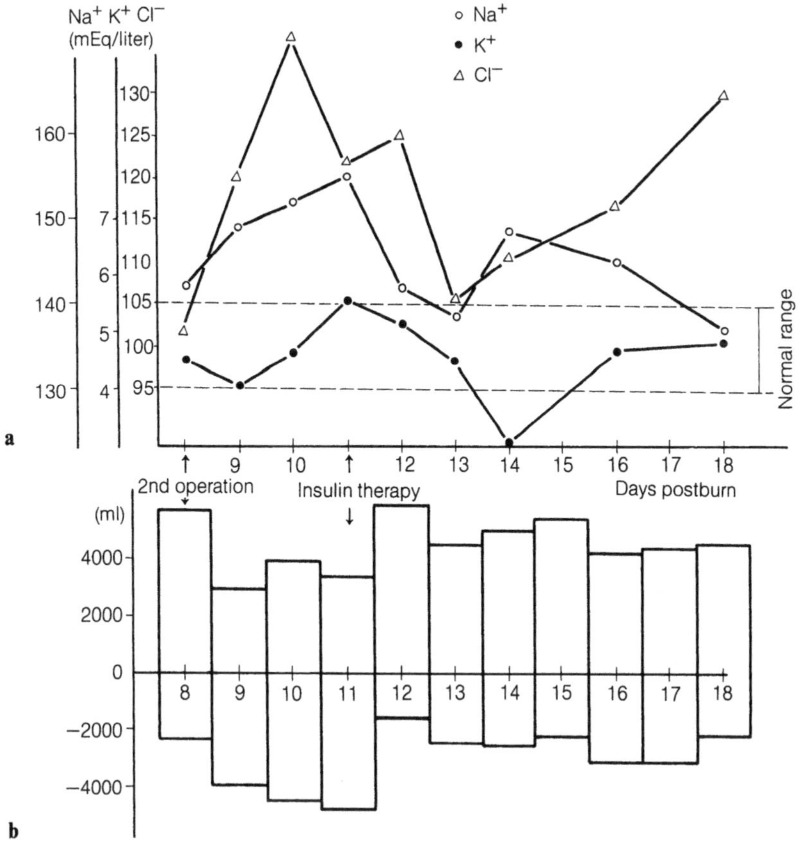

Fig. VI.3. Hypernatremia induced by uncontrolled diabetes in a patient with burns to 95% of the BSA, including third degree burns to 85%. Changes in **a** the levels of serium sodium, serum potassium, and serum chloride and **b** the water balance are shown

1.2.2.1 Sodium-Deficient Hyponatremia

Sodium-deficient hyonatremia is mainly due to insufficient intake or excessive loss of sodium. Sodium is chiefly lost through the kidneys and the gastrointestinal tract. Among patients with extensive burns, loss of sodium through the kidneys is more often observed (so-called sodium-losing nephritis). As it is frequently accompanied by the loss of a large quantity of potassium, it is also called salt-losing nephritis.

When the ability of the renal tubules to reabsorb sodium is impaired and there is an increase in the amount of urine and solutes passing through the renal tubules, sodium is still continuously being excreted by the kidneys even though at that time the level of sodium in the body fluids is lower than normal. Salt-losing nephritis is not a specific disease; it is the term applied to any renal tubular lesion which results in salt loss. It is mostly seen in patients with severe systemic infection, after long-term administration of aminoglycosides or polymyxins, or in the polyuric phase of acute renal failure.

During severe salt-losing nephritis, the daily amount of sodium excreted by the kidneys may be as much as 400–700 mEq. After antibiotics such as polymyxin and gentamicin are injected over a comparatively long time, daily excretion of sodium by the kidneys may reach 200–300 mEq (equal to 12 g–18 g sodium chloride). In patients with extensive burns an oral dose of 6 g sodium chloride should be administered routinely in order to make up such losses. Since 10 g sodium chloride are present in the diet, the daily intake is about 16 g. When oral intake is difficult, the patient should be given 1–2 liters of physiologic saline every day by intravenous infusion.

Case Illustration. Male, aged 55. The patient had burns to 91% of the BSA, including third degree burns to 11%. No past history of chronic illness was given upon inquiry. On the 4th day after injury, hemoconcentration with leftward shifting of Schilling's count appeared and infection of the wound was aggravated. Therefore systemic polymyxin B and kanamycin were administered. On the next day, *Proteus vulgaris* was found in the blood culture. On the 7th day fulminative infection of the wound caused progressive necrosis of the deeper tissue. At the same time, high fever, chills, raving, abdominal distention, and diarrhea developed. The serum sodium level on the 6th day following injury was 110 mEq/liter, and on the 7th, when the patient became irritable and disorientated, it was 94 mEq/liter. Urinary sodium excretion on the same day was still 99 mEq/liter (24-h total 118 mEq). Apart from the infusion of 835 mEq sodium in the first 2 days after injury, the patient received no salt, yet large amounts of sodium salt were lost continuously through the kidneys, and severe hyponatremia appeared. Therefore on the 7th day postburn 25 g sodium chloride were supplemented in the form of hypertonic solution. On each of the following days, 15 g were given, and at the same time the intake of water was limited. Urinary output increased significantly (from 1,000 ml–2,000 ml to 4,000 ml per day). Hyponatremia was thus rectified (Fig. VI.4), and the patient survived.

1.2.2.2 Dilutional Hyponatremia and Water Intoxication

Aside from the effect of intake of excessive water, hypersecretion of antidiuretic hormone or lesions of the kidneys per se may cause disturbances of renal function. Overhydration is more often seen in children, owing to the supplement of large quantities of water at a time when blood volume is decreased. When extracellular fluid volume decreases, the kidneys will still retain a large amount of water in spite of hypotonicity of the body fluid. That is to say, whenever blood volume is deficient the kidney will retain water rather than excrete it, even though the serum sodium level is lower than normal. In such a condition, the level of serum potassium may be normal or slightly lower than normal.

The rate of passage of sodium through the blood-brain barrier is very slow. If osmotic pressure of the body fluids drops suddenly and rapidly, water will be quickly transferred into the brain tissue, causing edema of the brain. Coma and convulsion may supervene. When the edema is severe, the patient may die. In patients with extensive burns, there is hypersecretion of antidiuretic

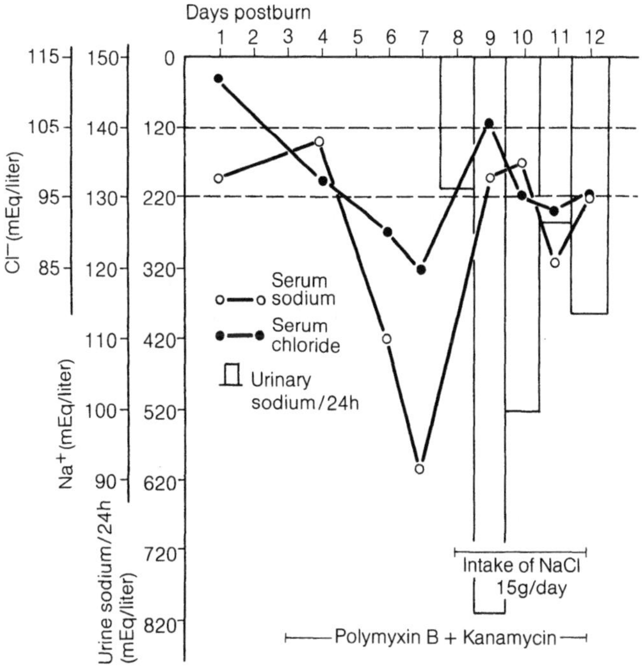

Fig. VI.4. Hyponatremia due to salt-losing nephritis in a patient with burns to 91% of the BSA, including third degree burns to 11%. Changes in the levels of serum sodium, serum chloride, and urinary sodium are shown

hormone during the shock stage. If, at that time, the blood volume of the patient is not adequate, he will be very thirsty and request water. Under such circumstances to administer water orally or glucose solution intravenously in an unlimited quantity would result in water intoxication.

In the treatment of water intoxication, one should first correct hypovolemia and then administer such solute diuretic agents as mannitol and sorbitol. If definite symptoms of central nervous system disorders appear or the serum sodium level is below 120 mEq/liter, 2.5%–5% NaCl solution may be infused (hypertonic salt solution per se is also a kind of solute diuretic agent; when sodium chloride is excreted by the kidneys, it will carry water with it).

Intravenous injection of glucocorticoid hormone can increase the glomeruli filtration rate as well as lessen the osmotic effect of the distal convoluted tubules, thereby promoting excretion of water from the kidneys. If convulsion occurs, barbitals should be given. Among the barbiturates, amobarbital sodium is the drug of choice. In children, the first injection of 5 mg/kg may be given intravenously. After that, a maintenance dose of phenobarbital 5 mg/kg at 4 h–6 h intervals should be given.

Case Illustration. Male, aged 10. The patient had second degree burns to 31% of the BSA. Within 20 h after injury, 5% glucose 2,000 ml, physiologic saline 500 ml, and low molecular weight dextran 500 ml were given intravenously. At that time, urine output was low, and the quantity was not recorded. Convulsion occurred 17 h postburn. The child was transferred to our hospital 20 h postburn, at which time he was very irritable. Pulsation of the dorsal artery of the foot was weak, and the pulse rate was 120–160/min. Twenty-two hours after injury the patient again went into a coma with intermittent cessation of respiration and cyanosis due to convulsions. Serum sodium was 106 mEq/liter; serum chloride, 76 mEq/liter; serum potassium, 4.2 mEq/liter; and carbon dioxide combining power, 17 mEq/liter. Based upon the above-stated principles for the treatment of water intoxication, phenobarbital was injected 22 h postburn to control convulsions, and, at the same time, 200 ml whole blood, 100 ml plasma, 50 mg hydrocortisone, and 200 ml 2.5% sodium chloride were infused in that order. After the use of these measures, urine output gradually increased (24-h urine amounted to 1,370 ml, with an intake of 1,300 ml water). Serum

Day

	0	1	2	3
5% glucose	2000ml		750ml	160ml
10% glucose			250ml	1000ml
LMD	500ml			
PS	500ml	150ml	200ml	500ml
2.5% saline			200ml	
Blood or plasma		200ml	250ml	100ml

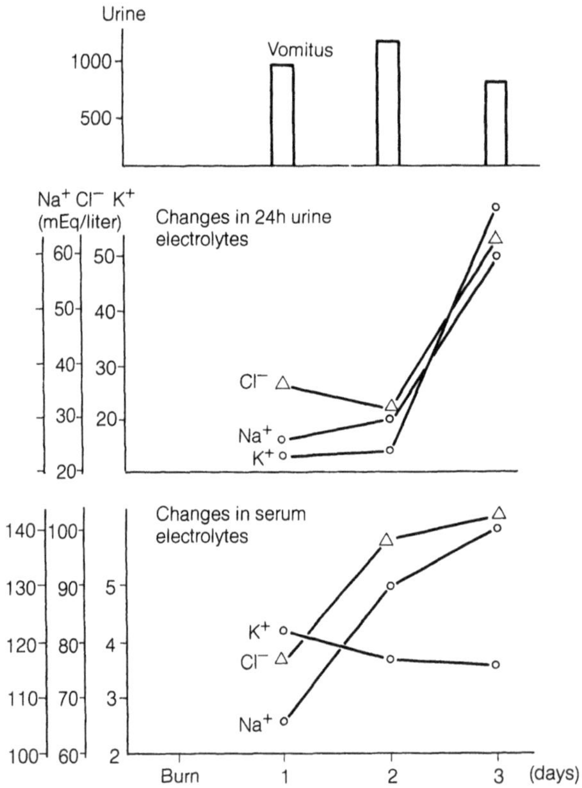

Fig. VI.5. Water intoxication in a 10-year-old boy with second degree burns to 31% of the BSA. *PS*, physiologic saline; *LMD*, low molecular weight dextran

electrolytes recovered to normal levels 32 h after injury. Urinary sodium increased from 26 mEq/liter on admission to 60 mEq/liter (Fig. VI.5), and the patient survived.

1.2.2.3 Hyponatremia During the Shock Stage After Extensive Burns

During the shock stage after extensive burns, urine output is sharply decreased; and both water and sodium are retained. Sodium enters the cells, especially those of the burned tissues, thereby causing lowering of the level of extracellular sodium (to 115–125 mEq/liter). However, due to the fact that hemoconcentration, retention of sodium, and enhanced potassium excretion take place after severe burns, serum sodium may be within the normal range, while the level of serum potassium may be normal or lower than normal. If the serum sodium level is less than 120 mEq/liter with symptoms of hyponatremia, hypertonic salt solution should be given (for adults, 200 ml–300 ml 2.5%–3% NaCl solution). After extensive burns, hemoconcentration and sodium retention with potassium excretion will generally begin to reverse on the 4th day postburn, yet excretion of sodium retained in the body will not be completed until the 7th–10th day.

Case Illustration. Female, aged 33. The patient had burns to 82% of the BSA, including third degree burns to 60%. Until 5 days postburn, the amounts of both urinary sodium and potassium excretion were low (Fig. VI.6). Beginning from the 5th day postburn, urinary excretion of sodium increased, and, owing

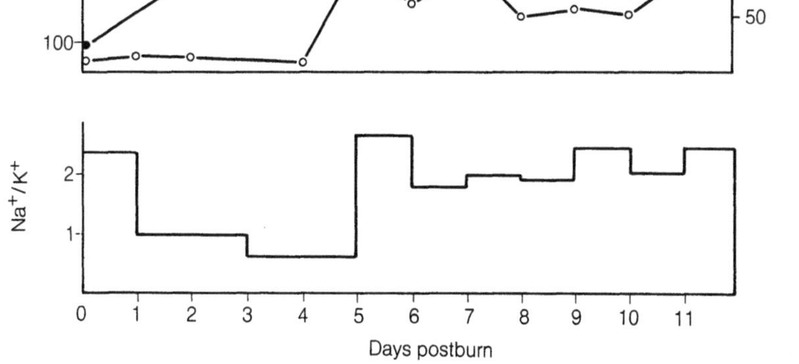

Fig. VI.6. Hyponatremia during the shock stage in a patient with burns to 82% of the BSA, including third degree burns to 60%. Changes in the levels of urinary sodium and potassium as well as in the ratio between them are shown

to the increase of urine output, urinary excretion of potassium was also increased. Although there was a good deal of sodium retention in the first 5 days after injury, serum sodium was at a comparatively low level (125–130 mEq/liter). Since no symptoms of hyponatremia appeared, no treatment was employed, and the patient survived.

1.3 Potassium Balance

The quantity of potassium loss from patients with extensive burns is very large. When estimating the amount to be supplemented, loss of potassium from the wound surface should be considered as well as potassium excreted in the urine.

After shock has passed, one should begin to supplement potassium salts if the level of serum potassium is not high and the daily urine output exceeds 1,000 ml. Our routine program of treatment is: oral administration of 3 g potassium chloride or potassium citrate and intravenous administration of 6 g potassium chloride, giving a total of 120 mEq potassium daily. If there is nausea, vomiting, diarrhea, or increase of urinary excretion of potassium, the intake of potassium should be suitably increased.

In adults, a reduction in the level of serum potassium by 1 mEq/liter means that there is already a potassium loss of 100–200 mEq. Since most potassium ions are intracellularly located and time is needed for potassium to enter the cells, the rate of supplementation of potassium should not be rapid, and in every 1,000 ml solution, the content of potassium ions should not exceed 40 mEq. The rate of infusion should be about 40 drops per minute. In adults, infusion of 40 mEq potassium may immediately increase the level of potassium in the serum by 2 mEq/liter. After the potassium ions have entered the cells, the level of serum potassium will drop again. If the serum potassium level is lower than 3 mEq/liter, in order to raise the level by 1 mEq/liter it is necessary to supplement 200–400 mEq potassium, given in divided doses over a period of several days.

Potassium chloride is irritating to the gastrointestinal mucosa and sometimes needs to be substituted by potassium citrate (1 g potassium chloride contains 13.4 mEq potassium, while 1 g potassium citrate contains 10 mEq potassium). Potassium glutamate may be used when potassium needs to be supplemented intravenously in patients with elevated serum chlorides (1 g potassium glutamate contains 5.4 mEq potassium).

Several days are needed for the adjustment of potassium, regardless of whether it is given orally or intravenously. For patients with potassium deficit associated with low serum calcium, symptoms of the latter may often be masked by those of the former. If low serum calcium is not corrected at the same time as low serum potassium, tetany due to low blood calcium may result.

1.3.1 Hypokalemia

When the serum potassium level is lower than 3.5 mEq/liter, clinically it may manifest itself as anorexia, abdominal distention, palpitation, apathy, general weakness, and reduction or even loss of tendon reflex. During severe acute hypokalemia, coma, muscular paralysis, and even respiratory collapse may appear. In such instances we observed on EKGs an increase in amplitude of the P wave, Lengthening of the Q-U interval, depression of the S-T segment, and inversion of the T wave. There was a prominent U wave. In advanced cases premature beats may progress to lethal ventricular tachycardia.

Case Illustration. Male, aged 24. The patient had burns to 12% of the BSA, including third degree burns to 7%. The wound healed 34 days after injury, but high fever persisted and was accompanied by vomiting, diarrhea, and abdominal distention. Routine blood and bone marrow smear examinations revealed signs of infection. The patient was then treated with polymyxin and other antibiotics, but supplement with potassium was neglected. On the 38th postburn day, serum electrolyte levels were determined, with the following results: sodium, 125 mEq/liter; chloride, 85 mEq/liter; potassium, 2 mEq/liter. The patient was in a coma with dyspnea, cyanosis, dilatation of pupils, and loss of light reflex. Emergency intubation was performed, and artificial respiration applied immediately. Within 5 h after intravenous infusion of 8 g potassium chloride (107.2 mEq), the serum potassium level was 1.9 mEq/liter and carbon dioxide combining power was 5 mEq/liter. Within the next 2 h, 2 g potassium chloride and 5 g sodium bicarbonate were infused. The patient gradually became conscious. He coughed frequently and could not bear the intubation. Although dyspnea was still present, intubation and the assistance of respiration were abandoned. On the 39th postburn day, 13 g potassium chloride were infused intravenously. At the same time, 11 g potassium citrate (K^+ totals to 284 mEq) and 15 g sodium bicarbonate (bicarbonate 180 mEq) were given by nasal feeding. The serum potassium level then rose to 3 mEq/liter and carbon dioxide combining power rose to 31 mEq/liter. Respiration recovered to normal 40 days after injury. Between 100 and 200 mEq potassium were administered intravenously and orally every day for 1 month. The patient survived.

The above case demonstrates that hypokalemic alkalosis does not necessarily appear in chronic potassium deficiency. But when the patient's general condition deteriorates and acute deficit of potassium occurs, complications related to metabolic acidosis may appear instead, and adjustment of both potassium deficiency and metabolic acidosis must be carried out.

1.3.2 Hyperkalemia

Hyperkalemia may be defined as a serum potassium level of more than 5.6 mEq/liter. When this level is reached, clinical symptoms which denote the toxic effect of potassium ions on the myocardium and striated muscles will appear. Acidosis often aggravates the injurious effect of hyperkalemia on the myocardium; thereby evident clinical symptoms may be produced at an early stage. Alkalosis, on the other hand, may mask the symptoms of hyperkalemia and confuse the changes appearing on the EKG. The clinical signs and symptoms of hyperkalemia include slow pulse, extreme tiredness, muscle pain, clammy extremities, pallor, even sudden cardiac arrest. Timely, complete adjustment is very necessary.

Electrocardiography reveals an increase in amplitude of the T wave and a narrowing of its base. In serious cases, a low and wide P wave appears or it is even lost; at the same time widening of the ventricular complex with low R and deep S and slowing of the ventricular rate may be shown. Finally the heart ceases to function.

Hyperkalemia is often accompanied by acidosis. Emergency treatment should include correction of acidosis besides intravenous infusion of glucose and insulin solution (i.e., GI solution: to every 5 g glucose, one unit of regular insulin is added; routine dosage is 500 ml 25% GI solution or 1,000 ml–2,000 ml 10% GI solution). In extensive burns catabolism is usually greatly enhanced, and after renal failure, the serum potassium level may rise very rapidly. Therefore, dialysis should be carried out immediately whenever the serum potassium level is above 6 mEq/liter.

In order to promote reabsorption of edema in extensively burned patients after the shock stage, we used to administer spironolactone on the 4th day after burn. However, since spironolactone causes retention of large quantities

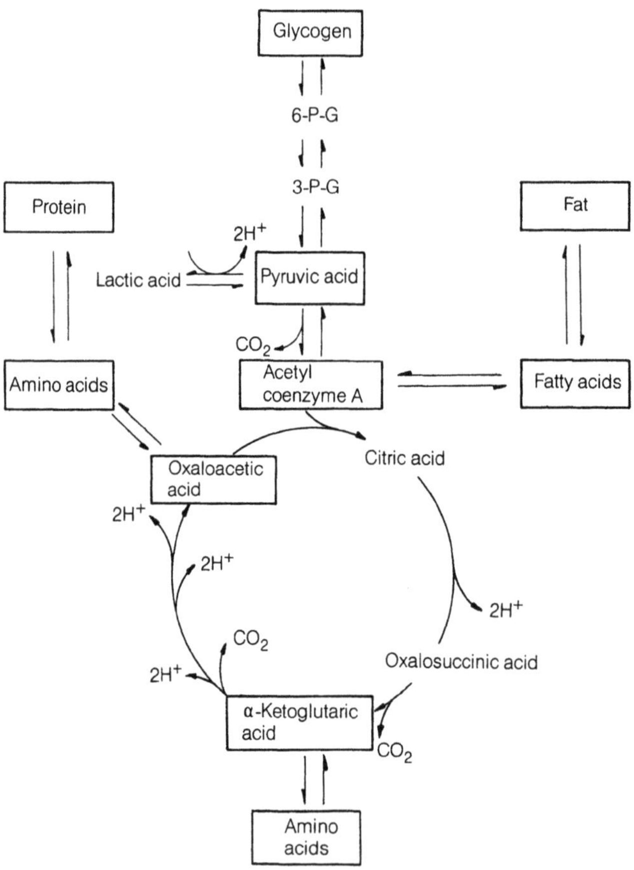

Fig. VI.7. Aerobic degradation of biologic substrates

of potassium and elimination of large amounts of sodium, certain patients developed hyponatremia and hyperkalemia. Consequently we have more recently been using dihydrochlorothiazide, 25 mg t.i.d., and triamterene, 50 mg t.i.d. (these two drugs are not used in combination for more than 5 days in order to prevent the development of hyperkalemia).

2 Acid-Base Balance

2.1 Introduction

2.1.1 Biologic Oxidation and Hydrogen Ions

Under normal conditions, the energy required for the survival of a human being depends upon the aerobic degradation of biologic substrates, such as carbohydrates, proteins, and fats. During the process of oxidation of these substrates, hydrogen ions, carbon dioxide, and other acid substances are released (Fig. VI.7).

After extensive burns, shock, infection, etc. may all cause disturbances of the Krebs' cycle as well as incomplete degradation of sugar, fat, and protein. The products of incomplete degradation, such as lactic acid, pyruvic acid, and ketone, are all acidic in nature, and when they become accumulated in the body, metabolic acidosis will result. For example:

$$\text{glucose} \rightleftharpoons 2\ \text{lactic acid}^- + 2\,H^+$$

$$\text{methionine} \xrightarrow{O_2} \text{urea} + CO_2 + H_2O + SO_4^{2-} + 2\,H^+$$

$$1/4\ \text{palmitate} \xrightarrow{O_2} 2\ \text{acetyl coenzyme A} + 2\,H^+$$

$$\updownarrows$$

$$\text{acetoacetic acid} + H^+$$

$$\downarrow O_2$$

$$CO_2 + H_2O$$

2.1.2 Pulmonary and Renal Compensation and Buffer Systems

The acids produced by degradation of substrates may be divided into two major groups:

1. Volatile acid: carbonic acid
2. Nonvolatile acids:

i) which may be further metabolized, i.e., lactic acid, pyruvic acid, acetoacetic acid, ketone bodies, etc.;

ii) which may not be further metabolized, i.e., acid phosphate, acid sulfate, etc.

2.1.2.1 Lungs

Volatile acids are mainly expelled by the lungs. Carbon dioxide produced by degraded substances is carried off by the blood and is expelled through the lungs. If the expulsion of carbon dioxide from the lungs is impeded, such as in cases of constrictive torso eschars, in the shock stage in children with burns of the head, face, and chest, and in patients with burns of the lower respiratory tract, accumulation of CO_2 causes the following reaction to proceed from left to right. Thereby, the hydrogen ions and bicarbonate ions are increased, resulting in respiratory acidosis. If the reaction is reversed, respiratory alkalosis will be the result.

$$CO_2 + H_2O \rightleftharpoons H_2CO_3 \rightleftharpoons H^+ + HCO_3^-$$

$$NaHCO_3 \rightleftharpoons Na^+ + HCO_3^-$$

The daily amount of carbon dioxide expelled by the human lungs is about 15,000 mEq. During functional disturbances of respiration, hydrogen ions may accumulate in the body at a rate of 10 mEq/min. If respiration is inhibited for only 30 min, blood pH will drop to below 7.0, and severe acidosis will be caused. The correction of respiratory acidosis depends mainly upon the improvement of ventilation and ventilative function, not upon the use of alkali.

Increase in arterial pCO_2 or excess of H^+ in the blood can stimulate directly the chemoreceptors of the respiratory center or indirectly through the carotid and aortic bodies, causing hyperpnea, and carbon dioxide will be quickly expelled. But if pCO_2 rises to above 65 mmHg, the respiratory center will be inhibited instead. The latter condition is called CO_2 narcosis.

2.1.2.2 Kidneys

When incomplete degradation of substrates is caused by shock and severe infection, the result is accumulation of mainly nonvolatile acids which may be further metabolized, e.g., lactic acid, pyruvic acid, acetoacetic acid, and ketone bodies. When shock is satisfactorily treated and severe infection controlled, the above-mentioned substances may be further metabolized to form carbon dioxide and water. Those nonvolatile acids which cannot be further metabolized are the degradation products of proteins and fats. These are excreted by the kidneys. Under normal conditions the amount excreted is about 50–75 mEq daily, of which 75% is excreted in the urine in the form of NH_4^+. When acidosis is severe, the amount of NH_4^+ excreted by the kidneys may even reach 700 mEq daily (10 times the normal value of hydrogen ions in the urine). According to our determinations, in the shock stage in extensively burned patients, the amount of hydrogen ions expelled by the renal tubules is decreased to only twice the normal value excreted in the urine. Incomplete degradation of substrates and the small number of hydrogen ions *expelled* by the kidneys are the cause of metabolic acidosis in the shock stage in extensively burned patients.

2.1.2.3 Buffer System

Besides the lungs and kidneys, the buffer system in the body fluids is an important means for the maintenance of acid-base balance in the human body. That is to say, at the time when changes of hydrogen ion concentrations take place, the buffer system is an important means for the maintenance of pH at a constant value. In the human body, the quantity of buffers is about 1,000 mEq. Among the nine buffer pairs, there are two principal pairs, namely, $H_2CO_3/B \cdot HCO_3$ and $H \cdot Hb/B \cdot Hb$. The former occupies 30%–35% of buffer capacity of the whole body, and the latter, about 20%. Due to the fact that red blood cells circulate all over the body, their oxidation-reduction process goes on perpetually; therefore their buffer capacity is very large. Consequently, after extensive burns, maintaining the hemoglobin level at above 12 g/100 ml will play a very important role in the maintenance of acid-base balance.

2.2 Symbols and Terms of Importance in the Expression of Acid-Base Changes

1. *pH* is the expression of hydrogen ion concentration $[H]^+$ and numerically it is equal to the negative logarithm of the hydrogen ion concentration expressed in moles per liter of solution. Normal plasma pH is 7.35 to 7.42, but that of children is lower than that of adults (normal pH of children is 7.32). pH of venous blood is slightly higher than that of arterial blood, but the difference is very small.

2. pCO_2 is the symbol for CO_2 partial pressure or tension. Plasma pCO_2 and pCO_2 in the lung alveoli are usually balanced. Maintenance of normal value is dependent upon the CO_2 exhaled during respiration. If respiration becomes deeper and its rate increases, pCO_2 is lowered owing to the expulsion of large quantities of CO_2. If disturbances of ventilation or ventilative function occur, CO_2 will be accumulated and pCO_2 is thereby increased. The normal value in men is 36 mmHg–44 mmHg, but it is somewhat lower in children and women (the normal pCO_2 value in children is 37 mmHg).

3. CO_2cp is the symbol for carbon dioxide combining power. When lactic acid is added into the plasma, CO_2 is released from HCO_3^-; determination of the volume of this released CO_2 denotes carbon dioxide combining power. In some laboratories the calculation unit of CO_2cp is volume percent, which can be converted into milliequivalents per liter by the following method:

$$CO_2cp = \text{vol.}\% \div 2.24 = \text{mEq/liter}$$

Normal value of CO_2cp is 22–28 mEq/liter

4. Standard bicarbonate is the content of HCO_3^- in the plasma under standard physical and chemical conditions. When the blood temperature is 38 °C, pCO_2 is 40 mmHg, and there is 100% oxygen saturation of hemoglobin, the normal value of standard bicarbonate is 21–27 mEq/liter. In the majority of adults it is about 24 mEq/liter, in children, 21 mEq/liter.

5. *Base excess or base deficit* denotes the amount of alkali or acid required to titrate the plasma to pH 7.40 under the following conditions: pCO_2,

40 mmHg; blood temperature, 38 °C; and 100% oxygen saturation of hemoglobin. A positive value means base excess, while a negative value means base deficit. Since pCO_2 of the specimen has been adjusted to 40 mmHg before the determination, and the changes of the level of blood HCO_3^- due to respiratory compensation are thus excluded, the condition of metabolic acid-base disturbances in the body is more accurately reflected. The normal value is 3 to −3 mEq/liter in adults and, 0 to −4 mEq/liter in children.

6. *Buffer base* includes the total base of all the buffer pairs. The main components are HCO_3^-, 26 mEq/liter; protein, 8 mEq/liter; and hemoglobin, 15 mEq/liter. The normal value is 45 mEq/liter–50 mEq/liter; the children's normal value is 45 mEq/liter. There is no relationship between buffer base value and pCO_2 or pO_2; therefore the value of venous and arterial blood is the same. If, on determination, it is found that the content of bicarbonate is normal, while buffer base is low, it shows that both plasma protein and hemoglobin levels are low. Supplementation of protein and whole blood is therefore needed to increase the amount of alkali reserve.

2.3 Signs and Symptoms of Acid-Base Imbalance

1. *Acidosis* ($pH < 7.2$): Constriction of peripheral vessels, cherry-red lips, weakness, somnolence, headache, nausea, vomiting, oliguria, sweating, papillary edema of optic nerves, disorientation and even coma, and deep and strong respiration.

2. *Alkalosis* ($pH > 7.5$): dilatation of peripheral vessels, headache, nausea, paresthesia, spasm of limbs, and feeble respiration.

2.4 Methods of Calculation

The extracellular fluids amount to about 23% of the body weight. The infused fluids, besides being uniformly distributed in the extracellular fluids, are partly excreted in the urine or eliminated from the body in the form of insensible water loss, and partly enter into the cells. Therefore, we usually assume extracellular-fluids to account for 30% of the body weight for the purposes of our calculations.

$0.3 \times$ body weight (kg) $\times$ (normal CO_2cp mEq/liter − CO_2cp mEq/liter determined) = the base deficit expressed in milliequivalents,
or $0.3 \times$ body weight (kg) $\times$ [mEq/liter base deficit (negative number) + 3 mEq/liter] = the base deficit expressed in milliequivalents,
or $0.3 \times$ body weight (kg) $\times$ (mEq/liter of normal standard bicarbonate − mEq/liter of standard bicarbonate determined) = the base deficit expressed in milliequivalents.
(When alkalosis is concerned, the value determined minus the normal value is the base excess expressed in milliequivalents.)

Clinically, the first administration should be between one-half and one-third of the quantity obtained by calculation and subsequent treatment ought to be decided according to clinical manifestations and laboratory results.

Example 1: The patient's weight is 70 kg. When metabolic acidosis appears clinically, the CO_2cp determined is 22 vol.%, i.e., 10 mEq/liter (22÷2.2):

$$0.3 \times 70 \times (22 \text{ mEq/liter} - 10 \text{ mEq/liter}) = 252 \text{ mEq base deficit}$$

Therefore, the amount of sodium bicarbonate to be supplemented is 252÷12=21 g (each gram of sodium bicarbonate contains 12 mEq HCO_3^-); alternatively, one might supplement 252 ml 11.2% sodium lactate solution (each milliliter of which equals 1 mEq HCO_3^-). The first injection should be one-half of the calculated quantity, i.e., 10.5 g sodium bicarbonate or 120 ml 11.2% sodium lactate solution.

Example 2: The patient's weight is 70 kg. When metabolic alkalosis appears clinically, the standard bicarbonate determined is 32 mEq/liter:

$$0.3 \times 70 \times (32 \text{ mEq/liter} - 27 \text{ mEq/liter}) = 105 \text{ mEq base excess}$$

Since 1 mEq H^+ equivalent to 6 ml 0.9% ammonium chloride solution, the amount to be supplemented is $105 \times 6 = 630$ ml. The first injection should be one-half of the calculated quantity, i.e., 315 ml 0.9% ammonium chloride.

Example 3: The body weight of the patient is 70 kg, the serum sodium determined is 150 mEq/liter, and base deficit is −10 mEq/liter. In such a case, THAM should be chosen for the adjustment of acidosis. Since THAM may be evenly distributed both in the intracellular and extracellular fluids, and the total amount of intracellular and extracellular fluids is 55% of the body weight, we usually calculate with 60% of the body weight. In this case:

$$0.6 \times 70 \times (-10 \text{ mEq/liter} + 3 \text{ mEq/liter}) = -294 \text{ mEq base deficit}$$

Since 1 mEq HCO_3^- equivalent to 3.3 ml 3.6% THAM, the amount of 3.6% THAM supplement is 294×3.3 ml=970 ml. For the first injection, the amount should be one-third of the calculated quantity, i.e., 320 ml.

2.5 Frequently Used Solutions

2.5.1 Sodium Bicarbonate Solution

For acute metabolic acidosis which is not accompanied by dehydration, infusion of 2.5% or 5% sodium bicarbonate solution (1.25% is approximately isotonic) is often employed. The principle of adjustment of metabolic acisosis is:

$$NaHCO_3 \rightleftharpoons Na^+ + HCO_3^-$$

$$\updownarrow$$

$$HCO_3^- + H^+ \rightleftharpoons H_2CO_3 \rightleftharpoons H_2O + CO_2\uparrow$$

HCO_3^- combines with H^+ to form H_2O and CO_2, sodium is retained in the body, CO_2 is expelled from the lungs, the H^+ level in the body fluids is thus lowered, and acidosis is corrected.

2.5.2 Sodium Lactate Solution

11.2% (1 *M*) solution is given, 1.8% (1/6 *M*) solution being isotonic.

$$NaC_3H_5O_3 \rightarrow Na^+ + C_3H_5O_3^-$$

$$\downarrow$$

$$C_3H_5O_3^- + H^+ \rightarrow C_3H_6O_3$$

Lactic acid ($C_3H_6O_3$) is either synthesized to form glycogen in the liver or undergoes aerobic degradation to form CO_2 and H_2O with release of energy. Since either forming of glycogen or the degrading reaction must proceed under aerobic conditions, sodium bicarbonate solution should be chosen in shock, anoxia, hepatic disease, and cardiac failure.

2.5.3 Sodium Lactate–Physiologic Saline or Sodium Bicarbonate–Physiologic Saline Solution

In order to prevent infusion of too much chloride, a better method is the use of sodium lactate–physiologic saline or sodium bicarbonate–physiologic saline solution. With the exception of patients with alkalosis or impending alkalosis, to supplement electrolytes with one or the other solution mentioned above is the most suitable method to fulfil the physiologic requirement of the patient.

The best way to supplement potassium intravenously is to add 2–3 g potassium chloride into every 1,000 ml of fluid administered.

1/3 (1/6 *M* sodium lactate)+2/3 (physiologic saline) forms sodium lactate–physiologic saline solution. One thousand milliliters of this solution contains 159 mEq Na^+, 103 mEq Cl^-, and 56 mEq $C_3H_5O_3^-$.

1/3 (1.25% sodium bicarbonate)+2/3 (Physiologic saline) forms sodium bicarbonate–physiologic saline solution. One thousand milliliters of this solution contain 153 mEq Na^+, 103 mEq Cl^-, and 50 mEq HCO_3^-.

2.5.4 Tromethamine (THAM)

If acute respiratory or metabolic acidosis occurs in patients for whom supplement of sodium is contraindicated, THAM may be given.

1. Tromethamine can penetrate into the cells and conjugate with CO_2, causing a fall in intracellular pCO_2. It will slow down the increase of the intra- and extracellular H^+ concentration due to acute respiratory acidosis.

2. It can be rapidly excreted in the urine (50%–76% in 24 h) and has a diuretic effect.

3. It can conjugate with CO_2 and H^+ simultaneously and cause a rapid rise in blood pH.

4. It dose not contain any Na^+ and, as stated above, is suitable for patients for whom sodium is contraindicated.

Tromethamine may, however, induce hyperkalemia, hypocalcemia, hypoglycemia as well as a fall in pCO_2, and thus causes inhibition of respiration.

Table VI.3. The common solutions used for adjustment of acid-base disturbances

	Osmolality	Concentration (%)	Gram-molecular weight	g/liter	mEq/liters of HCO_3^- or Cl^-	Conversion factor 1 mEq–*x* ml
Sodium lactate	Isotonic	1.8	1/6	18.7	167	6
$NaC_3H_5O_3$	Hypertonic	11.2	1	112	1,000	1
Sodium bicarbonate	Isotonic	1.25	1/6	12.5	150	6.6
$NaHCO_3$	Hypertonic	2.5	1/3	25	300	3.3
	Hypertonic	5	2/3	50	600	1.66
Tris(hydroxyl-methyl)	Isotonic	3.6	0.3	36	300	3.3
amino-methane	Hypertonic	7.2	0.6	72	600	1.67
(THAM)						
$NH_2-C-(CH_2OH)_3$	Hypertonic	36	3	360	7,000	0.33
Ammonium chloride	Isotonic	0.9	1/6	9	168	6
NH_4Cl	Hypertonic	2		20	374	2.67

Therefore, when it is used for metabolic acidosis, the rate and concentration of the infusion should be carefully monitored in order to avoid sudden respiratory arrest.

2.5.5 Ammonium Chloride (NH_4Cl)

NH_4^+ is transformed into urea $[O=C-(NH)_2]$ in the liver. Urea is excreted through the kidneys, and the following reaction is encouraged to proceed from left to right. Since Cl^- and H^+ will form highly dissociable H^+Cl^-, alkalosis is corrected.

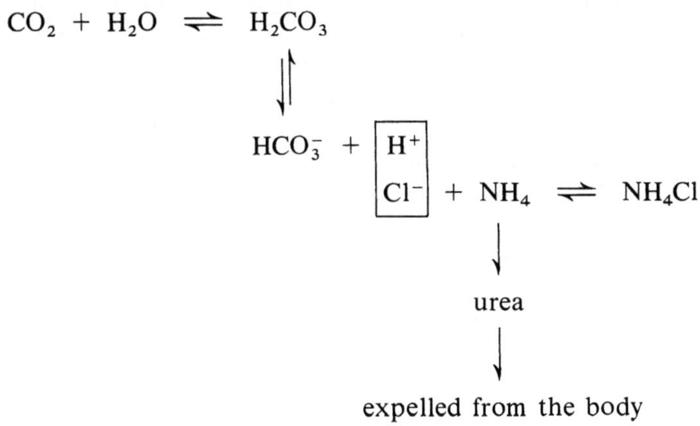

For calculations concerning supplementation of the above-mentioned solutions, see Table VI.3.

2.6 Frequent-Postburn Acid-Base Disturbances

2.6.1 Metabolic Acidosis

1. *Shock stage:* When the total burn surface area is more than 40% of the BSA or there are third degree burns to more than 10% (in children, a total burn surface of more than 10% of the BSA), metabolic acidosis may be induced owing to insufficient tissue perfusion within 24 h after injury with a tendency toward anaerobic degradation of the substrates and insufficient respiratory compensation. Forty-eight hours post burn, following improvement of tissue perfusion and increase of efficiency of respiratory compensation, acid-base levels in the blood gradually recover to normal. The degree of severity of metabolic acidosis during the shock stage is closely related to the extent of third degree burn. This is possibly due to the fact that in third degree burns there is a good deal of tissue destruction and shock is severe.

Figure VI.8 shows the acid-base changes (a) in adults with burns to an average of 42.6% of the BSA and third degree burns to an average of 20.8% and (b) in children with burns to an average of 42.5% of the BSA. Owing to the decrease of alkali reserve and deficiency of respiratory compensation, their pH values were lower than normal. Beginning from the second postburn day, their metabolic acidosis was gradually being compensated by respiration and at the same time alkali reserve also increased, and on the 4th day after injury their pH values recovered to the normal level. There was no evidence of acid-base disturbances in the shock stage in adults with burns to an average of 34.1% of the BSA and third degree burns to an average of 2.2% (Fig. VI.9).

If sodium bicarbonate–physiologic saline solution (i.e., 1/3 1.25% sodium bicarbonate solution + 2/3 physiologic saline) is used in adults with third degree burns to below 20% of the BSA, 0.75 ml electrolyte solution per kilogram body weight and per 1% BSA burned is administered on the 1st day postburn. On the 2nd day, only half of that amount is enough to compensate the alkali reserve lost on the 1st day. If there are third degree burns to more than 20% of the BSA in adults and 5% of the BSA in children, on the 1st day after injury the amount of sodium bicarbonate should be suitably increased [for adults, addition of 250 ml 5% sodium bicarbonate solution (containing 150 mEq bicarbonate ions)].

2. *Wound sepsis:* When the burn is complicated by wound sepsis, metabolic acidosis may occur. The amount of supplement should be calculated in accordance with the carbon dioxide combining power or standard bicarbonate determination.

3. Metabolic acidosis may also occur in patients with large burn surfaces *after Sulfamylon is used.* Sulfamylon (either hydrochloride or acetate) is absorbed from the wound surface and is transformed in the body into para-carboxyl-benzyl sulfonamide. Both Sulfamylon and para-carboxyl-benzyl sulfonamide can inhibit carboxyl anhydrase, and the bicarbonate radical excretion in the urine is thereby increased. The urine becomes alkaline with a loss of alkali reserve and metabolic acidosis is thus induced. Accumulation of hydrogen ions in the body plus the

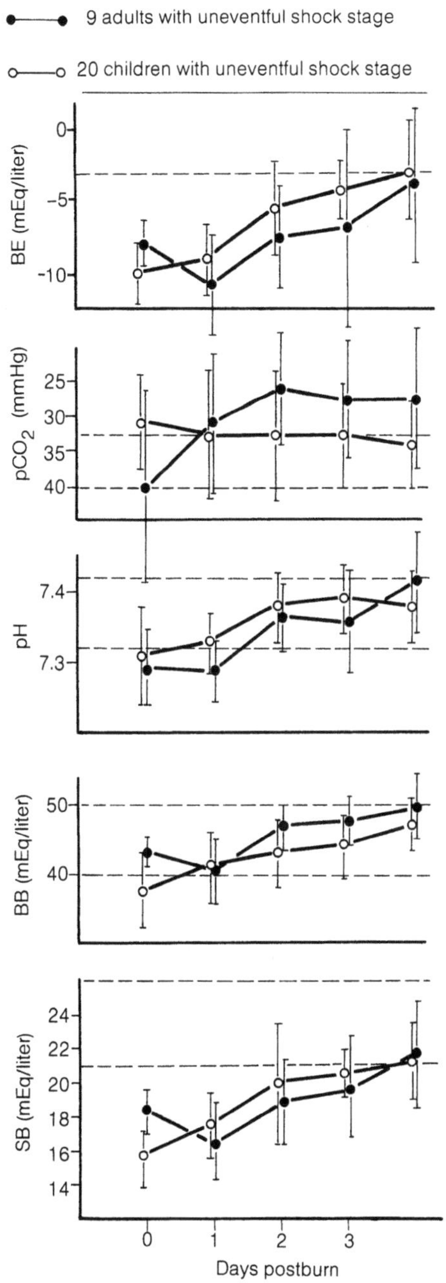

Fig. VI.8. Acid-base disturbances in adults (average BSA burned, 42.6%, with third degree burns to an average of 20.8%) and children (average BSA burned, 42.5%). *SB*, standard bicarbonate; *BB*, buffer base; *BE*, base excess

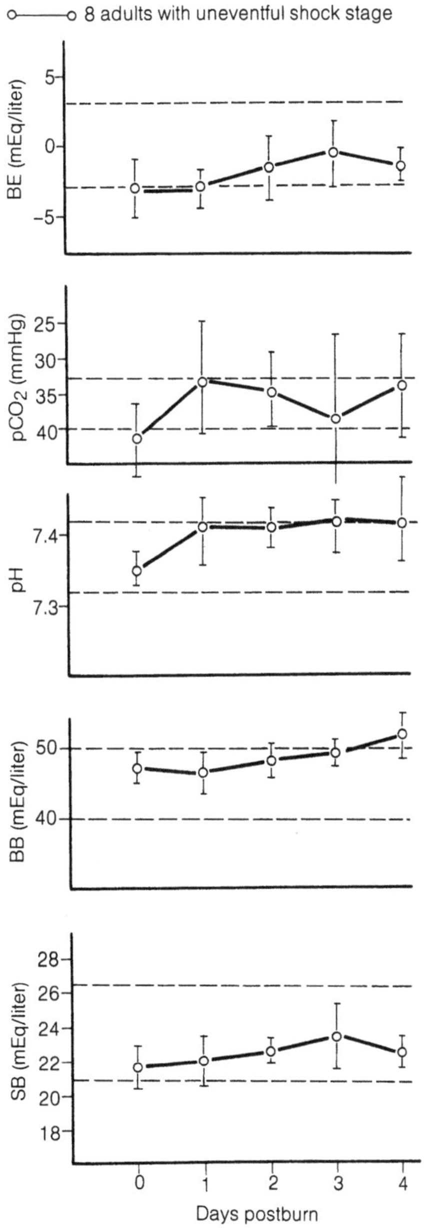

Fig. VI.9. Lack of evidence of acid-base disturbances during the shock stage in adults with burns to an average of 34.1% of the BSA and third degree burns to an average of 2.2%. Abbreviations as in Fig. VI.8

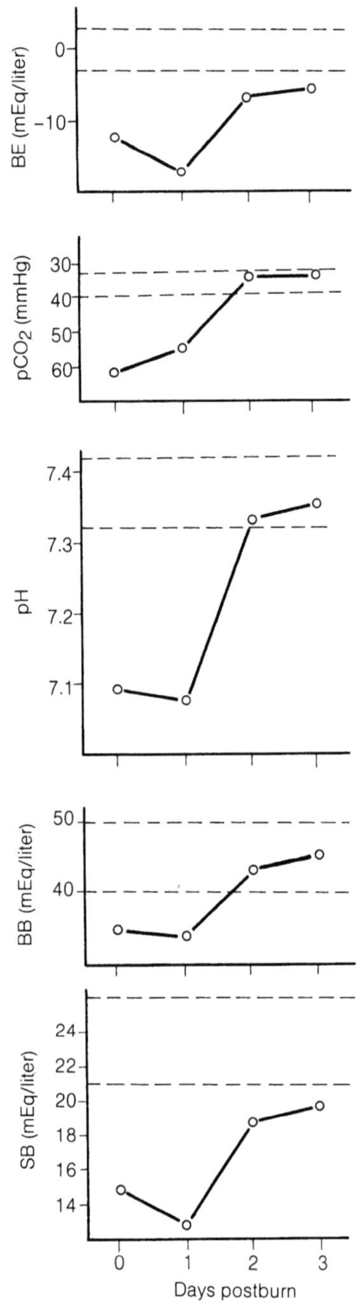

◁ **Fig. VI.10.** Combined metabolic and respiratory acidosis during the shock stage in a child (who survived). Abbreviations as in Fig. VI.8

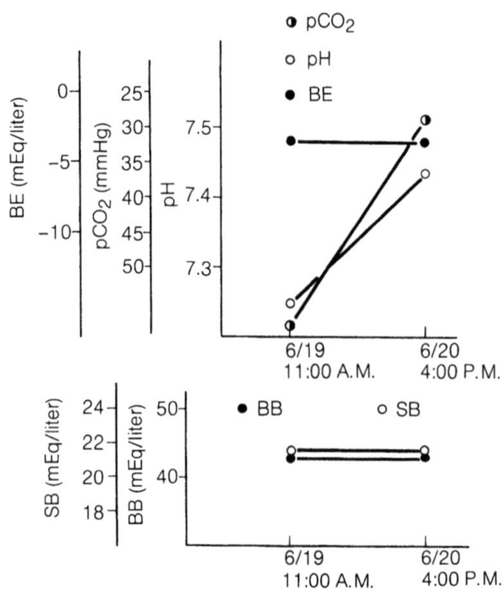

Fig. VI.11. Respiratory acidosis secondary to respiratory disturbance and paralytic ileus due to wound sepsis. Following control of wound sepsis, respiratory acidosis was corrected, and the patient survived. Abbreviations as in Fig. VI.8

inhibition of carboxyl anhydrase causes respiration to become deeper and more rapid. Symptoms of hyperventilation may appear clinically after the use of Sulfamylon for 1 h in patients with large burn surfaces. At that time, both carbon dioxide combining power and pCO_2 in the plasma will become lowered.

Sodium bicarbonate is supplemented intravenously in amounts in accordance with the laboratory reports. We usually supplement 250 ml 5% sodium bicarbonate for every 1,000 g 10% Sulfamylon cream used.

2.6.2 Respiratory Acidosis

Burns of the lower respiratory tract may cause ventilation and ventilative function disturbances, and pCO_2 may be increased to above 60 mmHg. In such a condition, at the same time as the accumulated exudation in the respiratory tract is being cleared, a respirator should be used to increase the amount of tidal air and the ratio between expiration and inspiration should be set to 2.5:1 or even 3:1 in order to expel CO_2 as quickly as possible. Hibernation–hypothermal therapy may be used in the shock stage when patients with minor burns have burns of the lower respiratory tract; oxygen consumption of the body is thus reduced, and accumulation of CO_2 in the body may also be diminished. If a burn of the respiratory tract becomes infected, disturbances of ventilation or ventilative function will be much more serious than those in the early period of injury, and the possibility of respiratory acidosis is also much greater.

During the early phase of the shock stage in children, peripheral vascular disturbances, cyanosis, lengthening of capillary refilling time, etc. often occur, and large quantities of CO_2 may be accumulated in the tissues. Therefore metabolic and respiratory acidosis may appear concurrently (Fig. VI.10).

Burn wound sepsis may also be the cause of central respiratory disturbances and paralytic ileus, effecting gaseous exchanges during respiration and causing respiratory acidosis (Fig. VI.II).

2.6.3 Acute Hypokalemic Alkalosis

In the cells, the content of K^+ ions is high while that of Na^+ is low. This phenomenon is mainly due to the expulsion of Na^+ and H^+ ions from the cell by the sodium pump. Extracellular K^+ ions enter the cells to maintain the osmotic balance. During acute potassium deficiency, intracellular K^+ ions are extruded while Na^+ and H^+ ions enter the cells. Therefore the concentration of the H^+ ions in the extracellular fluids is lowered, causing an increase in the pH value and alkalosis. When the K^+ ions in the renal tubular cells are decreased, while sodium–hydrogen exchanges are increased followed by the increase of urinary H^+ excretion, alkalosis is further aggravated. When the level of serum potassium ions is lowered and symptoms of alkalosis appear clinically, the only means of correction is to supplement potassium ions.

Case Illustration. Female, aged 26. A large area of skin on the patient's buttocks was necrotic. One and a half months after injury, anorexia, abdominal distention, palpitation, apathy, and weakness appeared. At that time, supplementation of potassium was neglected. Typical symptoms of alkalosis, such as extreme irritability, muscular spasms of face and limbs, and mental confusion, appeared within a few days. Serum potassium determination showed 1.41 mEq/liter. In 5 days a total of 744 mEq potassium was supplemented. Serum potassium then gradually recovered to the normal level, and symptoms of alkalosis disappeared (Fig. VI.12). The patient survived.

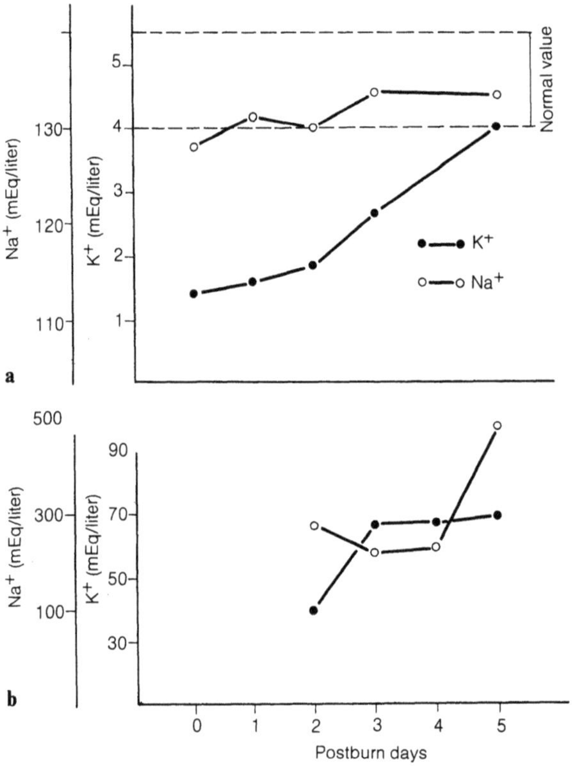

Fig. VI.12. Hypokalemia in a 26-year-old woman. Changes in the levels of **a** serum and **b** urinary sodium and potassium are shown

Chapter VII Burns of Special Sites

TANG SHEAN-SHII

Translated by LING LI-LI

Burns of special sites include burns of the head, face, eyes, ears, respiratory tract, hands, perineum, and bones. Since the anatomic and physiologic features of these parts differ from those of other parts of the body, burns with the same surface area and depth often run a more severe course and possess individual characteristics with regard to clinical manifestations and management. This chapter deals chiefly with the special features of clinical manifestations and management of burns of these sites.

1 Burns of the Head and Face

The head and face are sites of exposure and are easily burned. Very deep burns may involve the brain tissue, leading to cerebral edema, and are often associated with respiratory tract burns.

1.1 Characteristics

1. The subcutaneous tissue is loose and richly vascularized. Therefore exudation in the shock phase is greater than that in burns of other sites, and local edema is especially severe, usually reaching its maximum 48 h postburn (Fig. VII.1). The size of the head in second degree burns may swell enormously. In third degree burns, the external swelling may not be apparent owing to limitation of the local edema by the eschar, but the edema may spread inward, pressing on the upper respiratory passages or obstructing the pharyngolaryngeal region and leading to upper respiratory tract obstruction.

2. There is a rich nerve supply in this region. The severe edema appearing locally after burn is a strong stimulus to the body. Therefore, systemic reaction is particularly pronounced, and complications such as shock, acute gastric dilatation, high fever in the early stage, and cerebral edema frequently occur. These complications are especially common in children.

3. The eschar separates more quickly, and healing of the wound is more rapid: Healing in second degree burns of the head and face occurs 3–4 days earlier than in burns of the trunk and extremities, and separation of third degree eschar occurs 5–7 days earlier. In the hair-bearing areas, the hair follicles are deeply seated and part of them will remain even in deep burns. The epithelium

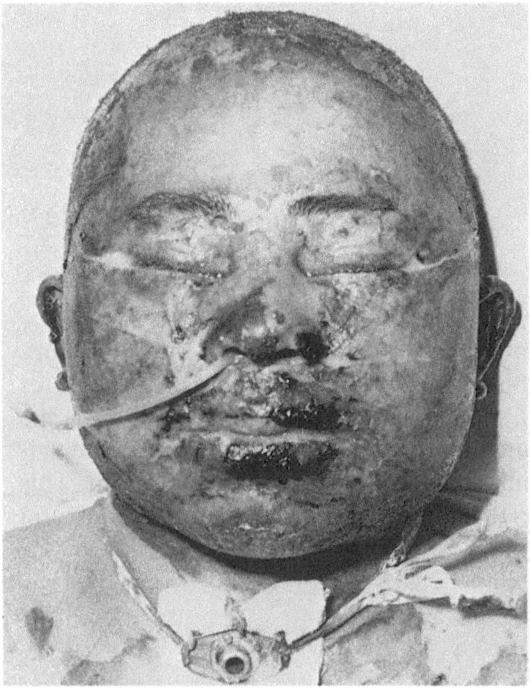

Fig. VII.1. Burns of the head and face. Edema reaches its maximum 48 h post-burn

spreads outward and covers the wound surface by itself; therefore skin grafting is not required.

4. Secretions from the orifices and food taken may contaminate the wound surface, causing infection around the orifices, especially the mouth, and leading to deepening of the wound, delay in healing, and marked cicatrization.

5. In deep second and third degree burns of the head and face, contracture due to scar formation often leads to such deformities as decrease in size of the mouth and nose and ectropion of the eyelids. The impairment of functions necessitates plastic surgery.

1.2 Problems Requiring Attention During Management in the Early Stage

1. Owing to the copious exudation in burns of the head and face, the amount of fluids that must be administered in the shock stage is greater than in burns of other sites. For burns of the head and face in children, the requirement for colloid and electrolyte solutions per kilogram body weight and per 1% of the BSA burned in the first 24 h usually exceeds 2 ml; half of the corresponding amount should be given in the second 24 h.

2. Severe local edema causes inconvenience in eating, and burns of the head and face often lead to such reactions as vomiting and acute gastric dilatation. Therefore it is better to let the patient fast during the 48 h immediately after injury.

3. Burns of the head and face may cause cerebral edema; therefore the supply of water should be limited, generally with a one-third to one-fourth reduction of the usual amount. It is especially important to pay attention to the sequential arrangement of fluid administration. The colloid and electrolyte solutions and water should be given alternately. One must not be given a large quantity of water parenterally or orally within a short period of time.

4. Reactive high fever and convulsions sometimes appear subsequent to burns of the head and face in children. The convulsions may be local, spread to the whole body, or involve the whole body from the very beginning. Besides prevention and treatment of shock, an appropriate anticonvulsant should be given. When blood volume is normal, artificial hibernation mixture may be used to reduce excessive reactions of the body. In order to stop convulsions rapidly, sodium amytal may be injected intravenously with good effect; appropriate amounts are 5 mg per kilogram body weight per dose for children and 0.5 g per dose for adults. This is followed by intramuscular injection of phenobarbital, 4–7 mg per kilogram body weight per dose for children and 0.2 g per dose for adults. Corticosteroids, e.g., hydrocortisone 100 mg or dexamethasone 5 mg may be used at the same time.

5. Burns of the head and face arouse an intense reaction with much exudation, and easily lead to shock and such complications as fever, cerebral edema, acute gastric dilatation, and convulsions in the early stage. The severe edema present in deep burns on the face and anterior part of neck may compress the trachea (upper respiratory tract), causing respiratory tract obstruction. Generally the patient, especially children, should be hospitalized for close observation. Even in second degree burns of a small surface area, death may ensue from neglectful observation or from improper management.

Case Illustration. Male, aged 15 months. A cup of hot water caused burns of the face, anterior neck, and chest. Six percent of the BSA was affected by superficial and deep second degree burns. The patient was brought to the emergency room 30 min after injury. Morphine 2.5 mg was given intramuscularly. After debridement of the wound, dressings were applied locally. Two hours after injury, the patient developed dyspnea followed by respiratory distress, cyanosis, and laryngeal stridor. Pulsation over the dorsal artery of the foot was very weak. Tracheotomy was performed immediately, and marked edema of the anterior part of the neck was found during operation. Cerebral edema, high fever, and convulsions appeared on the following day and the child died in spite of energetic treatment.

Case Illustration. Female, aged 17 months. The head, face, and neck were burned by hot water. Twelve percent of the BSA was affected by superficial and deep second degree burns. The patient was admitted 30 min after injury. The heart rate was 156/minute. Four hundred milliliters of oral electrolyte solution were given within 8 h. Intravenous fluids had not been given. The child was restless, and 13 h after injury she became very weak with coldness of the extremities and manifestations of shock. Fluids were given intravenously, but not fast enough. In spite of the administration of 100 ml each of blood and plasma, the blood volume could not be corrected efficiently, and shock persisted with progressive aggravation. The child died 14 h after injury.

It is apparent, therefore, that even in a second degree burn limited to the head and face (including the neck) fluid replacement in the stage of shock cannot depend entirely on oral administration. It is very important to give fluids intravenously. If signs of upper respiratory tract obstruction are found during the course of observation, tracheotomy should be performed immediately because of the rapid development of edema, which will lead to suffocation within a short time.

1.3 Local Management

1. One must first establish whether there are any burns of the respiratory tract (see Sect. VII.2).

2. Shave and expose the wound after debridement in the early stage. When the shock stage is over, generally on the 3rd day, elevate the head of the bed may accelerate the resorption of the edema.

3. Attention should be paid (i) to the prevention of secretions from the orifices and (ii) to the possible contamination, via food, of the exposed wound surface, which should be occasionally wiped with sterilized cotton balls or sticks. After eschar has been formed on the wound surface, it is important to examine frequently for any pus accumulation under the eschar. Purulent eschar should be removed as soon as possible.

4. Third degree eschar of the head and face should not be excised since it will separate quickly, the operation will involve much bleeding, and there will be difficulty in achieving hemostasis. But surgical excision may be considered if the burn is found deep to the muscular layer, or has become the focus of infection.

5. In order to prevent contracture of severe scarring from causing such deformities as ectropion of the eyelids or microstomia," large sheets of autograft should be used for the head and face in patients with plentiful donor sites.

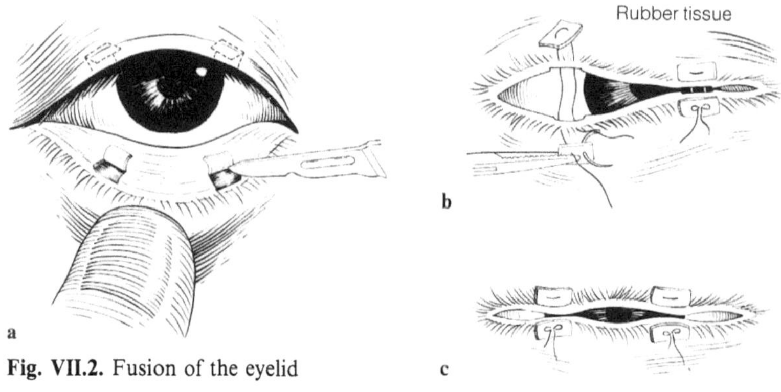

Fig. VII.2. Fusion of the eyelid

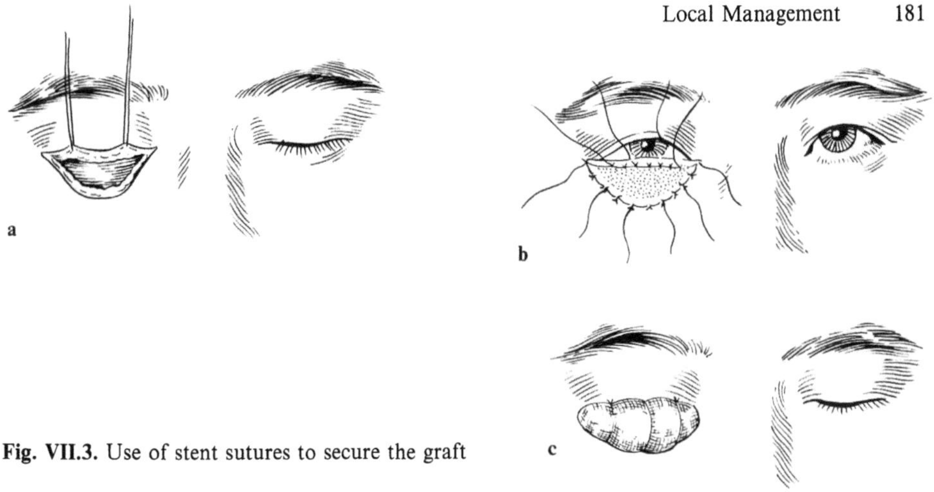

Fig. VII.3. Use of stent sutures to secure the graft

Margins of the grafts need not be sutured, and pressure dressings may be applied for 2–3 days. Nasal feeding is necessary for 2–3 days to prevent shifting of the grafts during chewing. If remnants of epithelial islands have been left in the recipient area, they should be excised during the operation, otherwise the autograft will be lifted away by the remaining epithelial islands. If the graft site involves the eyelids, the latter should be sutured for 3 weeks. Figure VII.2 shows the procedure. The graft may be fixed by stent sutures (Fig. VII.3).

If the site of grafting includes the areas surrounding the lips, the mucosa of the corners of the mouth should be everted to form a triangle (Fig. VII.4) to prevent "microstomia" following scar contracture.

6. In deep burns of the eyelids, ectropion due to edema of the palpebral conjunctivae occurs and cannot be reduced. Even incarceration may occur in

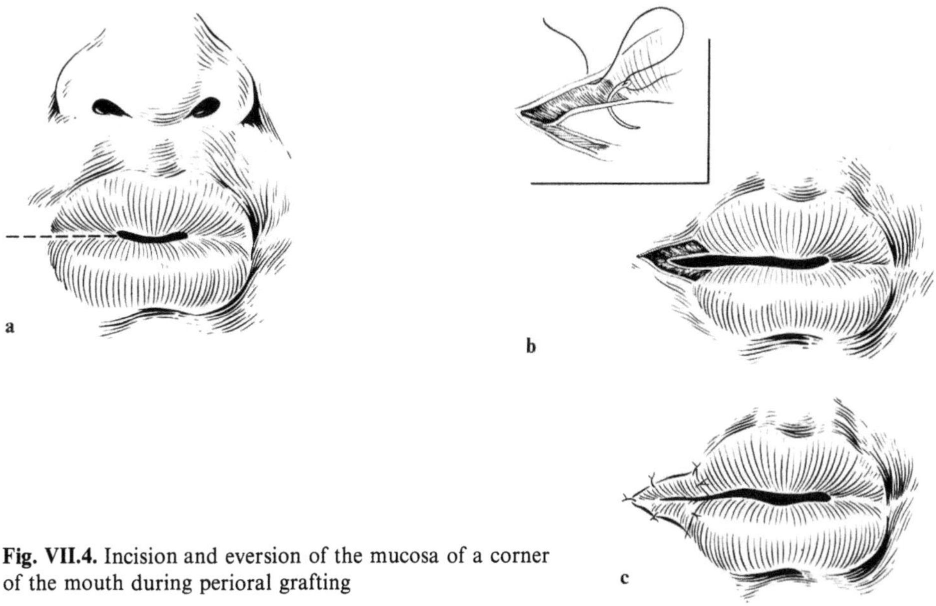

Fig. VII.4. Incision and eversion of the mucosa of a corner of the mouth during perioral grafting

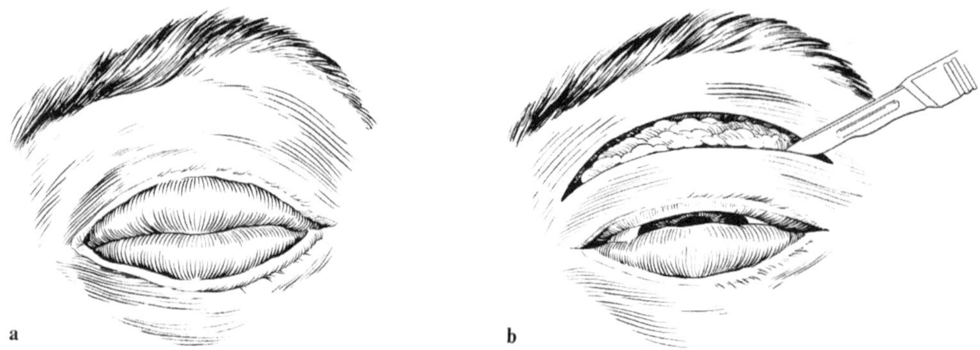

Fig. VII.5a, b. Decompression of the eyelid eschar. **a** Ectropion palpebrarum caused by massive edema. **b** Incision made for decompression

severe cases. The everted palpebral conjunctivae have a poor blood supply and may be ulcerated if not well protected. Early management consists of temporary suturing of the upper and lower eyelids or of incising the eschars of the eyelids during the early stage for decompression. (The incision should be deep enough to reach the normal tissue and should extend to the inner and outer canthi, Fig. VII.5.) If ectropion has occurred already, the everted palpebral conjunctivae should be reduced after the eschars have been incised and decompressed. Protection with ointment is only sufficient in mild cases. If the ectropion becomes more severe when the patient is in prone position, light pressure dressings on the eye may be applied temporarily.

7. The eyeballs may be involved when burns of the head and face become infected. Therefore it is necessary to protect the eyeballs against infection with antibiotics, e.g., 0.25% chloramphenicol may be used as an eyedrop, or 0.5% Aureomycin ointment may be applied three to four times a day. In infection of the head and face with gram-negative bacilli, especially *Pseudomonas aeruginosa*, 1% colistin or polymyxin B ointment may be applied.

8. Owing to the lack of elasticity of the eschars, third degree burns around the corners of mouth may cause difficulty in opening the mouth, thus preventing eating. Perioral incision of the eschar may be performed during the early stage.

2 Burns of the Respiratory Tract

Burns of the respiratory tract may result from: deep flame burns of the head, face, and neck; remaining in dense smoke for a long time during injury; crying loudly in an enclosed space while facing the source of heat; inhalation of hot steam, irritative chemical gases, or corrosive and irritative liquids.

An air way burn is followed by serious consequences and requires emergency measures both in first-aid care and early stage management.

Factors such as reflex closure of epiglottis, efficient cooling of the air by the upper airway, and the poor heat conducting power of the air itself will protect the part of airway below the larynx from burning. Therefore it is rare to encounter an actual burn of the lower respiratory tract. Such burns may be caused by inhalation of hot steam (with a heat conducting power 4,000 times the hot air) or gases with strong penetrating power. We have encountered patients with severe burn of the lower respiratory tract caused by falling into ammonia water and acidic ammonium sulfate solutions.

2.1 Classification

Burns of the respiratory tract may be classified into burns of the upper respiratory tract and burns of the lower respiratory tract according to their anatomical location. Burns of the upper respiratory tract denote those above the glottis (larynx), including the vestibulum nasi, nasal cavity, pharyngolarynx, and glottis. Burns of the lower respiratory tract denote those below the glottis (larynx), including the trachea, bronchi, and alveoli. These two kinds of burns differ markedly in their pathological processes, clinical manifestations, treatment, and prognosis.

The classification is, admittedly, arbitrary, because it is sometimes difficult to make a sharp delimitation. For instance, a burn may chiefly involve the upper respiratory tract, but there may be burns of a mild degree in the mucosae of the trachea and bronchi. On the other hand, a burn of the lower respiratory tract is always accompanied by burns of the upper respiratory tract.

2.2 Pathologic Changes

1. Burns of the upper respiratory tract: Mucosa of the pharnygolarynx is congested and edematous. The edema reaches its maximum 6 h–10 h postburn. Mucosal secretions increase during the edema stage. The edema subsides 48 h later, and the mucosa becomes dry with viscous secretions. The necrotic mucosa appears grayish-white. It desquamates in pieces and may be expectorated 3–7 days later.

2. Burns of the lower respiratory tract: Exudation, necrosis of mucosa, and secondary infection are principal changes and manifest as pulmonary edema, airway obstruction, and pneumonia. These changes represent the three stages of the disease but may be interchangeable.

2.2.1 Pulmonary Edema

Pulmonary edema begins immediately after burn and persists up to 48 h postburn. There is an increase in capillary permeability of the walls of trachea and bronchi, with a copious amount of exudate accumulating in the lumen. Heat and various kinds of chemical substance may injure the endothelial cells of the lungs directly, causing an increase in capillary permeability of the lungs and resulting in interstitial pulmonary edema. Clinically, typical symptoms of pulmonary edema appear with large amounts of pinkish, frothy sputum which is rich in protein.

2.2.2 Sloughing of the Necrotic Mucosa

Sloughing of the necrotic mucosa occurs 72 h to 2 weeks postburn. Necrosis of the columnar ciliated epithelium of the mucosae of the trachea and bronchi will interfere with the clearing up of secretions in the respiratory tract. The accumulated secretions, dust inhaled during injury, or the desquamated necrotic mucosa may form a coagulum obstructing the bronchi and bronchioles, leading to atelectasis. Clinical symptoms of respiratory distress and cyanosis appear. The respiratory distress may be ameliorated after suction or expectoration of the desquamated necrotic mucosa and mucous coagulum. If the sites of obstruction are widespread, massive atelectasis may be the result.

2.2.3 Pulmonary Infection

Pulmonary infection begins 24 h postburn and may last for months without resolution. It is often secondary to mechanical obstruction and atelectasis. It begins as bronchopneumonia, but may turn into interstitial pneumonia.

2.3 Early Diagnosis

Airway obstruction and pulmonary edema caused by respiratory tract burn call for urgent treatment. Early diagnosis and prompt management have a significant bearing on the prognosis.

1. In any flame burn of the head and face it is necessary to investigate the environment in which the burn occurs and the course of events in order to establish whether there is any possibility of respiratory burn. If the burn occurs in an enclosed space, the possibility of coexisting respiratory tract burn should be seriously considered and investigated. If corrosive and irritative chemicals such as ammonia water and lime enter the mouth and nasal cavity, they may cause respiratory tract burn without burn of the skin.

Case Illustration. Male, aged 45. The patient accidentally fell into 20% ammonia water. The entire body and the mouth were rinsed with large amounts of water immediately. The skin was not burned. Respiratory distress appeared 2 h later, with asthmatoid attacks and restlessness. Tracheotomy was performed immediately, and a large amount of fluid was sucked out. In spite of the tracheotomy, the patient was still in respiratory distress and coughed unceasingly. Five days later, a large amount of mucosal fragments and intact mucosal casts of the trachea and bronchi were expectorated. The respiratory distress was ameliorated, and the patient survived.

Similar cases have been encountered frequently. It is important to note that children are often brought to the pediatric emergency clinic and hospitalized under the diagnosis of aspiration pneumonia.

2. The physician should establish whether there is any burning off of the nasal hair and examine the oral and laryngeal mucosa with a laryngoscope.

Mucosal congestion, edema, vesicle formation, pallor, or desquamation point to the possibility of a deeper airway burn. Attention should be paid to the appearance of respiratory obstruction, and preparation for tracheotomy should be made beforehand.

3. Patients with upper respiratory tract burn may suffer from hoarseness, pharyngeal pain, a feeling of obstruction, and laryngeal stridor. The lungs often show negative findings, however. Tracheotomy should be performed immediately.

4. In lower respiratory tract burns, there may be a copious amount of pinkish frothy sputum in the early stage. There is no elevation of the central venous pressure. These changes should be differentiated from pulmonary edema caused by myocardial insufficiency or excessive fluid replacement. Chest roentgenograms in the early stage may show an increase of homogeneous densities.

Mucosal and submucosal edema may cause obstruction of various degrees, leading to respiratory distress. Wheezing sounds and diminished or even disappearance of breathing sounds may be found on auscultation.

Case Illustration. Male, aged 38. The patient accidentally fell into acidic ammonium sulfate solution. The skin was washed with water and was not burned. On arrival at the emergency clinic the patient's chief complaint was abdominal pain, and the vomitus consisted of blood-tinged food. Examination of the oral cavity revealed congestion of the pharyngeal mucosa. Pulmonary edema appeared 1 h later. Chest roentgenograms on the next day showed massive inflammatory consolidation of the right lung and small areas of consolidation scattered over the left lung field. On the 6th day, small areas of radiolucency were found on the left upper lung, while the rest of the lungs showed inflammatory consolidation. The patient died of pneumonia and acute renal failure on the 7th day postburn.

2.4 Management

The principles of management are: maintenance of patency of the airway and prevention and treatment of pulmonary edema and secondary infection of the lungs.

Tracheotomy should be performed as early as possible if there are definite signs of respiratory tract burn.

Resorption of edema is slow in patients with a large burn area because of the long duration of exudation. Respiratory obstruction might occur even after 48 h. During the course of observation, the oral cavity and pharyngolarynx should be examined frequently by laryngoscopy. Any blebs in the pharyngolarynx should be opened immediately to prevent obstruction.

Case Illustration. Male, aged 53. The patient had burns to 90% of the BSA, including third degree burns to 10%, caused by falling into a pool containing water at a temperature of 80 °C. There were burns of the oral cavity and pharynx. He was admitted 4 h postburn with hoarseness and congestion of the pharynx. There was no respiratory distress and the patient was kept on observation. Tracheotomy was not performed. Fifty hours postburn, dyspnea appeared, hoarsenss became more marked, and there were chest oppression and restlessness. Tracheotomy was performed at once, but the patient died of suffocation during operation. Postmortem examination of the oral cavity revealed a large bulla in the pharynx which caused complete obstruction, leading to suffocation.

2.4.1 Burns of the Upper Respiratory Tract

1. *Tracheotomy* not only prevents or relieves respiratory obstruction but also makes suctioning of sputum, secretions, and desquamated necrotic mucosa easy. Nursing after tracheotomy is very important. Besides strict observation of aseptic technique in tracheal suction, the respiratory tract should be kept moist by ultrasonic nebulization.

In patients with minor respiratory tract burn, the cannula may be removed 4–5 days postburn as the edema subsides. But in patients with severe respiratory tract burn, the mucosae of the pharnygolarynx or trachea and bronchi are necrotic, and the cannula should be removed after complete sloughing of the necrotic mucosa.

Preparation of nebulizing solutions: 1% neomycin 100 ml, isoproterenol 20 mg, prednisolone 25 mg. Other antibiotics and expectorants may be added according to the clinical condition.

2. *Corticosteroids* are used to ameliorate air passage edema. Intravenous injection of dexamethasone 10 mg–20 mg or hydrocortisone 100 mg–300 mg, followed by dexamethasone 5 mg or hydrocortisone 50 mg–100 mg every 4 h, may be given for 3 days.

3. Prevention of pulmonary edema by *regulating the fluid intake:* In upper respiratory tract burns, the trachea and bronchi may be burned in different degrees simultaneously. The secretions of the airway increase and even pulmonary edema may occur. The fluid intake should be properly regulated.

4. Use of *bronchial dilators.*

5. Preventive use of *antibiotics.*

2.4.2 Burns of the Lower Respiratory Tract

The more severe the burn, the earlier pulmonary edema appears. It may be followed by pulmonary infection with paroxysmal asthmatoid attacks. The necrotic tracheal and bronchial mucosa begin to slough off 3–5 days postburn, and the sloughing may continue for 2 weeks in patients with severe lower respiratory tract burns. Interstitial pneumonia in the late stage may last as long as 3–4 months. Before the sloughing of the necrotic mucosa, factors such as exudation, obstruction, and infection may interfere with gaseous exchange, causing anoxia and the risk of suffocation.

The principles of treatment are: maintenance of the patency of the airway, prevention and treatment of pulmonary edema, reduction of oxygen consumption, and prevention of secondary infection.

1. *Proper control of fluid administration:* This should be attended to especially during the first 48 h postburn in order to prevent aggravation of the pulmonary edema. It is at this time that the amount of water and sodium in the pulmonary parenchyma is at its maximum, and a large amount of plasma-like exudate is present in the airway. Measurement of the central venous pressure is very helpful in the estimation of fluid administration. Exudate in the lungs is rich in protein, which is approximately half the amount of plasma proteins. We treated a patient with lower respiratory tract burn from whose trachea 2,000 ml of frothy fluid, with a protein content of 81 g, had been sucked out during the first 24 h postburn. Fluid loss through this route should be considered in colloid replacement. The principle of fluid replacement in lower respiratory tract burn is one of strict control, keeping the central venous pressure at about 6 cm of water column.

2. *Reduction of oxygen consumption:* In patients with severe lower respiratory tract burn, the respiratory distress cannot be completely relieved even after tracheotomy. There are often signs of anoxia, such as gaping and depression of the intercostal spaces. In such conditions, artificial hibernation drugs and physical hypothermia may be employed for sedation and to reduce oxygen consumption. Artifical hibernation drugs are used first, followed by physical hypothermia. Physical hypothermia should not be applied until the ether test has turned to negative. The effect is even better if ice caps are applied. The rectal temperature should be maintained at 32 °C–34 °C continuously for 3–4 days so that the patient survives the severest stage of anoxia. Artificial hibernation mixtures No. 1 and No. 4 have the strongest actions; usually one dose (cf. Chap. II) is given every 3 h–4 h. The dose may be somewhat increased in patients with high tolerance, and the addition of diazepam or γ-sodium hydroxybutyrate may enhance the sedative effect of the artificial hibernation mixture. But we must consider the other side of the problem: one of the disadvantages of artificial hibernation is inhibition of the cough reflex. Therefore, during the stage with a large amount of secretion, intervals of 6 h–8 h should be allowed to elapse between administrations of artificial hibernation drugs. This will allow the patient to become conscious for some time, and the cough reflex will reappear. The latter will enhance expectoration of the secretions and desquamated necrotic mucosa. During sloughing of the necrotic mucosa, the dosage of Dolantin should be somewhat reduced to prevent inhibition of respiration.

3. *Intratracheal suction and washings:* This is an important measure in the management of lower respiratory tract burns. During the first 48 h postburn there is large amount of plasma-like exudate in the airway which may need continuous suction. Necrotic tracheal and bronchial mucosa begin to slough off on the 3rd day postburn, and suction will stimulate coughing and is therefore useful for the expectoration of the necrotic mucosa. The coagulum formed by viscous secretions and desquamated mucosa often causes obstruction of the trachea and bronchi and will aggravate respiratory distress and even lead to suffocation. Intratracheal washings should be carried out in addition to suctioning.

Preparation of solutions for intratracheal washings: 1% neomycin 50 ml, 2.5% sodium bicarbonate 50 ml, and epinephrine hydrochloride 8 drops.

Between 5 and 10 ml is used for each washing. Washing is carried out through the tracheotomy opening, and suction is performed simultaneously. These procedures will stimulate the cough reflex, and the secretions and necrotic mucosa will be so loosened and thinned as to be easily washed off. The bronchial suction tube may be used to introduce the catheter directly into the bronchi for suctioning, and will give a better result. These washings and suctionings should be done repeatedly, every 15 min–30 min in general. As the amount of secretion and desquamated necrotic mucosa decreases, the frequency of washing and suctioning may be reduced correspondingly. Aseptic technique should be strictly followed during the procedure. The time for each washing and suctioning should be sufficiently short to avoid anoxia. Postural drainage and patting the back may supplement suctioning. Occasionally, large pieces of necrotic mucosa slough off and obstruct the trachea and bronchi, and they should be removed under direct vision through a bronchoscope.

4. Preventive use of *antibiotics*.

5. *Assisted intermittent positive pressure respiration.* Respiratory support should be instituted when PaO_2 falls below 75 mm Hg. If PaO_2 still cannot be raised, PEEP initiated with 5 cm H_2O should be considered.

6. The heart should be taken care of during pulmonary edema. *Digitalis* may be given.

7. *Nasal feeding with gastric tube:* In patients with respiratory tract burns, the epiglottis is edematous and cannot close completely during swallowing; this will increase chance of aspiration pneumonia. Therefore the gastric tube for nasal feeding should be retained until the epiglottis can close completely.

Case Illustration. Male, aged 22. There were hot steam burns to 54% of the BSA, including third degree burns to 10%. They were distributed over the head and face, lower extremities, forearms, and hands, and were accompanied by severe lower respiratory tract burn.

The patient was admitted 3 h postburn. Upon admission, both lungs were normal on auscultation, but respiratory distress developed gradually and the tracheal secretions were pinkish and frothy. One and a half hours after admission, tracheotomy was performed and 100% oxygen was given. Chest roentgenograms 12 h postburn showed haziness all over both lungs. The amount of fluid administered was regulated according to the urinary output and central venous pressure. During the first 24 h, colloid solution 1,900 ml, electrolyte solutions 3,700 ml, water 2,000 ml, and 25% sorbitol 375 ml were administered. Urinary output was 762 ml. The central venous pressure was maintained at 2 cm–10 cm H_2O. During the first 24 h, 475 ml of hibernation mixture No. 1 (concentrated) was given to reduce oxygen consumption, and intratracheal suction was continued. During the 27th h postburn, secretions of the air passage suddenly increased, and bubbling sounds could be heard over both lungs. Cedilanid (lanatoside C) 0.4 mg was given, and the secretions decreased in amount 30 min later; 4 h later, a further 0.2 mg Cedilanid was given, and the pulmonary edema was essentially controlled. During the second 24 h, the total amount of fluid administered was 4,275 ml, including colloid 1,000 ml, electrolyte solutions 800 ml, and water 1,475 ml (including hibernation mixture No. 1 1,075 ml, 25%

sorbitol 375 ml, 20% mannitol 125 ml, and 5% glucose 900 ml). The urinary output was 1,724 ml.

Dyspnea appeared 50 h postburn, and there were wheezing sounds in the chest which disappeared after 100 mg hydrocortisone was given. Respiration became quieter, but sometimes there were gape, depression of the intercostal muscles, and dyspnea. These symptoms were ameliorated after suctioning of the secretions. Continuous tracheal suction and artificial hibernation were maintained. Artificial hibernation mixture No. 1 (concentrated) 1,000 ml was given daily, and the condition improved slightly. On the 4th day postburn, oxygen was not given for a time. From then on, the tracheal secretions were scanty but very viscous, and could not be easily sucked out. Bilateral pneumonia appeared. Starting from the 5th day postburn, respiratory distress became aggravated, and was accompanied by status asthmaticus. Breathing sounds were markedly decreased over both lungs, vesicular breathing sounds were masked by the wheezing sounds, and there were widespread moist rales. Treatment with corticosteroids and artificial hibernation mixture was useless. Bronchoscopy was performed on the 6th day postburn, and the mucosa of the trachea and bronchi were found to be swollen and eroded with narrowing of the lumen, which was obstructed by the desquamated necrotic mucosa and secretion coagulum. Eight pieces of these substances were picked out. The respiratory distress was not relieved after operation, and wheezing sounds persisted. Physical hypothermia was performed in addition to artificial hibernation, but there was no improvement of the clinical condition. Intratracheal washings and suction were started from the 7th day postburn, and more of the desquamated necrotic mucosa was sucked out (Fig. VII.6). Gape disappeared 6 h later, but sloughing of the necrotic mucosa continued and obstructed the airway, leading to intermittent dyspnea. It was noted that plugs were often sucked out with washings and suctioning whenever there was severe respiratory distress, and that the latter was thereby ameliorated. The characteristic chicken-foot bronchiolar casts sloughed off on the 8th day postburn (Fig. VII.7). The necrotic mucosa sloughed off almost completely on the 13th day postburn. From then on, only small pieces were occasionally sucked out. The tracheal cannula was removed on the 19th day postburn. The bilateral bronchopneumonia which appeared on the 4th day postburn lasted for more than 2 months and was gradually controlled. The patient was discharged in good condition.

In some patients with severe lower respiratory tract burns, the severity and extent of burns of the trachea and bronchi may prolong the duration of sloughing of the necrotic mucosa to more than 3 weeks, even though the alveoli have not been involved. After the pulmonary edema in the early stage has been resorbed, the large amount of necrotic mucosa in the trachea and bronchi may be secondarily infected; this will hinder the passage of air, especially in expiration. Diminished breathing sounds, and even absence of breathing sounds in some areas, will be found on auscultation. Chest X-ray findings are essentially negative, except for an increase in radiolucency. These physical signs and radiographic findings are characteristic of lower respiratory tract burns. Aggravation

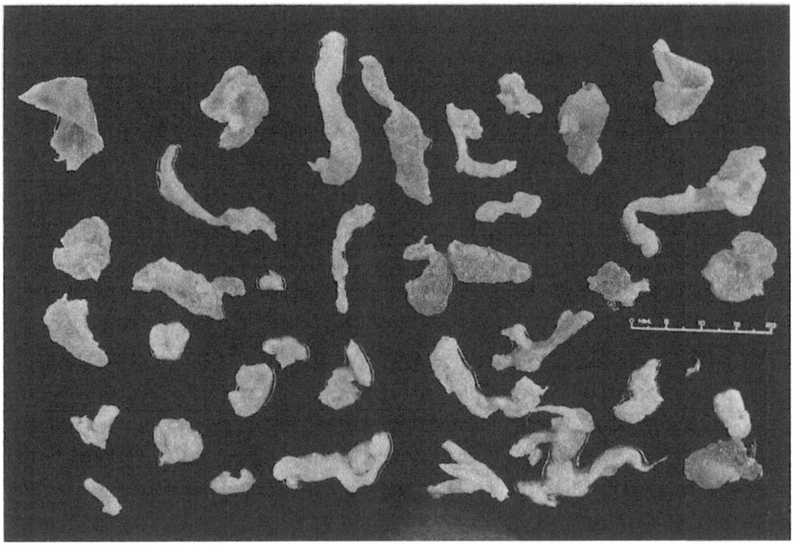

Fig. VII.6. Large amounts of necrotic tracheal endothelium were washed out 7 days postburn in this 22-year-old male patient with burns of the lower respiratory tract

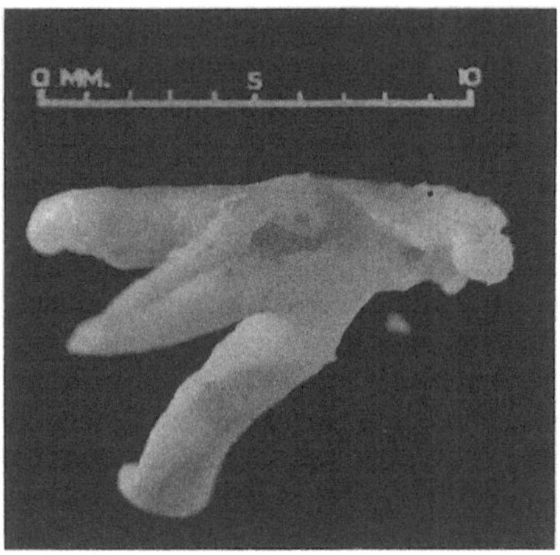

Fig. VII.7. A "chicken-foot" bronchiolar cast sucked out on the 8th day postburn from a patient with burns of the lower respiratory tract

of the infection may cause marked obstruction, and reflex bronchial spasm due to the necrotic mucosa and infection will further increase the mechanical obstruction already present. Wheezing sounds will then appear continuously, and the patient is in great distress during both inspiration and expiration. There may be severe anoxia and carbon dioxide retention. In this group of patients, even intratracheal washings and suction will not loosen and cause expectoration of the necrotic mucosa plugged in the trachea. At present, we still have difficulty in treating this kind of patient, and mortality is still high.

3 Burns of the Eye

The eyelids are usually closed by reflex, and therefore burn of the eyeball is rare. Even in third degree flame burn of the face, the eyeball is often unhurt. But in chemical burns, the eyelids cannot close promptly, owing to rapid splashing of the chemicals, and the eyeballs are often involved.

Burns of the eye may be classified into burns of the eye appendages and burns of the eyeball. The former denote burns of the eyelids and palpebral conjunctiva. Burns of the eyelids have been described in Sect. 1 of this chapter, and the present section chiefly concerns the burns of the conjunctiva and cornea.

3.1 Symptoms

The manifestations of burns of the eye are photophobia, lacrimation, pain, feeling of foreign body, increase of secretions, and decrease of eyesight. Minor burns of the conjunctivae cause edema and congestion only, but the conjunctivae may be necrotic and appear whitish in severe burns. Pain is more marked in corneal burn than in conjunctival burn. In mild cases, the corneal burn cannot be easily detected grossly, but with 2% fluorescein solution as an eyedrop the burned cornea will be stained yellowish-green. In severe cases, the cornea becomes opaque with ulceration and even perforation, causing extrusion of the contents of the eye. In the majority of patients, corneal burn will resolve spontaneously, but there may be scar formation affecting the eyesight. Daily examination is necessary for close observation of ulcer formation.

3.2 Management

1. In *chemical burn of the eye,* irrigation with a large amount of physiologic saline should be carried out immediately, followed by continuous irrigation at constant speed for 48 h. If physiologic saline is not available, tap water may be used instead. Any foreign bodies present in the conjunctival sacs should be removed as soon as possible.

2. In *mild conjunctival burn,* the following treatment is sufficient: 0.25% Chloromycetin solution for eye instillation every 2–4 h; Aureomycin ointment 0.5% four times a day. Secretions should be wiped off with sterilized gauze. Generally, healing will result in a few days.

3. *Corneal burn:* The principle of management involves prevention of infection, prevention of iridocyclitic adhesions, and expedition of resorption of the inflammation.

The cornea resists infection poorly, and severe consequences such as corneal perforation and panophthalmitis may follow infection. Besides the management stated above, polymyxin B or 0.5% colistin ointment four times a day may be used to prevent Pseudomonas infection. In deep corneal burn or burn with Pseudomonas infection, 100,000 units polymyxin B may be injected subconjunctivally once a day.

Iridocyclitic adhesions may be prevented by the use of atropine, 1% ointment or solution, as a mydriatic agent.

Vasodilators may be used to hasten resorption. Dionin, 1%–3% solution, may be used as an eyedrop three times a day; in severe cases, tolazoline 25 mg may be injected subconjunctivally and oral Dibazol 10 mg may be given three times a day.

Pantocaine 1% may be used as eyedrops for severe pain, but it should be used as little as possible because of its inhibitory effect on epithelial growth of the cornea. For deep corneal burn or progressive corneal ulcers, a piece of conjunctival flap should be raised to cover the injured cornea. Instillation or subconjunctival injection of corticosteroids may reduce tissue reaction and scar formation.

4. In *severe conjunctival or corneal burn* with local congestion, persistent edema, and much secretion, sterilized glass sticks should be used two to three times a day to separate the conjunctival sacs and thus prevent adhesions of the eyeball.

5. *Panophthalmitis* should be treated by ophthalmectomy.

6. *If, after deep burns of the eyelids* have healed, contraction of the scars makes it impossible to close the eyelids or causes ectropion, the cornea is exposed. The scar ought to be excised as early as possible and the wound covered with full-thickness autograft or medium split-thickness autograft for the correction of ectropion. Before the operation 0.5% Aureomycin ointment may be applied temporarily to protect the corneal epithelium.

4 Burns of the External Ear

The incidence of burns of the external ear is higher than that of burns of the eye.

4.1 Characteristics

The special features of the external ear are thinness of the skin and scantiness of the subcutaneous tissue. Therefore burns of the external ear often involve the auricular cartilage. The latter has a poor resistance to infection and is easily complicated with auricular chondritis, causing "small ear" deformity.

In the management of burns of the head and neck, prevention of auricular chondritis is an important objective. Although it will not appear until 2 weeks postburn, once it does occur the involved cartilages should, in many cases, be excised. Therefore attention should be paid to the prevention of auricular chondritis during the early stage after burn.

4.2 Management

After debridement in the early stage, pillows should not be used: the ear should be fully exposed and should not be submitted to pressure. The occurrence of auricular chondritis is closely related to local pressure. Any exudate should be wiped off with sterilized cotton swabs to keep the wound surface dry; the whole ear may be buried in silver sulfadiazine paste (Fig. VII.8).

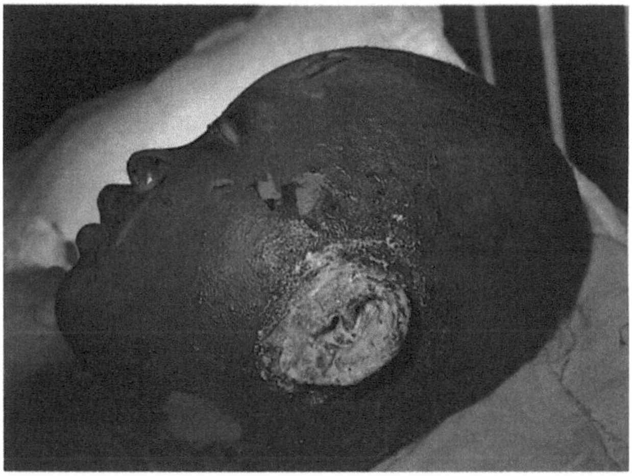

Fig. VII.8. Burying of the burned external ear in silver sulfadiazine paste

Once infection has occurred, the pus and the separated necrotic tissue should be removed. Effective antibiotics should be selected for dressings, which must be changed every day. The infection should be controlled promptly.

When the auricular eschar separates and sheds, small areas of auricular cartilage may often be exposed. The wound surface (including the cartilage) should be covered by autogenous skin grafts as early as possible. The cartilage has no vascular supply and the rate of take of the graft is low. During grafting, small pieces of exposed cartilage may be trimmed off.

4.3 Symptoms and Management of Auricular Chondritis

Severe pain and marked tenderness are present in cases of auricular chondritis. The pain may be so severe as to cause sleeplessness, and an analgesic is needed. On inspection, the auricle is red and swollen (Fig. VII.9). Fever of 39 °C or higher may be present. If the pain is not relieved or reappears after operative removal of the cartilage, incomplete removal of the necrotic cartilage or the re-formation of necrotic cartilage might be indicated; a second operation is

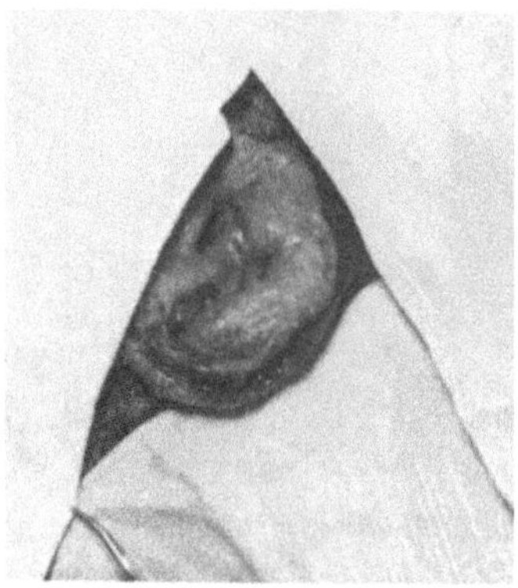

Fig. VII.9. Auricular chondritis

then required. Auricular chondritis may become the focus of infection of septicemia. Wound healing ointment No. 10 with an equal volume of 2% silver sulfadiazine may be tried in the early management of auricular chondritis. During application of the ointment, the auditory canal should be packed with sterilized cotton balls to avoid intraauricular infection caused by inward flowing of the pus. The area of application of the medicine should be broader than the area of local swelling. Dressings should be changed daily, and possibly twice a day when there is much pus. If the swelling becomes localized after application of the ointment, a sterilized No. 8 syringe needle may be used for aspiration of the pus at the site of the most marked swelling; alternatively a pointed knife may be used to incise and drain the pus. The ointment is then applied until the wound heals.

If conservative treatment fails, surgical drainage in combination with excision of all the necrotic cartilage is the only effective treatment. The operation should be performed with the patient under general anesthesia. The incision should be made at the site of most marked swelling of the auricle, and the necrotic cartilage, which appears grayish-white, lusterless, and brittle, is then excised (Fig. VII.10). In cases which have been treated conservatively, there will be marked proliferation of fibrous tissue around the necrotic cartilage, and the proliferated fibrous tissue should also be excised during the operation.

Gauze soaked with hydrogen peroxide may be applied with pressure to achieve hemostasis if there is much oozing of blood during the operation. Postoperatively, one or two layers of antibiotic gauze or petrolatum gauze should be packed between the two halves of the incised auricle and dressings applied. It is important to keep the auricle in normal position during dressing to maintain a free blood circulation and thus avoid ischemic necrosis. Dressings may be changed every other day until granulation tissue grows between the two halves of the auricle and the wound heals.

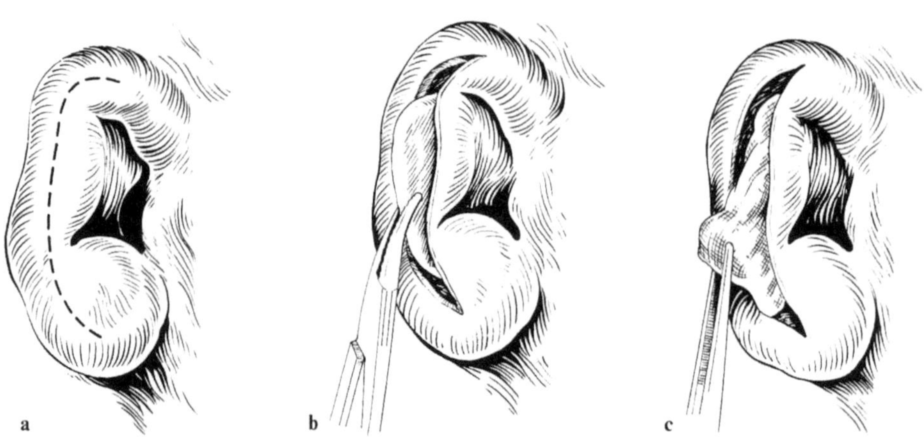

Fig. VII.10a–c. Excision of the necrotic auricular cartilage. **a** incision; **b** extraction of necrotic cartilage; **c** gauze packing

Both surgical excision of the necrotic auricular cartilage and liquefaction of the necrotic auricular cartilage following conservative treatment will lead to loss of the framework of the auricle, causing small ear deformity.

5 Burns of the Hand

The hands are easily burned because of their exposure. When there is a danger of burns of the head and face, the patient often protects his face with both hands with the dorsum facing outward, causing burns of the dorsum of hand. Children often grasp very hot objects, and thus the incidence of burns of the palm is higher than in adults.

5.1 Characteristics

The anatomic characteristics of the hand are as follows: The skin of the dorsum of hand is thin, with scanty subcutaneous fat, and the tendons lie immediately beneath the deep fascia. Deep burns of the dorsum of the hand often involve the tendons and bones, causing severe functional disturbances. The skin of the palm is thick, and there is little need for skin graft. The skin of the palm and subcutaneous adipose tissue are in close contact, and the latter is rich in blood vessels so that the anatomic cleavages cannot be distinctly discerned and there will be much bleeding during excision of the eschar. Burns are often deeper in the thenar and hypothenar eminences than in the midpalmar space; therefore these muscles may undergo necrosis.

5.2 Management

The hand is an organ for labor, and the most important consideration in the management of burns of the hand is to prevent or minimize disability. The deformities caused by deep burns of the dorsum of the hand are hyperextension of the metacarpophalangeal joints, flexion of the proximal interphalangeal joints, loss of the transverse arch of the palm, adduction of the thumb, and flexion of wrist. The damage caused by the deformities involve the skin, fascia, ligaments, tendons, lumbrical muscles, interosseous muscles, and joints. A deep second degree burn of the dorsum of hand, if not treated by grafting, will result in scar contracture after healing and cause disability of the hand due to the deformities.

In burns other than deep burns involving the tendon and bone, the principal causes of deformities are: persisting edema, infection of the wound surface, prolonged immobilization in a nonfunctional position, and delay of skin grafting. These problems should be seriously considered even in the early stage of management. The principles of management of burns of the hand are: meticulous debridement, prevention of infection, hastening the subsidence of edema, maintaining the hand in a functional position, early covering of the wound surface, and early mobilization.

The reader is referred to Chap. III with regard to debridement in the early stage. Any dirt in the skin furrows should be wiped off and nails cut. No matter what method (exposure or application of dressings) is used after debridement in the early stage, the position of the hand should be maintained at dorsiflexion of the wrist joint, 80° flexion of the metacarpophalangeal joint, extension of the interphalangeal joint, and abduction and apposition of the thumb. Every joint should be placed in a proper position: Dorsiflexion of the wrist joint will counteract the flexor muscles; the purpose of 80° flexion of the metacarpophalangeal joint is to maintain the collateral ligaments at their full length (shortening of these ligaments will cause hyperextension and inability to flex the metacarpophalangeal joint); and extension of the interphalangeal joint will prevent flexion deformities of this joint. The involved extremity should be elevated to reduce edema.

5.2.1 Superficial Second Degree Burns

Superficial second degree burns will heal without scarring and disturbances of function. To prevent deepening of a superficial second degree burn after infection, silver sulfadiazine cream may be applied or one may expose the burn wound to induce scab formation immediately after debridement with the purpose of obtaining primary subscab healing.

5.2.2 Deep Second Degree Burns

In deep second degree burns of the hand, scar formation and contracture after healing may cause deformities and functional disturbances. In order to obtain a good function it is necessary to perform tangential excisions in the early stage, to transplant large sheets of autologous skin without suturing, and to apply dressings for immobilization.

5.2.3 Third Degree Burns

The most ideal treatment of a third degree burn is early excision of the eschar and grafting of large sheets of autologous skin (Figs. VII.11, VII.12). The operation is generally performed 3–5 days postburn, while there is no obvious infection of the wound. Even if the wound has been infected already, operation is not contraindicated. The method of excision of the eschar of the hand is similar to that of other sites (cf. Chap. III), but the following additional remarks should be noted.

1. The operative field should first be scrubbed with sterilized soap water with the patient under anesthesia, and then disinfected.
2. A tourniquet should be applied during operation to reduce blood loss and to guarantee the complete excision of the dead tissue.
3. If the third degree burn is shallow, better function may be obtained if the excision is made down to the plane of the superficial fascia.
4. If there is burn of the finger web, the web should be incised during operation and a triangular skin inserted to the palmar side to prevent shallowing of the finger web or formation of a false web (see Chap. XIV).

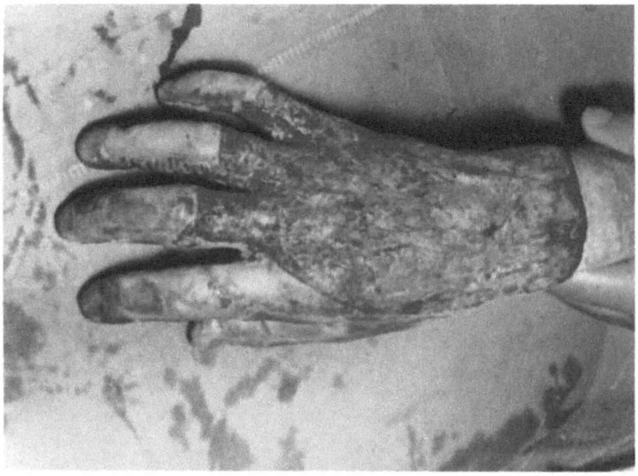

Fig. VII.11. Third degree burn of the dorsum of the hand. The eschar has been excised, and grafting of a large sheet of autoskin onto the deep exposed fascia is planned

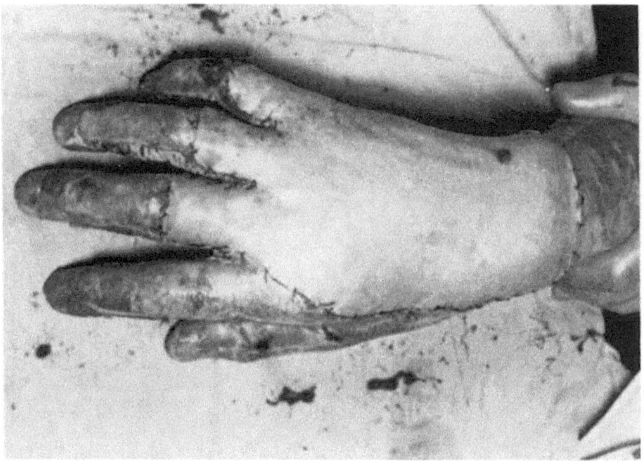

Fig. VII.12. Same patient as in **Fig. VII.11.** The autoskin has now been grafted

5. If the eschar is obviously infected, incision should be through the part not yet infected or less severely infected. The eschar should be removed en bloc by gradual separation along the plane of the deep fascia. It is not feasible to perform autologous skin grafting immediately after excision of the eschar.

6. After excision of eschar of the hand, large sheets of autograft may be grafted immediately if there is no infection, but the grafting may also be postponed. The method for delayed grafting is to use single-layer antibiotic dressings or artificial skin wrapped up under pressure after excision of the eschar. Since there are large amounts of exudation from the wound after excision of the eschar, the dressings should be thicker. These dressings may be removed 48 h later, and large sheets of skin transplanted. When antibiotic dressings are used, there will be a very thin layer of granulation tissue by this time. Any remnant of the necrotic tissue should be removed. The necrotic tissue must be excised thoroughly and hemostasis should be complete because any hematoma or remnant necrotic tissue will influence the viability of the skin graft. Delayed grafting does not have the drawbacks cited above. If the preoperative preparation is

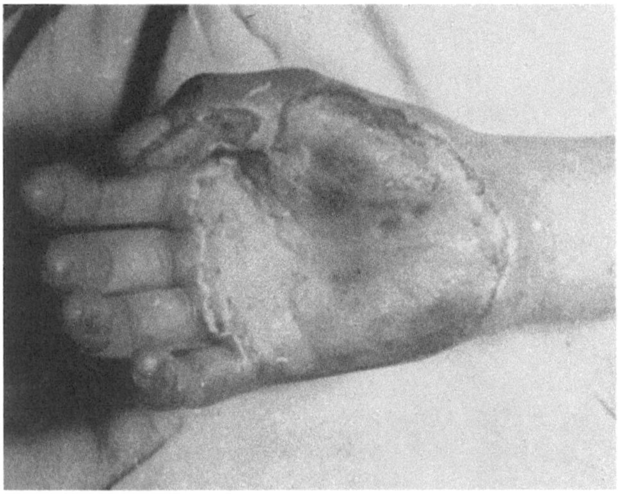

Fig. VII.13. Deep burn of the palm

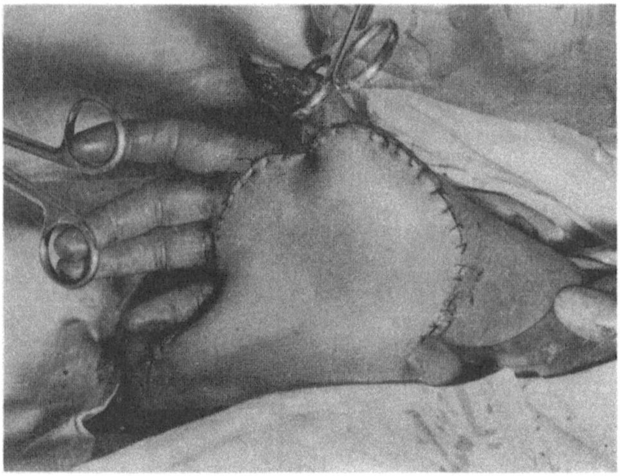

Fig. VII.14. Same patient as in **Fig. VII.13.** An abdominal pedicle flap has been applied to the wound after excision of the eschar

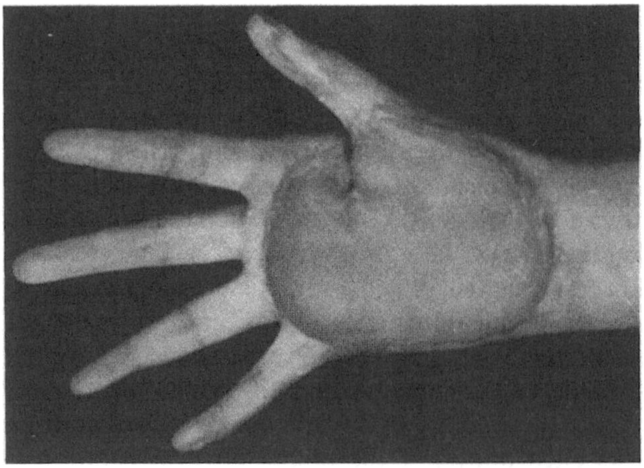

Fig. VII.15. Same patient as in **Fig. VII.13**; final result

meticulous, aseptic technique is strictly observed during operation, and antibiotic dressings or artificial skin is used to cover the wound, there will generally be neither wound infection nor any ill-effect on the skin graft owing to it being wrapped up for 48 h. The viability of autograft is good in delayed skin grafting. The purpose of early excision of the eschar of the hand and grafting of large sheets of autoskin is to achieve a better function after healing, and therefore all of the grafted skin is expected to survive. In some of the functional parts of the hand, failure of even a small area of skin graft to survive will affect the function.

7. In patients with massive burn and poor resources of autografts, large sheets of allograft may be used with intermingled transplantation of autograft after excision of the eschar of the hand in the early stage. This achieves better restoration of function than does grafting of postage stamp-sized grafts on the granulating wound surface.

8. Sutures may be removed 1 week after skin grafting, and exercises for restoration of function started.

9. Excision combined with the use of mesh grafts will give satisfactory functional results if the expansion of the meshed skin is less than 3:1.

10. In patients with deep burns of the palm or burns of the dorsum of hand down to the tendons, bones and surrounding tissue are suitable for a pedicle flap, which may be applied to cover the wound surface in the early stage (Figs. VII.13, VII.14, VII.15). With the protection of the well-vascularized skin flap, some of the remnant necrobiotic tissue may regenerate.

In patients with burns as deep as the tendons, the necrotic tissues may be excised in the early stage if severe infection has not occurred. Dead bones should be chiselled off, and metacarpophalangeal joints should be fixed with Kirschner wires. If the burn is extensive and suitable pedicle flaps or free flaps cannot be found, grafting of skin flaps may be delayed. If the wound is already severely infected, skin grafting should be performed on the granulating wound surface after the eschar has sloughed off spontaneously. The necrotic tendons and sequestrum must be removed. This kind of hand burn is often complicated by phalangeal and metacarpal osteomyelitis, and the swelling may last as long as 2–3 months. Severe deformities occur after healing of the wound owing to prolonged local swelling and fibrous contracture.

6 Burns of the Perineum

Perineal burn is most often seen in children. Healing of deep second degree and third degree burns will result in deformities due to scarring, and plastic surgery is necessary in the late stage.

The management of perineal burns chiefly involves meticulous nursing. The exposure method of treatment may be employed. After spontaneous sloughing of the third degree eschar, skin may be grafted on to the granulating wound surface. Surgical removal is required if the wound has become a focus of infection. The postoperative management is similar to that in ordinary anorectal operations.

Case Illustration. Female, aged 4. There were flame burns of the lower extremities, lower abdomen, perineum, and buttocks. The burns involved 40% of the BSA and included third degree burns to 26%.

On the 4th day postburn eschar excision was performed on both lower extremities, and the wound surface was covered with large sheets of "punched" allograft. The perineal eschar burst, and the necrotic adipose tissue was exposed and infected. The body temperature rose to 39 °C, the heart rate was 150/min, and there was loss of appetite. During excision of the eschar of the lower abdomen and buttocks on the 9th day postburn, the perineal eschar and the partly burned external sphincters were excised too, since the perineal eschar had been a focus of infection. Large sheets of punched allografts were used to cover the wound surface, and the postoperative management was the same as in ordinary anorectal operations. The body temperature fell to 38 °C 2 days after operation, the patient's appetite improved, and the allograft was taken.

There had been severe prolapse of the rectum at one time postoperatively. The patient was placed in the Trendelenburg position, and the prolapsed rectum was reduced after defecation and supported with bandages. Several months later, following restoration of the function of the remaining anal sphincters and local formation of fibrous tissue, the rectum was no longer prolapsed. Follow-up for 2 years showed neither anal stricture nor abnormality in defecation.

7 Burns of the Bones and Joints

Burns of the bones most often occur in the tibia, followed by the olecranon, the ulnoradial styloid processes, the patella, and the cranial bones. Deep burns of the hand and foot involving bones of the fingers and toes are not rare. Wound infection around superficial joints may be complicated by suppurative arthritis. Electric injuries involving bones and joints are especially common.

After a burn, the bone appears black and dry or yellow and lusterless. The sequestrum will persist for several months without separation if left alone – consequently surgical removal is required. Removal of the sequestrum will enhance the growth of the granulation tissue from the medullary cavity and helps the spread of surrounding granulation tissue toward the viable bone surface. The granulation tissue surrounding the sequestrum is unhealthy, pale, edematous, and exuberant. Grafting on this granulation tissue always fails. Sequestrectomy should be performed after the wound surface around the sequestrum has been covered with skin, generally 1 month postburn. Premature removal of the sequestrum will expose the medullary cavity, in which the neighboring infection might spread, with serious consequences.

7.1 Management

7.1.1 Tubular Bones

There are two ways of dealing with the sequestrum: either chiseling or drilling may be used according to the extent and location of the sequestrum.

1. *Chiseling* is indicated when treating small or thin sequestrum. A bone chisel or rongeur is used to chisel or bite the sequestrum until bleeding occurs. Bleeding is a quite reliable index of the viability of the bony tissue. Generally, skin grafting is performed after the appearance of granulation tissue; alternatively the skin flap is directly transplanted upon the bleeding viable bony surface. Sometimes the exposed medullary cavity will undergo further necrosis after the cortex has been chiseled off; therefore it is better to cover it with allograft after chiseling. The necrotic bones of the fingers and toes may be bitten off simply with a rongeur.

2. *Drilling:* The bone is drilled with the bone drill until bleeding occurs. There is still some sequestrum left between the holes, and the granulation tissue will grow out through the holes. The small pieces of sequestrum between the holes generally separate off 2–3 weeks later. The granulation tissue grows more slowly after removal of the sequestrum by means of the drilling method. Therefore the method we use at present is to chisel off or bite off the small bits of sequestrum left between the holes as much as possible during drilling, so as to leave a cribriform framework with only a thin layer of sequestrum. In this way separation of the sequestrum is faster and the extent of bone to be chiseled can be more easily regulated. Especially when the area of burn of the long tubular bones is large, this method will prevent fracture due to excessive bone chiseling.

If the joint cavity is exposed after sequestrectomy, the synovial membrane and the exposed articular cartilage must be excised to allow growth of granulation tissue from the joint surface and closure of the joint cavity. If this is not done, there will be exudation of the synovial fluid and necrosis of the articular cartilage leading to persistent infection.

7.1.2 Cranial Bones

The cranial bones consist of the internal and external diploë. The dura mater lies immediately beneath the internal diploë, and any improper management of cranial burns will lead to infection of the brain. If the dura mater is accidentally perforated during surgery, the cerebrospinal fluid may leak out and there will be infection of the subarachnoid space followed by very serious consequences. Therefore the depth of chiseling of necrotic cranial bone should be well regulated. Special personnel should hold the head during surgery to avoid fracture of the base of the skull during the operative maneuver.

Small necrotic cranial bone may be chiseled off with a bone chisel. If all the layers of the cranial bone are necrotic, they should be chiseled off completely; this should be followed by immediate transplantation of autograft or allograft on the dura mater without waiting for the growth of granulation tissue.

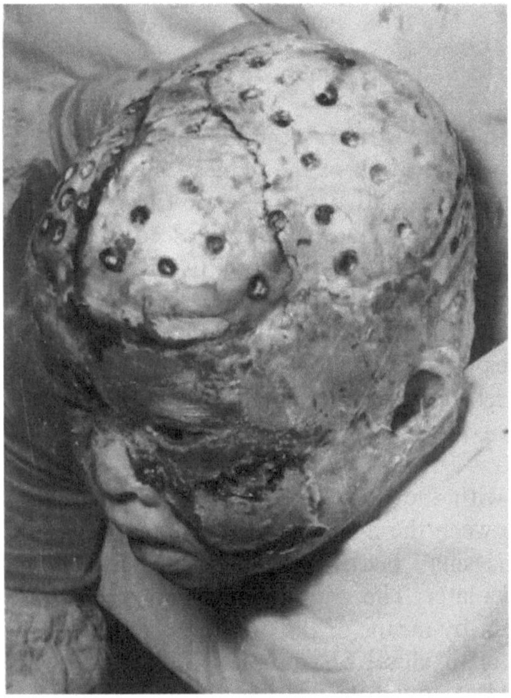

Fig. VII.16. One-year-old female with electric burns of the cranium. Drilling was performed on the 37th day postburn

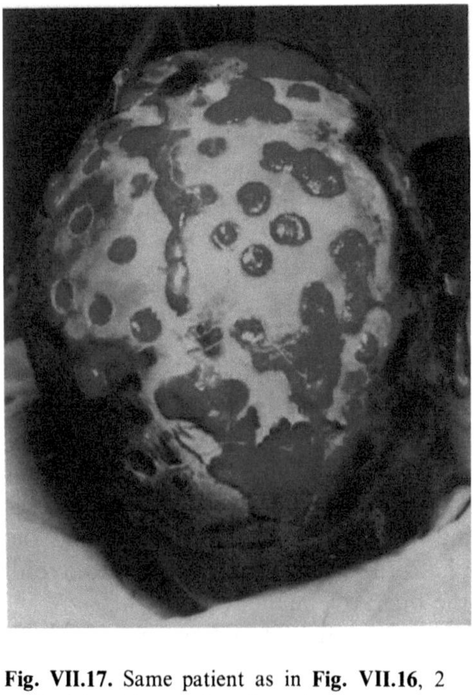

Fig. VII.17. Same patient as in **Fig. VII.16**, 2 weeks later. Granulation tissue has grown out through the holes

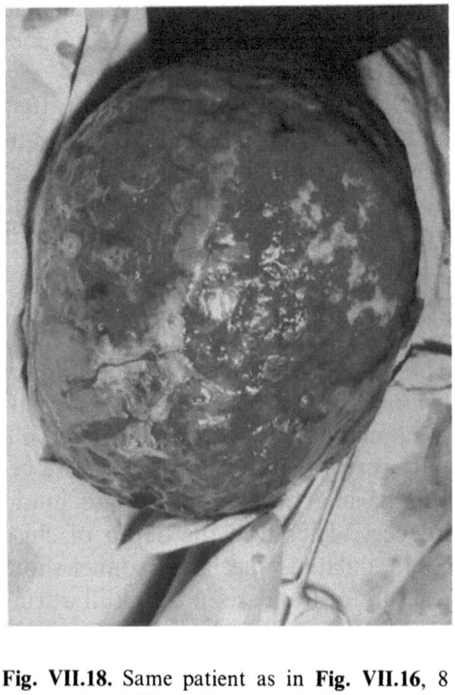

Fig. VII.18. Same patient as in **Fig. VII.16**, 8 weeks after drilling. The granulation wound is ready for grafting

If necrosis of the cranial bones is extensive, in order to determine the depth of drilling during operation the bone may be drilled until bleeding occurs. If all layers of the cranial bones are necrotic, the drilling should reach the dura mater. After drilling, the remnant cranial bone between the holes should be further chiseled off. The remnants generally slough off 2–3 weeks later, and grafting may be done after growth of the granulation tissue (Figs. VII.16–18). After operation, signs of meningeal irritation should be closely watched for.

If the dura mater is accidentally perforated during operation, the site of perforation should be covered with allograft, autograft, or a transposed skin flap or repaired with sutures. Antibiotics should be selected according to the findings of bacterial sensitivity tests of the wound surface. The antibiotics of choice should be those capable of penetrating the blood-brain barrier.

7.1.3 Joints (cf. Chap. VIII)

The principles of management of joint burn are: excision of the surrounding necrotic tissue, free drainage of the joint cavity, and immobilization of the joint in functional position. If amputation is necessary but the stump lacks healthy soft tissue for coverage, disarticulation may be performed to prevent exposure of the medullary cavity.

Chapter VIII Electric Injury

LIU YUE-LIANG

Translated by NYI PAO-CHUN

The electric injury to be discussed in this chapter concerns the direct contact of the human body with electric current, with one or more inlet and outlet through the body.

Apart from a direct electric contact burns, both those injuries inflicted by high voltage electric arc and those caused by flames induced by electricity can involve deep burns: the former because of the very high temperature (about 2,500 °C) generated, and the latter because the victim may be in coma for some time and consequently be burned by the flames for a corresponding period.

The degree of severity of injuries inflicted by electric shock is depend upon the electric voltage, the type, amperage, and pathway of the electric current, the electric resistance on the path of the electric current, and the duration of contact.

When electric current passes through the human body, the degree of heat generated is in direct proportion to the square of electric amperage, tissue electric resistance, and the duration of contact.

Joule's law: $P = 0.24 I^2 Rt$

(P, heat generated; I, amperage; R, tissue electric resistance; t, time in second)

The greater the electric resistance, the greater the heat transformed by the electric energy and the more severe the burn. The epidermis has no blood vessels. When the skin is dry, the electric resistance may reach 100,000 Ω per square centimeter. As the corneous layer of the palm and plantar surfaces is rather thick, the electric resistance is also rather high. (The degree of electric resistance ranges from low to high in nerves, blood vessels, muscles, skin, tendons, fat, and bone respectively.) The thicker and drier the skin, the higher the electric resistance. After the electric current enters the human body, it follows the path of least resistance (i.e., the nerves and blood vessels). The tissue at the outlet of the electric current is also burned by the heat produced by the resistance of the tissue. When the resistance of the skin is high, the local burn is severe; when it is low, the local insult is milder, but the systemic damage may be very serious.

The body is less tolerant of alternating current than of direct current. Electric currents of low frequency (15 Hz–150 Hz), especially alternating currents of 50 Hz–60 Hz (city current) involve the greater risk, because the ions in the cells move back and forth following the pace of the alternating current, and the integrity of the cell is thus destroyed.

When electric current of 8 mA–12 mA enters the body, contractions of the muscles are induced. At that moment, the body may break away from the source of the current. When the current is above 20 mA, the skin may be carbonized very quickly if it is dry. If the current continues to increase, tetanic contractions of the muscles will be produced; if the current is still held by the hand there is no way to break away from it, and the consequences will be very serious (Fig. VIII.1a). Tetanic contractions of the muscles may also cause fracture of bones and dislocation of joints. When alternating current of above 25 mA passes through the heart, ventricular fibrillation or cardiac arrest may be induced. Cardiac arrest may also be caused by reflex of the vagus nerve or spasm of the coronary arteries. Besides the lesions mentioned above, atrioventricular block, ectopic cardiac rhythm, and supraventricular or ventricular tachycardia may also be caused. When electric current of above 100 mA passes through the brain, the victim will lose consciousness immediately. If the current is still larger, convulsions of the whole body may occur, and partial, transient, or permanent damage may be produced. When the current is between 200 mA and 1,200 mA, paralysis of the respiratory and circulatory centers may be produced directly. When the electric current passes through the abdomen, hemorrhagic necrosis of the viscera or even perforation of the hollow viscera may be caused.

1 Pathologic Features

1. The area of electric burn on the body surface may be small, but the extent of destruction of the deep tissues (especially the muscles) is much greater.

2. Electric burns usually have one inlet and one outlet (on rare occasions there may be more than one). The injury of tissues at the inlets is often more serious than that at the outlet(s) (Fig. VIII.1b), manifesting as carbonization of the skin and necrosis of large pieces of muscle. Large amounts of sodium and water sequester under the skin and into the necrotic muscles, forming massive edema around the inlet. Owing to the fact that the body serves as a volume conductor, at regions where the cross section is small (such as extremities of limbs), the density of the electric current is higher and the heat generated greater than in the regions with larger cross sections (such as the trunk). Consequently, the injury inflicted is more serious. As dispersion of heat of the deep tissues is slower than that of the superficial layer, "sandwich necrosis" is produced. That is to say, blood circulation of the superficial muscle belly is good, while the deep muscle belly, in contrast, is necrotic; or on the same muscle, the proximal end of the muscle belly is necrotic, while blood circulation of the distal end is good (Fig. VIII.2). Electric injury is usually accompanied by electric arc or electric flash burn.

3. As the electric resistance of the blood is low, electric current may easily pass through the blood vessels, and necrosis of the endothelial and muscular layers may be caused. In such an instance, the lumen of the vessel may be dilated or ruptured, causing hemorrhage. Angiography may show irregular stenosis or dilatation and even thrombosis of the vascular lumen. The latter may

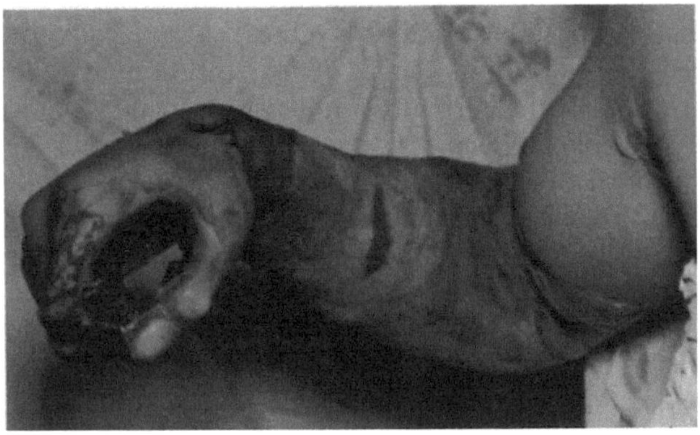

a

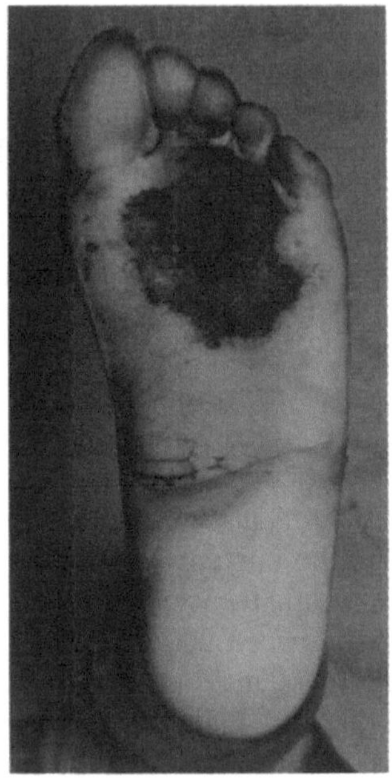

b

Fig. VIII.1. a Inlet of high tension electric burn. Since the current is held by the contractured hand, there is no possibility of breaking away from it. **b** Outlet in the same patient; injury here is less serious

extend toward the proximal end to cause secondary necrosis. This is the basis for resection of the involved blood vessels and replacement with autovascular grafts at the same time as the burn wound is repaired with pedicle skin flaps (replacement of burned radial and/or ulnar artery with great saphenous vein graft).

4. When electric current passes through the peripheral nerves, reversible injuries of the motor fibres may be caused. If the whole nerve is destroyed, the damage is permanent. Lesions of the peripheral nerves in the late stage are usually secondary to thrombosis and fibrosis of the tissues surrounding the nerves.

5. When the electric current passes through the head and face, especially around the eyes, unilateral or bilateral cataract and optic nerve atrophy may occur.

2 Treatment

Electric injuries are more often seen in young adults. Of 198 cases of electric injury admitted from 1958 to 1978, 42.9% of the victims were between 20 and 30 years old, with skin burns of 0.5%–70% of the BSA. In accordance with the limitation of civilian electric consumption to below 380 V in this country, electric injuries may be divided according to whether voltage was low or high. In this series, there were nine patients with low voltage injuries caused by alternating currents of 220 V–280 V and 18 with high voltage injuries inflicted by 380 V. The other 171 cases were injured by electricity of 1,060 V–

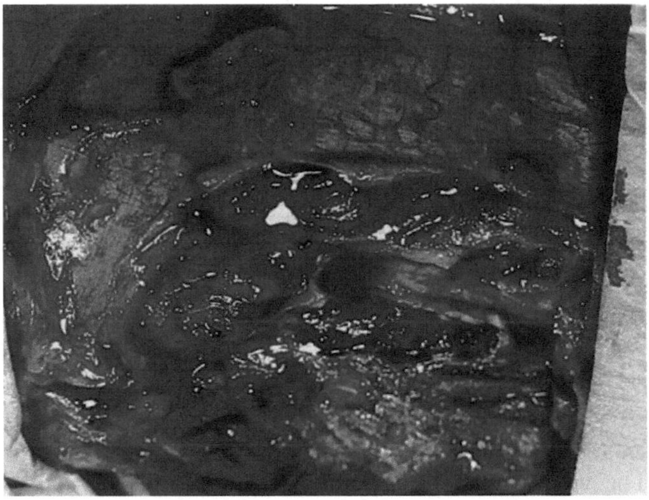

Fig. VIII.2. "Sandwich necrosis" of the muscles of an electric burn victim

35,000 V. In the low voltage group the average burn area was 2.56% of the BSA, with an average third degree burn area of 2.25% of the BSA. In the high voltage group the average burn area was 10.67% of the BSA, with an average third degree burn area of 7.5% of the BSA (Table VIII.1).

This denotes that so far as the surface area of the burn is concerned, there is not much difference between the high voltage and low voltage currents, but in regard to the destruction of deep muscles, high voltage injuries are far more serious than low voltage injuries.

Electric injuries of the upper limbs were more frequently seen: there were about 300 sites in our series (including one or more inlet and outlet), of which 152 were on the hands and 148 on the arms and forearms. There were 89 sites on the thighs and legs, 54 on the feet, 67 on the trunks, and 54 on the heads and faces.

Of the 198 cases of electric injury mentioned above, four died. One was an 8-year-old boy with high voltage injury involving third degree burns to 70% of the BSA. He died of wound sepsis 4 days postburn. Another case was a 45-year-old male whose head and face were injured by high voltage

Table VIII.1. Levels of amputation in 84 electric burns

No. of cases	Level									
	Disarticulation of shoulder; partial resection of scapular	Disarticulation of shoulder	Arm	Disarticulation of elbow	Forearm	Disarticulation of wrist	Thigh	Disarticulation of knee	Leg	Foot
84	1	14	45	3	34	3	5	0	9	1

current. Exploration by craniotomy revealed a subdural hematoma and disseminated hemorrhage in the brain tissue. He died 11 days after injury. The third case was a 34-year-old female with high voltage injury of the head, accompanied by burns of the cranium and damage to the brain tissue. She died 2 days after injury. The last case was a male of 63. Before the injury he was afflicted with cor pulmonale. He died of respiratory failure 9 days after injury.

The majority of the electric injuries were accidents caused by contact with electric utensils. In children, most of the injuries were caused by accidental contact with high tension wires or induced by kite flying near high tension wires.

2.1 Early Care

2.1.1 Resuscitation

The victim must be separated from the electric current as soon as possible. After this is done, mouth-to-mouth resuscitation and cardiac massage should be performed immediately if respiratory and cardiac arrest have occurred.

For the purpose of separating the victim from the electric current, the main switch may be turned off or the current may be cut off using any available insulated instruments or other means on hand, but the victim should never be pulled off by hand before the current is cut off.

Since the central nervous system is stimulated strongly and injured by the electric current, respiratory and cardiac disturbances may be induced, resulting in electric shock. If the shock is light, only transient loss of consciousness or apnea will take place. If the shock is severe, respiratory arrest followed by cardiac arrest may occur. For respiratory arrest, mouth-to-mouth resuscitation is most effective. In cardiac arrest, immediate resuscitation by extrathoracic cardiac massage and artificial respiration should be performed simultaneously. The pulse rate should be taken on the carotid or femoral artery. When the pulse becomes palpable and the lips of the patient turn pink, it shows that cardiac massage is effective. If extrathoracic massage produces no effect, open cardiac massage should be performed. As soon as the patient is admitted to the hospital, tracheal intubation should be performed and respiration should be maintained on a respirator.

Artificial respiration and cardiac massage may sometimes take 3 h–6 h or even longer. If EKG shows ventricular fibrillation, defibrillation should be carried out.

All of the above-mentioned patients in whom electric shock had occurred were admitted to the hospital after resuscitation had been performed at the place of injury.

2.1.2 Fluid Replacement in the Shock Stage

The amount of early fluid replacement depends upon the extent of the muscles burned. For patients with small low voltage burns, replacement of fluids is not necessary. When the patient is burned by high voltage current, large pieces of muscles are destroyed and large amounts of hemoglobin and myohemoglobin are released, causing serious hemoglobinuria and myohemoglobinuria. In such a case, an hourly urinary output of more than 50 ml is required; consequently solute diuretics may be given to promote rapid urinary excretion of hemoglobin and myohemoglobin.

2.1.3 Prevention of Tetanus and Other Anaerobic Infections

Owing to the fact that there is necrosis of deep tissues as well as cutaneous lesions of inlets and outlets in electric injuries, tetanus occurs much more easily than in thermal burns. Therefore routine tetanus antitoxin and toxoid should be administered. Among five cases of electrically injured patients, anaerobes were found in four. Mainly for the effective control of anaerobic infection, large doses of penicillin should be injected for 7–10 days following electric injury until all necrotic tissue has been cleared.

2.1.4 Early Decompression Incision of the Deep Fascia

As there is necrosis of large pieces of muscle under the deep fascia, the subfascial tension is exceedingly high owing to the accumulation of *sequestered* fluid and will easily cause compression necrosis. Therefore on admission decompression incision of the eschar and the underlying deep fascia should be made down to the muscle layer. Incision of the deep fascia will not only improve local circulation but also facilitate direct observation of the extent of necrosis. If the whole limb is edematous, yet the skin burn wound is small, a longitudinal incision needs to be made on the normal skin through the inlet.

The wound should be exposed after debridement.

2.2 Management of the Wound

We insist on early excision of the necrotic tissue. The appearance and elasticity of the tissue, the contractility of the muscle, and the condition of bleeding may be used during the operation to judge the viability of the tissues. Immediate tissue section using a cryostat and observation by means of a light microscope may also be used to assess the tissue viability and thus determine the amount to be excised. Pale edematous muscles with contractile response and bleeding on cutting and showing the presence of transverse striae on biopsy should not be excised: They may gradually recover to normal under the cover of healthy tissues. Sometimes, in order to avoid exposure of joints or important nerves and vessels, the necrotic tissue is not excised all at once. It is possible to wait for the formation of basal granulations, and skin may be transplanted after the necrotic tissue has spontaneously separated and cast off.

In the series of 198 cases of electric injuries mentioned above, debridement was performed 345 times and transplantation of skin 404 times. In patients admitted during the early stage, the first debridement was usually performed within 1 week after injury. The wounds were covered with autografts, allografts, or xenografts. Electric injuries of the hand, wrist, forearm, or elbow were repaired with pedicle skin flaps (including adjacent flaps, abdominal flaps, and cross-over forearm flaps; abdominal flaps were most frequently used). If, in electric injuries of the wrist, the extent of muscle excised is not large and the proximal end of the radial or ulnar artery is intact, the wound may be repaired by transplantation of free skin flaps.

2.2.1 Electric Injuries of the Hand

The hand is the most frequent site of electric injuries. In the series of 198 cases, there were 141 cases of hand injuries (71%), most of which were caused by contact with high voltage electricity. In such cases the finger and the wrist became spastically flexed and the source of the current was so tightly grasped that it was not possible for the victim to break free. The current arced through the wrist and the palm, and necrosis of the carpal flexor muscles was produced in many patients (necrosis of musculus pronator quadratus was not uncommon). The median nerve was also injured. After emergency debridement the defect was first repaired with an abdominal flap; tendon was transplanted at a second stage. In this way the function of the hand may be preserved to a certain extent.

2.2.2 Electric Injuries of the Limbs

Owing to necrosis of large pieces of muscle, the incidence of limb amputation was very high. Amputation at various levels was performed in 84 of the 198 cases (excluding amputations of fingers and toes). The indication for the amputation of limbs is total destruction of the limb or abundant necrosis with infection or wound sepsis threatening the life of the victim. When there are many inlets in an injured limb, debridement should be commenced from the most proximal inlet before a decision with regard to amputation is made. Furthermore, if amputation is needed, the level can only be finally decided after the most proximal inlet is explored. Of course, if amputation is not indicated after debridement of the most proximal inlet, other inlets should be debrided in order until a decision can be made.

After electric injury, the level of muscle necrosis far exceeds the level of skin burned. If palpation shows the consistency of the area proximal to the skin burn to be hard, edema has occurred following necrosis of the muscle. An incision should then be made at the uppermost point of the skin injury for the exploration of deep tissues. As progressive thrombosis often takes place in the blood vessels after electric injuries, progressive necrosis of the tissues may also occur. Even after amputation or after debridement with complete excision of the local necrotic tissue, progressive tissue necrosis may still occur if transplantation of skin flaps or vessels was not performed. Debridement then has to be performed once more.

If the brachial artery is already exposed or buried in the necrotic muscles after electric injury of the upper limb, the axillary artery and vein should be ligated: A sloping incision is made from the lateral third of the clavicle toward the anterior axillary fold and is carried down to the greater pectoral muscle. The muscle fibers are separated by transverse splitting. The lateral border of the smaller pectoral muscle is then identified. The axillary artery and vein are found posterior to the smaller pectoral muscle and are ligated separately after careful dissection.

If the axillary artery has been destroyed and the peripheral soft tissues are necrotic, the subclavicular artery and vein have to be ligated. For the operation, the head of the patient is turned to the contralateral side, with the arm adducted. The shoulder is depressed. Pulsation of the subclavicular artery can then be felt at the junction of the posterior border of the sternocleido-mastoid muscle and the clavicle. This is the third, most superficial portion of the subclavicular artery. An incision of about 6 cm in length is then made along the clavicle down to the periosteum from 1 cm medial to the posterior border of the sternocleidomastoid muscle to the junction of the middle and lateral third of the clavicle. An H-shaped incision is made in the periosteum to secure subperiosteal exposure of the clavicle. Four inches of the clavicle is then resected with a Gigli's wire saw. The subclavicular muscle is transected. On the upper border of the resected clavicle, the pulsation of the subclavicular artery can be felt easily. The sternocleidomastoid muscle is pulled upward and inward with a right-angled retractor. The subclavicular artery is exposed by blunt dissection and double ligated with no. 7 silk by the use of an aneurysm needle. The vein is ligated below the superficial portion of the artery. The operative wound is closed in appropriate layers. In some patients, the supra-scapular vein is rather large and can be seen crossing the operative field. Sometimes it may be mistaken for the subclavicular vein. The suprascapular vein should be ligated and sectioned to expose and ligate the subclavicular vein.

2.2.3 Electric Injuries of the Thoracic and Abdominal Walls

If electric injuries of the thoracic wall involve the ribs and intercostal muscles, debridement should not be performed in the early stage in order to avoid open pneumothorax. It is better to wait for the spontaneous separation of the eschar and the appearance of new granulation tissue; transplantation of skin is then performed to eliminate the wound surface. If the whole layer of the thoracic cage is necrotic and open pneumothorax has already occurred, the wound should be tamponed with vaseline gauze. Air in the chest should be aspirated by puncture in the uninjured region. After the pleural cavity has adhered to the thoracic wall and necrotic tissues have been gradually removed, skin may be grafted onto the granulation surfaces of the lung, the diaphragm, and even the perirenal adipose tissue.

When the cutaneous and muscular layers of the abdominal wall are necrotic, skin may be grafted onto the peritoneum after debridement. If the peritoneum is also necrotic, it may be excised and replaced with omentum, on which skin may be grafted.

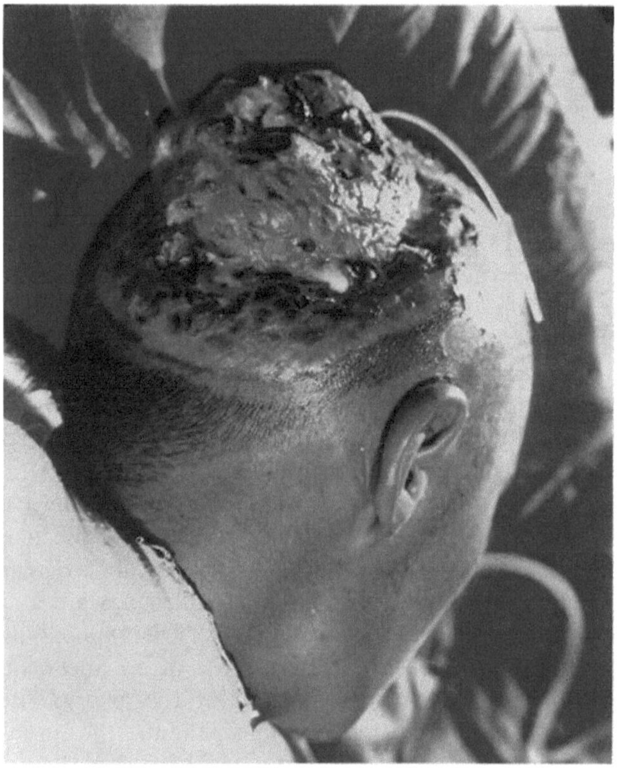

Fig. VIII.3. High tension electric injury; the cranium, dura mater, and part of the brain tissue were burned. Herniation of the brain occurred, and the right lateral ventricle is exposed. Autoskin was grafted onto the brain. The patient survived

2.2.4 Electric Injuries of the Cranium

When the cranium is injured by electric current, the entire layer of soft tissue becomes necrotic and dead bones are exposed. After excision of the necrotic bones, adjacent skin flaps may be transposed to eliminate the wound surface (cf. Chap. VII).

When the entire layer of the cranium is necrotic and there are burns of the dura mater, the necrotic dura mater should not be excised during the acute stage. If excised, herniation of the damaged brain will inevitably occur, leakage of the cerebrospinal fluid and infection of the cerebral parenchyma will take place, and the life of the patient will be threatened. If decompression is required to bring down the elevated intracranial pressure, the site must be in the uninjured region. If brain parenchyma is already adherent to the normal dura mater, and there is already infection underneath the necrotic dura, then the necrotic dura together with the necrotic tissue beneath it should be excised and free skin grafts transplanted to seal the wound surface (Fig. VIII.3).

Case Illustration. Male, aged 22. There were third degree electric burns to 3% of the BSA. Symptoms of elevated intracranial pressure appeared: headache, vomiting, etc. Solute diuretics produced no effect. On the following day the necrotic cranial bones were removed, and pus accumulation was discovered beneath them. After the purulent fluid was drained off, the necrotic tissue was excised. There was extensive leakage of cerebrospinal fluid with herniation of the brain tissue. Hemiplegia of the right side appeared between the 26th and 29th day after injury, and aphasia occurred on the 30th day. The patient was transferred to our hospital on the 32nd day, at which time the defect in the cranial bones measured 9 cm in diameter, crossing the median line. There was a large amount of cerebrospinal fluid leakage. Thirty-seven days postinjury the amount of herniated brain tissue increased, and headache was very severe. Papillary edema of the optic nerves was observed. After removing the herniated brain and freeing the dura mater, the defect was repaired with fascia of the temporal muscle, and the cranial defect was covered with a transposed skin flap from the frontal region. Hemiplegia and aphasia gradually disappeared and the patient survived.

2.2.5 Electric Injuries of the Joints

When electric injuries involve the joints (with the exception of joints of the fingers and toes), peripheral soft tissue, muscles, bony elements, and articular bursa are destroyed by burns. The joints are exposed and pyogenic arthritis may occur. If the necrotic tissues are completely excised, the drainage of the joints is adequate, and intraarticular infection is not severe, then the joints may preserve a certain degree of functional movement after healing takes place.

Case Illustration. Male, aged 24. There was electric injury of the right hand and left knee, with 5% of the BSA affected by third degree burns. On admission the femoral condyle was exposed and the articular bursa was ruptured with an outflow of cloudy fluid. During debridement the eschar of the knee and the necrotic m. vastus medialis were excised. The necrotic medial condyle of the femur was chiseled off down to normal bony elements. During exploration of the cavum articulare, edematous and congested synovial membrane was observed and the semilunar cartilage was found to be intact. The cavum articulare was irrigated by continuous dripping of antibiotic solution. By the time 18 days had elapsed granulations had flourished around the knee, and split-thickness graft was transplanted onto the granulation tissue. In a follow-up study 1 year later the movement of the knee joint was found to have totally recovered.

---

3 Complications

In this section we wish to discuss some specific or common complications of electric injuries. Of the 198 cases mentioned above, the following complications occurred in 140, i.e., 70.7% (Table VIII.2).

Table VIII.2. Complications in 198 cases of electric burns

Complication	No. of cases	Complication	No. of cases
Loss of consciousness	102	Cardiac arrest	5
Respiratory arrest	33	Premature beats	3
Brain edema	4	Intestinal obstruction, perforation	2
Brain hemorrhage	1	Acute renal failure	1
Cerebral herniation	1	Tetanus	1
Spinal injury	1	Gas gangrene	3
Peripheral nerve injury	18	Severe anemia	2
Secondary hemorrhage	20	Cataract	1

3.1 Complications Involving the Central Nervous System

Of 136 patients with central nervous system complications (patients may suffer from more than one symptom or sign), 102 suffered from transient unconsciousness and recovered spontaneously. Thirty-three patients had respiratory arrest and loss of sensibility at the time of injury; this was usully for a short time only, but in individual cases respiratory arrest lasted as long as 6 min. The condition of four patients with electric injuries of the head was complicated by brain edema, and the longest time required for complete elimination of the edema was 7 days. There was one case of cerebral hemorrhage. In this patient, disseminated hemorrhage of the parenchyma of the right frontal lobe and subdural hematoma of the right frontal portion were demonstrated by surgical exploration on the 3rd day after injury. The patient died 11 days after injury. One case was complicated by cerebral herniation, resulting in infection, hemiplegia, and aphasia. One patient suffered paraplegia induced by spinal medullary trauma and gradually recovered after 1 month.

3.2 Secondary Hemorrhage

In the above-mentioned series of patients, 20 suffered from secondary hemorrhage. The main cause was postinjury necrosis and infection of the intimal and medium layers of the arteries. The hemorrhage often occurred during the 3rd week after injury. At this time the necrotic tissue gradually separated from

Table VIII.3. Sites of secondary hemorrhage

Sites	No. of cases
Axillary artery	1
Radial artery	13
Ulnar artery	2
Digital artery	2
Brachial artery	1
Artery of the abdominal wall	1
Total	20

the wound surface and the blood vessels surrounded by the infected necrotic tissue or exposed were easily ruptured. As such arterial hemorrhage may cause loss of a large amount of blood, it must be managed by emergency treatment. Table VIII.3 shows the arteries involved in secondary hemorrhages after electric injuries.

In order to avoid exposure of the blood vessels in the necrotic tissue during the initial debridement, they should be *embedded* in the healthy tissue. If no healthy tissue can be found around the blood vessels, they should be ligated at the level of the healthy tissue. If oozing of blood is noticed afterward, the dressings should be removed for careful examination and the bleeding vessels ligated.

3.3 Peripheral Nerve Injuries

Electric injuries are often seen in the median, radial, and ulnar nerves.

3.4 Anaerobic Infection

In this series, there was one case complicated with tetanus and three with gas gangrene. When gas gangrene is encountered, debridement must be performed promptly, and large doses of penicillin, Chloromycetin, or clindamycin should be injected. The wound should be treated with hydrogen peroxide, Dakin's solution, or zinc peroxide. Serious cases should be treated by hyperbaric oxygen.

We found that use of the evacuation replacement technique for culturing anaerobic bacteria significantly increased the incidence of positive cultures from the deep necrotic muscles: of five cases cultured, four were positive. Besides various species of *Clostridium*, which are most often encountered, we have also isolated various species of *Peptostreptococcus*, and Propionibacterium.

3.5 Cardiac Arrest and Arrhythmia

Cardiac arrest and arrhythmia after electric injuries are related to direct electric stimulation of the myocardium. In our series, all patients with cardiac arrest and premature beats recovered after emergency treatment.

3.6 Ileus and Perforation of the Intestines

One patient with electric injury of the abdomen complicated by ileus and perforation of the intestine was cured surgically. A fecal fistula, which healed spontaneously, was found in another patient with electric burn of the abdominal wall.

3.7 Acute Renal Failure

The one patient in whom acute renal failure occurred was cured by thorough debridement of the electric injury wound and excision of the necrotic tissue followed by allograft coverage and peritoneal dialysis.

3.8 Severe Anemia

There were two cases of severe anemia. In one of them anemia occurred 2 months postinjury. Although repeated blood transfusions were given, the hemoglobin level could only be maintained at 7 g%. It was not until more than 100 days afterward that it recovered to 10 g%.

3.9 Cataract

There was one case of cataract, which occurred between 3–6 months after injury. The patient's eyesight was partially restored after surgical intervention.

Chapter IX Chemical Burns

LIU YUE-LIANG and TANG SHEAN-SHII

Translated by LING LI-LI

Chemical substances may damage the skin and tissues, causing chemical burns. If heat is produced during a chemical burn, the severity of burn of the tissues will be aggravated. However, this kind of burn differs from the thermal burn caused directly by flames or burning hot liquids.

The degree of severity of chemical burns depends upon the nature, concentration, quantity, penetrative power, mode of action, and duration of contact of the causative chemical substances and upon any absorption of the chemicals from the wound surface leading to poisoning. Locally, there may be oxidation, reduction, erosion, cytotoxic action, dehydration, and blister formation.

Over a period of 20 years 427 patients with chemical burns were admitted to our hospital, accounting for 10.04% of burn patients admitted during this period. Among these 427 patients, there were 112 cases of acid burns (26.22%), 235 cases of alkali burns (55.04%), 68 cases of burns by other chemicals (15.93%), 3 cases of chemical burns associated with explosive injury (0.70%), and 9 cases of chemical burns of unknown nature (2.11%). Four hundred patients (93.7%) were cured, and 27 (6.3%) died. The main causes of death were wound sepsis (16 cases), chemical poisoning (5 cases), and burn shock (3 cases). The average surface area of burn in the fatal cases was 59.16% of the BSA, including third degree burns to 22.21% (Table IX.1).

Sometimes chemical burns display discoloration of the skin with the appearance of a superficial burn, but actually the whole layer of skin is damaged and even the subcutaneous tissue may be involved. The incidence of complications is high in patients with chemical burns; the fatality rate of cyanide poisoning is exceedingly high. In the present series of burn patients there were 11 cases complicated by acute renal failure, five of which were caused by chemical poisoning.

Table IX.1. Cause of death in 27 cases of chemical burn

Cause of death	No. of cases
Wound sepsis	16
Septicemia	1
Cemical poisoning	5
Shock in the early stage	3
Acute renal failure	1
Respiratory (lower respiratory tract burn) failure	1

Washing with a large amount of running water is necessary in acute chemical burns, except when the causative agent is one of a few particular chemicals. The washing will remove or dilute the poisonous substances and prevent the chemicals from further damaging the skin and being absorbed through it. Some chemicals may produce a certain amount of heat when in contact with water, but the heat often disperses with the washing. It is therefore much better to wash continuously with a large amount of running water than to use neutralizing agents alone. The duration of continual washing depends on the nature of the burn. For ordinary chemical solvents, it is necessary to wash for at least 10 min; in burns by chemicals with strong actions, washing for 30 min or longer is required. Neutralizing agents may be applied locally after the washings; they should be washed off with water immediately after their application. In burns of the head and face, cleansing of the eyes, nose, ears, and oral cavity demands especial attention, and the eyes, in particular, should be washed first. Isotonic saline may be used if available. Special drugs for emergency management of burns caused by the common chemicals are listed in Table IX.2. Debridement demands removal of exogenous dirty substances and trimmed off the broken epidermis. Titanium tetrachloride (a fumigant) may cause burns if it contaminates the skin. After hydrolysis, titanium tetrachloride will form hydrochloric acid and liberate a large amount of heat. Therefore skin splashed with titanium tetrachloride should not be washed with water immediately after injury. The contaminating liquid should be soaked up with cloth (or paper) as quickly as possible; the wound may then be thoroughly washed with water; if this procedure is not followed, the surface area of the burn will be enlarged.

Measures for detoxication should be taken immediately after burns by poisonous substances. Special emphasis should be placed on diuresis in burns by poisonous substances which are excreted through the kidneys in order to enhance their elimination and prevent damage to the kidneys.

The amount of fluid administration in the shock stage of chemical burns is about the same as that in ordinary burns. The amount of fluids replaced in acid burns should be less than the standard amount, while in alkali burns, it should approach or should be more than the standard amount. If it is necessary to expedite the elimination of poisons through the kidneys, the amount of fluids administered may be increased, and, at the same time, diuretics should be given to increase the urinary output for rapid elimination of the poisons.

1 Acid Burns

Burns by sulfuric acid and nitric acid account for 76% of acid burns; the others are caused by hydrofluoric acid, phosphoric acid, chromic acid, perchloric acid, chlorosulfonic acid, nitrous acid, and acetic acid.

Different kinds of acid react with the skin to form different kinds of proteinaceous coagulum; therefore the color of the scab or eschar in acid burns varies with the nature of the acid involved. For example, nitric acid burn gives a yellow color; sulfuric acid, black or brown; hydrochloric acid, white or grayish-brown; and carbolic acid (phenol), light gray or light brown. Following contact

Table IX.2. Special drugs for emergency treatment in chemical burns

Chemical substances	Specific medication for emergency
Sulfuric acid, nitric acid, hydrochloric acid, trichloroacetic acid	2%–5% sodium bicarbonate solution, magnesium oxide, soap water
Chromic acid	5% sodium thiosulfate solution and ointment
Hydrofluoric acid	5% sodium bicarbonate solution, magnesium oxide paste, calcium salts
Oxalic acid	Calcium salts
Ammonia water, sodium (potassium) hydroxide	0.5%–5% acetic acid, 5% ammonium chloride, 10% citric acid
Lime	0.5%–5% acetic acid, 5% ammonium chloride, 10% citric acid (used after the powder has been wiped off and washed with running water)
Yellow phosphorus	Washing with potassium permanganate 1:5,000 solution, wound surface lightly washed with 1% copper sulfate, removal of the phosphorus particles
Cyanides	Washing with potassium permanganate 1:5,000 solution, wet dressing with 5% ammonium sulfide
Bichromates	2%–5% sodium bicarbonate solution, 10% calcium disodium edetate, 7% potassium monohydric phosphate aqueous solution, 18% disodium phosphate, water
Phenol	Washing of wound surface with 10% ethyl alcohol, or ethylene glycol, wet dressing with saturated solution of sodium sulfate
Metallic sodium	Local excision and covering with oil
Mustard gas	Covering with oil

with the skin, the acid may cause cellular dehydration and coagulation of proteins; therefore in an acid burn the wound surface is dry with clear demarcation and less swelling.

Owing to the coagulation of proteins caused by acid burns, the pathologic changes usually do not involve the deeper layers (except in hydrofluoric acid burn), and scab, essentially of a deep second degree, is usually formed. Of the 112 cases of acid burn, only three had a third degree burn area exceeding 30% of the BSA, while in the majority of cases it was below 5%. The second degree scab in an acid burn resembles the eschar in gross appearance, color, and consistency, and this special feature of acid burns must be kept in mind before operation. However, third degree burns are also easily formed when a long period of contact with concentrated sulfuric acid or nitric acid occurs in sites with scanty subcutaneous tissue, such as the anterior part of the tibia, the dorsum of the foot, and the toes. Even bone necrosis may occur. Generally speaking, if the scab is dark colored, firm like leather, and markedly dehydrated, the burn is third degree.

Table IX.3. Comparison between 12 cases of acid burn and 11 cases of thermal burn in terms of the amount of colloid and electrolyte solutions administered and urinary output during the first 24 h postburn (all patients were cured)

	Average total BSA burned (%)	Average BSA with III° burns (%)	Amount of colloid and electrolyte solutions given (ml/1% BSA burned/kg)	Hourly urinary output (ml)
Acid burn	42.1 ± 18.8	11.8	1.23 ± 0.39	97.8 ± 49.8
Thermal burn	38.7 ± 13.8	6.7	1.75 ± 0.37	59.7 ± 35.4
P value			$P < 0.01$	$P < 0.05$

In acid burns, the wound surface is dry, the infection is mild, and the scab does not undergo lysis or slough off readily. In occasional cases the duration of sloughing of the scab may be as long as 2 months. Wound-healing Ointment No. 10 may be applied to the wound surface to accelerate sloughing of the scab (see Chap. III).

Swelling is mild in acid burns, and there is very little exudation from the wound surface; therefore the amount of fluid administration in the shock stage should be reduced accordingly. The required amount of colloid and electrolyte solution administered during the first 24 h postburn is generally only 1 ml per 1% of the BSA burned per kilogram body weight. (Table IX.3.)

After swallowing strong acids by accident, there are usually traces of burn in the vicinity of the lips, and there may be edema and ulceration of the buccal, esophageal, and gastric mucosae, and even perforation of the esophagus or stomach. Egg white, milk, soybean milk, starch porridge, and milk of magnesia may be taken orally. However, gastric lavage is forbidden, and sodium bicarbonate should not be given by mouth as this can cause gastric distension and subsequent perforation. If vapor or smoke dust of strong acids is inhaled, 2%–3% sodium bicarbonate solution may be used to wash the buccal and nasal cavities and to rinse the mouth. Tracheotomy should be performed in patients with respiratory distress.

1.1 Sulfuric Acid, Nitric Acid, and Hydrochloric Acid

Sulfuric acid is a rather strong dehydrating agent. When it comes into contact with the skin, sulfuric acid will form a "dry, hard, and coagulating eschar" differing from the "liquefying eschar" of alkali burns. Furthermore, sulfuric acid may form an indolent erosive surface, damages the tissues, and produces a considerable amount of heat during the burn reaction, causing severe pain. The systemic complications of taking sulfuric acid by accident consist of shock, edema of the glottis, suffocation due to laryngeal edema, and perforation of the viscera.

Concentrated sulfuric acid will produce heat when in contact with water; therefore it must be particularly emphasized that the amount of water used in washing must be copious to dilute the sulfuric acid and to disperse the heat produced.

1.2 Hydrofluoric Acid

Hydrofluoric acid may cause progressive tissue necrosis locally. In severe cases, ulcers may fail to heal; if not promptly treated, the damage may penetrate deep into the bones, leading to aseptic necrosis. Usually there is no sensation of pain at the time of contact, but unbearable pain appears several hours later. Therefore, the burn is often neglected in the early stage. 10% calcium gluconate may be administered intravenously, or calcium may be introduced by local galvanic current ion transfer. The calcium ions will react with hydrofluoric acid to form calcium fluoride. This will not only alleviate the pain, but also prevent tissue destruction and damage to the bone. Paste made of glycerin and magnesium oxide (2:1) may be used for topical application.

1.3 Oxalic Acid

Oxalic acid may combine with calcium to cause devitalization or "poisoning" of the cytoplasm of cells. Following contact with oxalic acid, the skin and mucosa will show white, indolent erosions. Besides immediate washing with running water, calcium gluconate should be injected locally and intravenously. Hypocalcemia may appear if oxalic acid burns over a considerable surface area are not treated in time.

1.4 Chromic Acid

Chronic chromic acid poisoning may cause erosion and perforation of the nasal septum. When taken by accident orally, chromic acid may cause severe gastroenteritis, muscular spasm, cyanosis, respiratory distress, shock, coma, and toxic nephritis with glycosuria. The skin contaminated by chromic acid will show proteinaceous coagulation with erosions and blister formation, and the skin surface appears yellowish. In improperly treated burns caused by chromic acid and dichromates, the chromium ions will be absorbed through the wound surface, leading to systemic poisoning. Treatment consists of washing with water, 5% sodium thiosulfate, or monophosphate and diphosphate buffer solutions

$$[7\%\ KH_2PO_4\ (70\ g):18\%\ Na_2HPO_4\ (180\ g):H_2O\ (850\ ml)].$$

A 10% solution of calcium disodium edetate may also be used for washing the wound surface to lessen the absorption of chromium ions.

There were three cases of chromic acid burn in this series. The largest burn area was 85% of the BSA. There were no symptoms of poisoning in any of these cases, and all the patients survived.

1.5 Chlorosulfonic Acid

Chlorosulfonic acid is dissociated into sulfuric acid and hydrochloric acid when it comes into contact with water; this will cause more severe burns than the ordinary strong acids.

2 Alkali Burns

The commonly seen alkali burns are those due to caustic alkali (potassium hydroxide or sodium hydroxide), lime, and ammonia water. We admitted 235 patients with alkali burns (55.04% of all chemical burns). Of these 235 cases, 48 were caused by caustic alkali, 167 by lime, and 20 by ammonia water.

The alkali can dissolve protein and collagen, forming alkaline protein compounds; it can also saponify fat and causes cellular dehydration of the tissues. The heat produced during saponification will cause further necrosis of the deeper tissues. Consequently the depth of burn in the early stage is often underestimated, and when it is reestimated in the late stage the surface area of third degree burn is often found to be greater than originally estimated.

Edema is marked during the shock stage of an alkali burn, with extensive loss of fluids. Of the patients with chemical burns, 17 showed hypovolemic shock on admission, and 15 of these patients had alkali burns. Their average total burn area was $53.6\% \pm 23.8\%$ of the BSA. Therefore, if the total burn area exceeds 30% of the BSA in patients with alkali burns, attention should be paid to the possible occurrence of shock due to insufficient fluid replacement. The clinical condition and urinary output must be kept under close watch.

In the first-aid management of alkali burns, the use of neutralizing agent should be avoided before washing with running water in order to prevent aggravation of the burn by the heat produced by neutralization. After washing with a large amount of running water, weak acids, such as vinegar, lemon juice, or orange juice, may be used for neutralization. Early tangential excision of eschar and grafting should be performed in deep burns.

2.1 Caustic Alkali

Owing to the strong penetrative power of the caustic alkali, burns are usually deep and edema is marked. There is more chance of infection and wound sepsis.

2.2 Lime

The depth of burns caused by lime usually exceeds deep second degree, and the wound surface is rather dry. In the management of such burns, the lime powder must first be wiped clean; washing with a large amount of running water may then be carried out. This will prevent aggravation of the burn by the heat produced by the contact of lime with water.

When the buccal or nasal cavities are involved in an alkali burn, 0.5%–5% acetic acid, 2% boric acid, or 5% ammonium chloride solutions may be used for rinsing the mouth or cleansing the nasal cavities.

2.3 Ammonia Water

Ammonia is an irritative gas and belongs to the category of strong alkali. Ammonia water is the aqueous solution of ammonia, i.e., ammonium hydroxide.

It is alkaline, with ammonia forming approximately 20% of its content. Prolonged contact with mucosa or skin will produce burns. The cause of burn is usually an accidental fall into an ammonia water reservoir which is not well equipped for protective purposes. Skin burn caused by ammonia water is usually superficial second degree. Seventeen of the 20 cases in this series belonged to this category. With one exception (an adult), all were children from 1 to 8 years old. Burns caused by ammonia water may also occur in factories producing chemical fertilizers; three cases in this series (young workers aged 18–24 years) belonged to this category.

Of the 20 patients burned by ammonia water, only seven had superficial burns of their body surfaces. The largest burn area was 12% of the BSA.

Ammonia water is highly volatile and irritative. Inhalation of a large amount of highly concentrated ammonia water may cause laryngeal spasm and burns of the respiratory tract. The clinical manifestations of mild respiratory tract burns are hoarseness, increase of respiratory rate, mild "depression triad," scanty secretions from the mouth and nose, and dry rales over the lungs. The respiratory distress usually ameliorates 24 h later; the pathologic changes are mild and limited mainly to the upper respiratory passages. The majority of burns by ammonia water (13 cases) were respiratory tract burns of moderate degree with signs of respiratory distress. The depression triad is marked, dry rales of the lungs are widespread, and there is a large amount of secretion in the respiratory tract. Between 3 and 6 days postburn a large amount of frothy secretion and desquamated necrotic mucosa may be aspirated through the opening created by tracheotomy. At the same time, edema of the bronchiolar mucosa subsides, followed by amelioration of the respiratory distress. Severe cases of respiratory tract burn have the following manifestations: abrupt increase of respiration rate to 50–60 per minute, cyanosis of the lips, toes, and fingers, dry and moist rales scattered all over the lung fields, wheezing sounds, extreme respiratory distress which cannot be relieved by tracheotomy, and a large amount of frothy secretion in the respiratory passages. Chest roentgenograms reveal "pulmonary edemalike" shadows of infiltration. Continuous use of artificial hibernation mixtures is often needed, supplemented by physical hypothermia measures for 3–7 days to reduce oxygen consumption during this period. Usually the respiratory distress shows gradual improvement as the necrotic tracheal mucosa sloughs off, but there may be an increase in the respiration rate because of residual pulmonary inflammation. This kind of dyspnea usually alleviates after 1–2 weeks.

Intravenous administration of dexamethasone 5 mg–20 mg daily after burns of the respiratory tract caused by inhalation of ammonia may be of some help in reducing the edema of the mucosa of respiratory passages and in decreasing the secretions.

In cases with a history of inhalation of concentrated ammonia, signs of respiratory tract burn in the buccal, nasal, and pharyngolaryngeal mucosae, and marked respiratory distress, tracheotomy should be performed as early as possible. After inhalation of ammonia the patency of the airway should be maintained, and a large amount of secretion in the airway and sloughing pseudomembrane may be sucked out through the tracheotomy opening. If this is not done, the necrotic intratracheal pseudomembrane will slough off 2–5 days postburn, causing obstruction of the airway and subsequent asphyxia. Furthermore, frequent aerosol inhalation may help in humidification, dilution, and drainage of the sputum. Continuous aerosol inhalation may be performed if necessary.

Case Illustration. Male, aged 2. The child fell into a boat loaded with ammonia water. There were burns of the buccal and nasal mucosae, conjunctivae, and cornea. He was admitted 3 h postburn, at which time the respiration rate was 60 per minute and the heart rate, 174 per minute. The child was fretful and had difficulty in inspiring. Depression triad was marked, there was a large amount of secretion from the mouth and nose, and moist rales and wheezing sounds were widespread over both lungs. Tracheotomy was performed immediately, but there was no amelioration of the depression triad. Tracheal secretion was still abundant, requiring frequent suctioning. The child was still fretful, and corticosteroids, artificial hibernation drugs, and inhalation from an ultrasonic nebulizer were given. On the 4th day postburn the respiratory distress was extremely severe, with the appearance of nodding and elevation of shoulders, and there was a large amount of tracheal secretion. On the 4th and 5th days, three pieces of desquamated mucosal fragments of the trachea were sucked out and the respiratory distress was reduced with disappearance of the depression triad on the 6th day. The tracheal cannula was removed on the 12th day. Chest roentgenograms still showed chemical pneumonia. The patient was discharged in good condition on the 15th day postburn.

---

3 Agents Causing Chemical Burns Associated with Systemic Poisoning

Some chemicals can be absorbed through the skin or respiratory tract, thus causing systemic poisoning. Among the 427 cases in this series, there were 31 cases of burns caused by poisonous substances; 13 cases in this category (41.95%) were associated with chemical poisoning, and six (19.36%) ended fatally. The poisonous substances causing systemic poisoning are: phenol, yellow phosphorus, organic phosphorus, carbon disulfide, cyanides, diazodiisobutyl nitrile, and ammonium sulfide.

3.1 Phenol

There were seven cases of phenol burn, with four cases associated with systemic poisoning; two case ended fatally. The cause of death in both cases was phenol poisoning, and the burn surface areas were 13% and 50% of the BSA. Phenol is corrosive. Light gray or light brown scab may be formed following contact of the skin with phenol, and the skin becomes firm and thickened. The wound surface is dry with well-defined margins, and swelling is not marked. Pain and numbness may be felt locally. Phenol can be absorbed through the wound surface, causing tubular necrosis of the kidneys, and may be complicated by acute renal failure.

The wound surface should be wiped repeatedly with 10% ethyl alcohol, or ethylene glycol immediately after burn until the smell of phenol on the wound surface disappears completely. 5% sodium bicarbonate or saturated sodium sulfate solutions may then be used for neutralization, and the local wound surface should be covered with vaseline gauze. Simultaneously with the management of the wound surface, energetic measures should be taken to enhance rapid elimination of the phenol with the urine. Solute diuretics may be used in addition (mannitol 3 g per kilogram body weight within 24 h) to the administration of large amounts of fluid. The hourly urinary output during the 1st day postburn should be maintained at about 200 ml.

Case Illustration. Female, aged 19. The patient had a phenol burn to 50% of the BSA. She was transferred to our hospital 1 h and 45 min after the injury. On admission, the catheterized urine was brownish and smelled of phenol. The estimated amount of urinary phenol was 1,665 mg per liter (the normal value being 12.4 mg per liter). Rapid intravenous instillation of 500 ml dextran and 250 ml of 20% mannitol was performed. The wound surface was wiped repeatedly with alcohol immediately after admission until there was no smell of phenol on the wound surface and on the gauze used to wipe it. Wet dressings of saturated sodium sulfate solution were then applied. The wound surface was once more lightly wiped with soap water 16 h postburn, followed by the application of wet dressings of saturated sodium sulfate solution. During the first 24 h postburn the amount of fluid replaced was 6,290 ml, and the urinary output, 5,992 ml. The total amount of phenol excreted within 24 h was 14.4 g, and the color of the urine gradually turned from brown to pink. At the end of the first 24 h the color of the urine was already light yellow, and the estimated amount of urinary phenol was 11.66 mg per liter. On the 2nd day postburn, liver function and kidney function tests were performed. Except for a 37% excretion of phenolsulfonphthalein in a 4-h PSP test, the other results were all within normal ranges. The patient survived.

In cases of phenol burn complicated by renal failure, early peritoneal or blood dialysis may be a life-saving measure.

Case Illustration. Female, aged 20. The patient sustained phenol burns to 39% of the BSA; there were associated burns of the lower respiratory tract and phenol poisoning. A large amount of alcohol was used for wiping the wound surface immediately after the burn. Upon admission, dry rales and wheezing sounds could be heard over both lungs. Tracheotomy and catheterization were performed, and the catheterized urine smelled of phenol.

The patient had oliguria after the injury. The specific gravity of urine was fixed at 1.013–1.015, and blood urea nitrogen increased. The diagnosis of acute renal failure was made. Peritoneal dialysis was started from the 2nd day postburn

Table IX.4. Relationship of fluid replacement and urinary output during the first 3 days postburn in the above-mentioned case

Days postburn	Fluid replacement			
	Amount of coloid (ml/1% BSA burned/kg)	Electrolyte solution	Average hourly urinary output (ml)	Amount of 20% mannitol or 25% sorbitol used (ml)
1	0.6	0.7	60	450
2	0.31	0.5	28	550
3	–	–	12	510

and stopped on the 8th day postburn. The polyuric phase started on the 14th day. One month after the burn, serum NPN and urea nitrogen levels were 26.9 mg% and 16.5 mg% respectively. The patient survived.

Table IX.4 illustrates that although the hourly urinary output reached 60 ml during the 1st day, it was still not sufficient to eliminate the phenol accumulated in the body. Therefore, in order to save a patient burned by phenol, large amounts of fluid should be replaced with a large dose of solute diuretics. The hourly urinary output should be maintained at about 200 ml during the 1st day.

3.2 Yellow Phosphorus

There were 11 cases of burns caused by yellow phosphorus, including one fatal case. (This patient was burned by phosphorus in its gaseous form; 99% of the BSA was burned, including third degree burns to 94.5% of the BSA. The cause of death was septicemia.) Three of the cases were complicated by toxic hepatitis, but all were cured.

Yellow phosphorus is insoluble in water, but it is soluble in various kinds of oils. It will undergo spontaneous combustion when exposed to an atmosphere of 34 °C. Bluish-green phosphorescence may be seen in a dark environment. The burning phosphorus granules may be incarcerated in the skin and continue to be oxidized and to combust. Therefore phosphorus burns are usually rather deep. Phosphorus is oxidized in the air into phosphorus pentoxide, and the latter will hydrolyze to form phosphoric acid. Consequently a phosphorus burn causes damage to the tissues through the joint action of chemical and thermal forces. A second or third degree burn wound is usually formed. The patient experiences severe pain. Absorption of yellow phosphorus through the wound surface may result in severe damage to the liver and kidneys.

In first-aid management at the site of accident, the wound should first be washed with a large amount of water followed by meticulous removal of the phosphorus granules, which should be placed in water after removal to prevent recombustion. The wound surface should be dressed with wet cloth before transfer of the patient to medical units. On the way to hospital it is important not to allow any contact between the wound surface and the air. On arrival at the hospital the dressings should be removed and the wound surface should be immediately washed once more with 1:5,000 potassium permanganate solution and then wiped lightly with 1% copper sulfate solution. The surface of the residual phosphorus granules will react with copper sulfate to form black cupric phosphide granules. The latter will form a coating on the surface of phosphorus so that the phosphorus is isolated from the air. The cupric phosphide granules should be removed from the wound surface as soon as possible. Lastly, it is necessary to use physiologic saline to wash off any copper sulfate solution remaining on the wound surface; if this is not done, copper sulfate may be absorbed through the skin, causing copper poisoning. The manifestations of the latter are vomiting, diarrhea, acute hemolytic anemia, and acute hepatic or renal failure in severe cases. Therefore copper sulfate should not be used in large amounts, and it is even more important not to use copper sulfate solution for wet dressings to the wound surface. If copper sulfate solution is not available, the phosphorus granules with their bluish-green fluorescence may be removed in a dark room.

The wound surface of minor phosphorus burns may be excised or tangentially excised in the emergency room, but wounds with a large surface area should be exposed or dressed with dry gauze. Oily dressings are prohibited to prevent dissolving and absorption of the phosphorus.

Case Illustration. Male, aged 42. The patient had yellow phosphorus burns to 55% of the BSA, including third degree burns to 2% of the BSA. The burned part was immersed in water immediately after injury, followed by washing and soaking in a large amount of 2% copper sulfate solution. The patient was admitted 2 h postburn. After admission, the necrotic epidermis was trimmed off with scissors and the wound surface was dressed with dry gauze. On the next day the sclerae became icteric, and the patient complained of discomfort over the upper abdomen. He had nausea, vomiting, and enlargement of liver to one finger's breadth below the costal margin. The liver continued to enlarge to two fingers' breadth below the costal margin on the 2nd day postburn. The cephalin-cholesterol flocculation test, thymol turbidity test, zinc sulfate turbidity test, and serum glutamic pyruvic transaminase test were all normal. The direct van den Bergh reaction was positive. The total bilirubin was 8 mg%. Under local anesthesia, the second and third degree wounds were tangentially excised and allograft was transplanted. The clinical condition improved on the 4th day postburn, and jaundice disappeared on the 7th day postburn. The acute hemolytic jaundice in this patient was due to the prolonged use of a large amount of 2% copper sulfate solution.

In an experimental study of animals with phosphorus burn, Ben-Hur (1972) reported on the local application of a mixture composed of 2% copper sulfate, 5% sodium bicarbonate, and 1% hydroxyethyl cellulose with the addition of 1% 12-lauryl sulfate. The chemical reaction is as follows:

$$H_3PO_4 + NaHCO_3 + CuSO_4 \rightarrow CuHPO_4 + NaHSO_4 + H_2O + CO_2.$$

Following the aforementioned treatment, the phosphorus granules were coated with the black $CuHPO_4$ or $CuPO_3$. The addition of 12-lauryl sulfate will reduce the surface tension of the phosphorus granules, thus achieving complete coating. The use of hydroxyethyl cellulose is to prevent the precipitation and absorption of copper salts. The various biochemical data (blood phosphorus, blood urea nitrogen, creatinine, electrolytes, glutamic pyruvic transaminase, urea clearance test, etc.) in animals with experimental phosphorus burn gave similarly good results to those in the control group.

Shortly after absorption of phosphorus through the skin, all patients show vomiting and severe gastrointestinal symptoms. Melena is frequently seen. The liver may show fatty degeneration and even acute atrophy.

Poisoning due to absorption of the phosphorus may also cause signs of renal damage such as hematuria, oliguria, cylindruria, and increase of amino acid and lactic acid in the urine. The liver and kidneys should be protected by the following measures: use of appropriate medicinal herbs; administration of a high caloric, high protein, low fat, and high vitamin diet; and use of vitamin K, γ-aminobutyric acid, glucose, and an appropriate amount of solute diuretics.

In very extensive burns caused by yellow phosphorus, the vomitus and feces of the patient should be properly disposed of and measures regarding isolation of the medical personnel taken. Failure to do so may lead to absorption of the phosphorus in vapor phase (with a garlic-like odor) through the mucosa of the respiratory passages, causing symptoms of poisoning in the attending medical personnel. Improper disposal of the phosphorus granules removed may also contaminate the bedding.

Case Illustration. Male, aged 28. The patient was burned by yellow phosphorus. The wound was covered with a wet sheet immediately, but no further measures were taken. He was hospitalized 30 min after the injury. On admission the patient was extremely restless (shouting with terror), with tremor of the extremities. White smoke fumed from his clothing, hair, and skin unceasingly, producing a foul smell of garlic. There were massive burns of the skin of the head, face, neck, trunk, and extremities. The burned area appeared pale and leatherlike in consistency. Eighty percent of the BSA was burned, including deep second degree burns to 10% and third degree burns to 70%. After admission, the whole body was immediately washed with soap and water, 4% sodium bicarbonate solution, and 1% copper sulfate solution. The phosphorus granules were removed. However, the skin still fumed white smoke continuously, and fire balls of the size of a fist sprang up twice in succession. Wet dressings of 4% copper sulfate solution were applied to the whole body. The wound was exposed on the next day. The patient died on the 4th day after injury.

During the course of resuscitation some of the medical personnel suffered from dizziness, salivation, oppression of the chest, and vomiting. The bedding still gave off a foul garlic smell after the death of the patient. One of the nurses also showed symptoms of phosphorus poisoning while she was disposing of the bedding. (The aforementioned information was kindly furnished by the Shao Kuan District People's Hospital, Canton Province.)

3.3 Organic Phosphorus

There were two cases of burns caused by organic phosphorus in this series; one of these cases (in which 89% of the BSA was burned) was associated with poisoning. Both patients were cured.

The wound surface contaminated by organic phosphorus should be lightly wiped several times with soap and water and then flushed with a large amount of physiologic saline. Hot water and rubbing with alcohol must be avoided. Contamination of the eye should be treated by continuous irrigation with 2% sodium bicarbonate solution or physiologic saline for at least 10 min.

Case Illustration. Male, aged 21. The patient sustained burns caused by organic phosphorus of 100 °C; 89% of the BSA was burned, including third degree burns to 24.5%. There was associated poisoning by organic phosphorus, and the patient suffered from vomiting. Fluid administration and intravenous injection of 2 mg atropine were performed, and the patient was admitted during the 14th hour postburn. After admission, 1 mg atropine was given every 30 min intravenously. During the 19th hour postburn, respiratory distress occurred. The neck was rigid, there were convulsive contractions of both upper extremities, the pupils were dilated, heart beat and respiration stopped. Extrathoracic cardiac massage, artificial respiration, and intravenous injection of atropine were carried out, with restoration of heart beat and respiration. Before each attack of convulsive seizure or stoppage of respiration, contraction of the pupils appeared; and there was then an increase of laryngeal secretions and rales over the lungs, followed by irregular breathing and subsequent stoppage. A total amount of 47 mg atropine and 1 g pralidoxime chloride had been given between the 14th and 34th hour postburn. The patient's face was flushed, the pupils were 0.8 cm in diameter, the tongue was dry and curled, and the patient was fretful. The rales over the lungs disappeared on auscultation, and the clinical condition became stable. The dosage of atropine was reduced to 0.5 mg every 2 h by intravenous injection. A total amont of 57 mg atropine and 3 g pralidoxime chloride was given within 80 h postburn. The patient became quiet. The diameter of the pupils was 0.5 cm, with positive light reflex. The use of antidotes was then discontinued. Antishock treatment and energetic management of the wound surface were employed simultaneously during the course of resuscitation. The patient survived.

3.4 Cyanides

The cyanides enter the body through the alimentary tract, respiratory tract, and the burn wound. They combine with the oxidized form of cytochrome oxidase and interrupt its reduction, thus inhibiting the redox mechanism of the cytochromes, causing the so-called cellular asphyxia. The blood still has a bright red color because cyanides only inhibit the usage of oxygen, not its content. Paralysis of the respiratory center is the usual cause of death. The cyanides are extremely poisonous. The greater part of the cyanides absorbed by the human body is expired from the lungs in the form of hydrogen cyanide, which gives the expired air an odor of bitter almonds; the rest is transformed in the liver to form thiocyanates which are eliminated through the urine.

Following contact with cyanides, the patient shows symptoms of irritation of the upper respiratory tract, dizziness, headache, tinnitus, and weakness. These symptoms are followed by oppression of the chest, palpitation, dyspnea, hypertension, arrhythmia and heart block, constriction of pupils followed by dilatation, exophthalmos, a sensation of terror, and indifference. Very soon the patient becomes comatose, with convulsions, syncope, both fecal and urinary incontinence, hypothermia, loss of sensation and reflexes, shallow and slow breathing, and, finally, cessation of respiration and cardiac arrest. Timely and efficient resuscitation may prevent aggravation of the condition.

Cyanide poisoning runs a very rapid course and death occurs within a few minutes. To achieve resuscitation, the patient may be forced to inhale amyl nitrite repeatedly at the site of injury and during transport. After admission, 3% sodium nitrite 10 ml–20 ml may be slowly injected intravenously (at a rate of 2 ml–3 ml per minute; excessively rapid administration may cause a fall in blood pressure). Following administration of sodium nitrite, 25 ml–50 ml of 25%–50% sodium thiosulfate may be injected intravenously, and injection of these drugs (at half or full dose) may be repeated within 1 h if necessary.

The wound surface of the burn may be washed initially with 1:1,000 potassium permanganate, followed by application of wet dressing with 5% ammonium sulfate solution.

The purpose of using amyl nitrite and sodium nitrite is to reduce the hemoglobin to methemoglobin, which combines with the cyanide ions to form the relatively stable cyanomethemoglobin. But the cyanomethemoglobin is again decomposed gradually in a few minutes to liberate cyanide ions. In order to form the less toxic thiocyanates by the combination of cyanide ions with sulfur, sodium thiosulfate should be injected simultaneously as an antidote.

There were four cases of cyanide burn in this series; one was associated with poisoning and ended fatally. The fatal case involved burns to 20% of the BSA. The patient was admitted to the hospital 15 min postburn with cessation of respiration and loss of reflexes. After emergency endotracheal intubation had been performed, assistance of respiration was started. After intravenous injection of 10 g sodium thiosulfate, 6 ml of 1% methylene blue, and 10 ml of 3% sodium nitrite, the patient's respiration again become spontaneous. His weak and slow heart beat became stronger, and the heart rate increased to 100–120 per minute. The dilated pupil constricted to 3 mm in diameter. Urinary volume increased after mannitol infusion and some of the reflexes recovered. Another 10 ml of 3% sodium nitrite and 2 g sodium thiosulfate were injected 2 h 45 m postburn. After the second injection the terminals of the extremeties turned cyanotic. No further antidotes were given. The patient's condition deteriorated, and he died 11 h and 20 min after the injury.

From the above case we can see that the cyanides can be absorbed from the burn wound and cause acute poisoning. The chief drugs used, sodium nitrite and sodium thiosulfate, seemed effective. The cyanosis appearing after the second injection of sodium nitrite cannot be regarded as a contraindication for the further application of antidotes: we certainly made a wrong decision in this respect in this case.

In the present series there were two cases of burns caused by organic cyanides, and both were associated with poisoning. One of the patients died. The burn was due to an explosion accident which caused inhalation of diazo-diisobutylnitrile, tetramethyldinitrile (product of the former after heating), and hydrogen cyanide. The patient who survived was a male aged 41 with burns to 77% of the BSA, including third degree burns to 15%. The patient who died (27 h after injury) was also a male (aged 40); he had burns to 70% of the BSA, including third degree burns to 10%. The poison acts chiefly on the nervous system. In the early stage the patient showed excitement manifested as muscular tremor, convulsions, and spastic contracture: he then showed mental inhibition with respiratory distress, finally leading to coma. Both of these patients were male, and the surface area and depth of burn were similar; however, the amount of poison inhaled by the patient who died was greater, and the symptoms of poisoning were considerably more severe. It should be noted that the organic cyanides may be decomposed continuously during the explosive combustion, producing a small amount of inorganic cyanides. The result of estimation of the urinary thiocyanate suggested that the amount of inorganic cyanides in the body was small. Analysis of the poisonous substances in the skin and necrotic tissue also indicated that there was no further absorption of the poison through the skin and no clinical manifestations of exacerbation due to reabsorption of the poisonous substances.

Antidotes should be given as early as possible after the injury. If hypovolemic shock is already present clinically, sodium nitrite should not be used because of its hypotensive action. Sodium thiosulfate should be used as the chief antidote during the shock stage. Sedatives should also be used as early as possible although, artificial hibernation mixtures are more effective and their adminstration may be repeated 6 h later if it is necessary to keep the patient quiet.

3.5 Carbon Disulfide

Carbon disulfide is mainly absorbed by inhalation, but it can also be absorbed through the skin and the alimentary tract. After inhalation, 5%–10% of the inhaled carbon disulfide is transported to various organs via the blood circulation. Between 70% and 90% of the carbon disulfide in the form of inorganic sulfates participates in metabolism. Less than 1% is eliminated with the urine in its original form and 10%–30% is eliminated from the respiratory system in its original form.

The symptoms of mild cases of acute carbon disulfide poisoning are rather similar to drunkenness: headache, dizziness, nausea, staggering gait, etc. In severe cases, excitement appears first, followed by delirium, coma, and even death. After a severe episode of acute poisoning there may be such sequelae as headache, insomnia, nightmare, and weakness, constituting the neurasthenic syndrome; in some patients there may be neurologic symptoms.

There is still no specific antidote for acute carbon disulfide poisoning. The patient should first be placed in a well-ventilated location to accelerate elimination of the poison from the respiratory passages. The wound surface of the burn should be washed immediately with soap and water and physiologic saline. Hypertonic glucose, mannitol, or sorbitol may be given intravenously to enhance excretion of the metabolic products (inorganic sulfates) from the urine and to prevent the possible occurrence of cerebral edema. If respiratory failure and cerebral edema appear, appropriate emergency measures should be taken.

Case Illustration. Female, aged 38. The patient was burned and poisoned by carbon disulfide. There were burns to 50% of the BSA, including third degree burns to 18%. On admission the patient complained of dizziness and oppression of the chest which was ameliorated the next day after administration of a large amount of vitamins and coenzyme A. The patient developed a cough on the 4th day. Starting from the 5th day, she had nausea, intermittent vertigo, nightmares, insomnia, and muscular tremor. Starting from the 9th day postburn, shouting, psychic symptoms, convulsions, and increase of muscular tension developed. The pupils contracted during convulsions. The traditional Chinese medicine, "calculus bovis balls," and γ-aminobutyricum were given, and the patient became mentally clear and survived.

3.6 Mercury

Mercury itself does not cause burn but painting of the wound of extensive burns with mercurochrome by mistake may cause acute renal failure. We encountered a case of this nature. The urinary mercury estimated quantitatively amounted to as much as 610 mg per liter, and the urine showed yellowish-green fluorescence. The main antidotes for mercury poisoning are:

1. Sodium dimercaptopropansulfonate: The mercapto radical will combine firmly with the mercury ions and they may be excreted together. In acute poisoning, the initial dose in adults is 2 ml–3 ml of 5% solution by intramuscular injection. It is followed by 1 ml–2.5 ml every 4 h–6 h; 1–2 days later the dosage may be reduced to 2.5 ml once or twice a day. The course of treatment depends on the clinical condition of the patient and the quantitative estimation of the urinary mercury content. Usually the treatment should last for about 1 week.

2. Sodium dimercaptosuccinate: 1 g–2 g may be given daily intravenously (slowly) or intramuscularly. The whole course of treatment lasts for 3–5 days. Another course may be given after an interval of 3–4 days. The aqueous solution of this drug is unstable, increasing in toxicity when left to stand for a long period. Consequently it should be freshly prepared before use.

4 Other Chemical Burns

4.1 Magnesium

Burns caused by magnesium are rarely seen. The magnesium may penetrate into the deep-lying tissues if it is not removed from the skin in time. It reacts with the tissue fluids in the subcutaneous tissue to form magnesium oxide and liberates hydrogen, causing local formation of emphysematous herpetic lesions and massive necrosis simulating gas gangrene which heal slowly. The ulcers formed by the magnesium are small initially, but they enlarge gradually several weeks later. Some ulcers are undermined with irregular bases; red granulomatous nodules may appear, and the ulcers heal slowly. After a magnesium burn, the wound surface should be tangentially excised or excised under local anesthesia so as to remove the magnesium together with the necrotic tissue, thus preventing delayed healing of the wound surface. If the magnesium is absorbed through the skin or inhaled, respiratory symptoms, nausea, vomiting, chills, or high fever may occur.

4.2 Tar

The greatest surface area in 11 cases of burns caused by hot tar was 90% of the BSA; not one case was associated with poisoning.

Tar is the residue after fractional distillation of coal tar and petroleum. There are four kinds of tar, namely coal tar, petroleum tar, oil-shale tar, and natural tar. Coal tar contains the greatest amount of volatile substances and causes the greatest damage; petroleum tar and oil-shale tar contain the least amount of volatile substances and cause less damage; natural tar does not contain any volatile substance and is not harmful to the human body.

Burns caused by attachment of hot liquid tar to the skin are not associated with chemical injuries; strictly speaking, they are thermal burns. However, hot liquid tar attached to the skin is not easily removed. If a large amount of gasoline or ether is used for washing, not only will the wound surface be damaged, but the gasoline or ether may also be absorbed and cause poisoning. Therefore, removal of the hot tar may be delayed until the shock condition is more or less rectified. The best method of removal is to wait until natural cooling or hardening of the tar occurs after the application of ice; the hardened tar may then be removed with the burned epidermis en bloc. The part of the epidermis which has not been burned and the wound surface of a first degree burn may be wiped lightly with gasoline or ether for a longer period.

5 Chemical Burns of the Eye

When chemical substances (solid, liquid, or gaseous) come into contact with the eye, chemical reactions with the tissue of the eye will occur, causing damage. Varying degrees of damage to the tissue of the eye may be produced according to the nature, concentration, and duration of contact of the chemical substances.

Besides the acid and alkali burns most commonly seen, other organic chemical compounds such as alcohol, ether, aldehyde, and benzene and inorganic chemicals such as ammonia, sulfur, cyanide, mercury, and arsenic may also cause burns of the eye.

1. *Acid burn:* After contact of acidic substances with the tissue of the eye, the tissue protein coagulates to form a pseudomembrane. The latter may prevent the residual acid from permeating into the deeper layers of the tissue; therefore burns of the eye caused by acids are usually milder than those caused by alkali.

2. *Alkali burn:* After contact of the alkali with the tissue of the eye there will be saponification of the fat of the latter, with lysis of protein and liquefaction necrosis of the tissue. The residual alkali may continue to permeate into the deeper layers, causing damage to the inner part of the eyeball. Animal experiments have indicated that alkali of high concentration may cause desquamation of the corneal epithelium, edema, and turbidity of matrix, followed by ulceration and even perforation. The alkali may also enter into the anterior chamber after passing through the conjunctiva, cornea, and sclera and causes change in the composition of the aqueous humor. It may also cause iritis, with the production of fibrinous exudate which covers the posterior surface of the cornea, corners of the anterior chamber, the iris, and the surface of the lens.

It is important to give immediate treatment after a chemical burn of the eye. Every second counts. Generally, irrigation should be performed for 10 min, with the eyeball rotating during irrigation. Any solid remnants, such as small particles of lime, should be removed. Topical anesthetics may be given for alleviation of pain.

In severe cases of acid or alkali burn, the anterior chamber may be aspirated to remove the chemicals which have entered the anterior chamber together with the aqueous humor. The aqueous humor may be aspirated repeatedly if necessary. In cases with severe conjunctival burn but without necrosis of the sclera, the burned conjunctiva may be excised and autografted with healthy bulbal conjunctiva or mucosa of the mouth. This operation can serve to remove the residual chemical substances which are impregnated in the burned conjunctiva, to improve the blood supply of the pericorneal vascular network, and to prevent adhesions of the palpebral conjunctiva. For control of infection, polymyxin B or gentamicin solution in the form of eye drops or ointment may be used. A mydriatic may be necessary to prevent iritis and iritic adhesions. Subconjunctival injection of autoblood, instillation with autoserum, or instillation with cystine and cysteine may be carried out.

If it is necessary to remove calcium ions from the cornea after a lime burn, 1%–2% edetate (EDTA) solution may be used as eyewash or for instillation.

Local instillation of cortisone may be used for inhibition of inflammatory reaction. Subconjunctival injection of vasodilators may improve the local blood circulation.

Chapter X Burns Complicated by Trauma

LI YING-YU

Translated by YANG CHIH-CHUN

Sometimes burns are complicated by other traumas. A comprehensive case history must be taken immediately after admission. If a history of suspected trauma is given or evidence of concomitant injury is revealed by corresponding symptoms or signs or the severity of the patient's general condition does not coincide with the burned area and the depth of burns, further investigations, including close observation and various diagnostic measures, should be taken.

Certain traumas (e.g., intracranial injury or internal hemorrhage) have an insidious onset. Diagnosis is usually made too late in the middle of the course of disease. Thorough and comprehensive physical examination followed by repeated checks are necessary for early diagnosis. Blast injury, electric injury, and falling from a height constitute the three main causes of trauma (Table X.1). With regard to the consequences, fracture and soft tissue injury are the most frequently encountered (Table X.2).

There are a lot of therapeutic paradoxes when trauma is encountered. It is impossible to perform open reduction and internal fixation of unstable fractures through deep burn wounds. It is also impossible to turn the patient prone to expose his burned back when continuous perpendicular traction of multiple fractured ribs is needed. The amount of resuscitation fluid estimated according to budget formulae is always beyond the endurance of patients who have sustained coexisting intracranial injuries, etc. Dealing properly with these contradictions will ensure successful management of this category of patients.

Table X.1. Cause of trauma in 100 cases of burns

Cause	No. of cases
Blast injury	26
Electric injury	16
Fall	16
Others	42

Table X.2. Classification of 100 cases of burn complicated by trauma

Type of trauma	No. of cases[a]
Fractures	41
Soft tissue injury	41
Spinal cranial injury	24
Chest injury	3
Abdominal injury	2

[a] Some cases were complicated by more than one trauma.

1 Blast and Gas Explosion Injuries

1.1 Blast Injuries

Besides the fractures and intracranial and soft tissue injuries which may result from the blast, the blast wave itself can cause a series of pathologic changes. Much more fluid than normal is needed to help the patient survive the shock stage. Resorption is usually delayed. During the resorption period toxemia is extraordinarily severe, accompanied by a sudden fall in the white blood cell count with a marked leftward shift of the Schilling's count, and the incidence of onset of early fulminating septicemia is exceedingly high. These characteristics must be recognized beforehand in order to gain time with regard to treatment. Hypovolemic shock should be avoided. Systemic broad-spectrum antibiotics should be instituted at the beginning of the 2nd postburn day. Large doses of vitamins B_4, B_6, and B_{12}, and folic acid are recommended. The wound must be protected by silver sulfadiazine cream or by thorough exposure; deep wounds must be excised and grafted.

1.2 Gas Explosion Injuries

A 2,000 °C air current is usually generated after gas explosion. Owing to the high speed of the exploded gas, the period of contact of the hot air current with the human body is very short. Gas explosion usually creates a second degree burn. The blast wave may cause concussion of the brain, bone fracture, internal hemorrhage, or even rupture of the viscera. When a gas explosion occurs in a coal mine, large amounts of coal dust may be inhaled, causing asphyxia in severe cases. Emergency tracheotomy must be performed at the site of injury. During gas explosion, carbon monoxide, carbon dioxide, nitrous oxide, nitric oxide, and other trace noxious gases may be generated. Owing to the lower specific gravity of carbon monoxide, the heavier carbon dioxide and nitrous oxide usually sink to the bottom. Therefore carbon monoxide poisonings are rarely encountered in gas explosion disasters.

Burns caused by gas explosions in coal mines are far more severe than other blast injuries. Apart from the similar clinical manifestations to those of blast injury, gas explosion possesses several specific characteristics of its own: The burn wounds are usually badly contaminated, most of the patients reveal significant mental disturbances, and not a few patients have respiratory distress or even respiratory arrest. This kind of respiratory distress may be caused by brain concussion or brain tissue anoxia due to intoxication by noxious gases. The peripheral white blood cell count drops precipitously and the bone marrow picture shows transient suppression of the maturation of the marrow cells. The principle of treatment is the same as in the case of blast injuries. Owing to varying circumstances, the content and amount of noxious gases generated are different, and due to different methods of management the progress and the prognosis of various gas explosion injuries will also be different.

2 Craniocerebral and Spinal Injuries

Burns complicated by craniocerebral injuries are more commonly seen than burns complicated by spinal injuries. In the case of head injuries, mild cases only involve hematoma, contusion, or laceration of the scalp with slight concussion of the brain. In moderate cases, fracture of the cranium and contusion of the brain may occur. Open brain injuries, fracture of the base of the skull, subarachnoid hemorrhage, and intracranial hematoma etc. are found in very severe cases.

2.1 Diagnosis of Craniocerebral Injuries

Whenever intracranial injuries are suspected, meticulous observation and thorough neurologic examinations should be performed. Early diagnosis can only be made after repeated continuous and well-considered examination, observation, and analysis. X-ray of the skull, ultrasonic scan, computerized tomographic scan, or even an angiogram may be taken if the patient's general condition permits. The items of observation include:

1. The mental state of the patient. Is there a "lucid interval" following initial unconsciousness? Generally speaking, the level of consciousness reflects the severity of the craniocerebral injuries.
2. Pupillary changes, expecially the symmetry of pupillary size.
3. Sudden and pronounced changes of body temperature, pulse rate, respiration, and blood pressure.
4. Presence or absence of hemiplegia.
5. Presence or absence of pathologic reflexes.

After the diagnosis of craniocerebral injury has been established, the dynamic clinical situation should be assessed in order to infer the extent of intracranial pathologic changes.

2.2 Treatment of Craniocerebral Injuries

There are many problems in the early treatment of traumatic craniocerebral complications of burns. Whether the treatment of the burns or that of the craniocerebral injury is to receive priority should be decided only after concrete analysis. For instance, fluid infusion must be restricted in cases of craniocerebral injury to avoid brain edema. However, overrestriction of fluid infusion will be harmful if the burn area is extensive, fluid loss is tremendous, or the patient has hypovolemic shock or reveals symptoms of impending shock. Generally speaking, an extensively burned patient is not in a suitable condition to undergo major operation during the shock stage. But if there is progressive impairment of the state of consciousness, progression of neurologic signs, or evidence of increased intracranial pressure, which lead to the deterioration of the patient's general condition, emergency exploration should be performed. Blood volume should be maintained to guarantee a good tissue perfusion and at the same time the fluid administered should be restricted to prevent postoperative brain edema.

2.2.1 Early Treatment

1. Except in laceration of the scalp and in mild concussion of the brain, craniocerebral injuries are always accompanied by brain edema of varying extent. During the shock stage the principle of treatment is to restrict suitably the fluid intake, especially salt-free water, and to increase the proportion of the colloids accordingly. The guidelines in this respect are urinary volume, heart rate, blood pressure, and CVP. Sometimes posttraumatic brain edema will result in decrease of heart rate and increase of blood pressure, which may give the attending surgeon a false impression. Solute diuretics are usually prescribed to prevent and to combat brain edema.

2. The state of consciousness is an important criterion for assessment of the patient's clinical condition in craniocerebral injuries, but the use of analgesics during the early stage of treatment and the shock stage may impede observation of the mental state. If analgesics are mandatory, observation of other neurologic symptoms and signs is necessary. Morphine is contraindicated because it is too strong a central nervous depressant.

2.2.2 Principles of Treatment of Various Craniocerebral Injuries

1. *Simple fracture of the skull:* Unless it is complicated by extradural or subdural hemorrhage, a simple skull fracture is usually treated conservatively. Surgery is not indicated for closed depressed skull fractures unless localized untoward neurologic signs are revealed.

2. *Open brain injuries:* The principle of treatment of an open brain injury is to debride, repair, and close the wound as soon as possible. If there is no evidence of infection, the wound can be closed or partially closed by sutures. If there is evidence of infection the wound must be drained after simple debridement. Thorough debridement of a severely infected wound will inevitably lead to the spreading of infection. Systemic treatment is given to lower the intracranial pressure, to prevent infection, to protect the central nervous system from further injury, and to prevent the occurrance of various other complications.

3. *Fracture of the base of the skull:* Basilar skull fractures which extend into the nasal sinuses or mastoid cells are really compound fractures. Therefore prevention of infection in basilar fractures is of prime importance. CSF rhinorrhea and otorrhea indicate the existence of a pathway for spreading of infection into the subarachnoid space. If the leak does not seal spontaneously within 2 weeks after the institution of systemic antibiotics, surgical intervention may be considered.

4. *Concussion of the brain:* Concussion is the most frequent of the craniocerebral complications in burns. It produces no demonstrable permanent pathologic changes in the brain; only transient impairment of neural function is observed. Treatment *should* involve no more than analgesics and tranquilizers.

5. *Cerebral contusion or laceration:* Positive localized signs may appear (e.g., pyramidal signs, aphasia). Severe cerebral contusion or laceration is usually accompanied by fracture of the skull and secondary intracranial hemorrhage. Patients with such a condition must be placed under close observation. In

order to protect the central neurons from further damage, dehydrants are used to prevent and treat edema of the brain. Tracheotomy may be performed to ensure an adequate airway for unconscious patients or for those patients with sluggish coughing and laryngeal reflexes.

Case Illustration. Male, aged 32. During a blast accident at a furnace, a red hot steel bar hit the patient's midocciput region. The patient sustained burns to 20% of the BSA, including third degree burns to 4.5%. A history of transient loss of consciousness for a few minutes and bleeding from the mouth and nostrils was given. The patient was admitted 1 h after the injury. Immediately after admission the patient became extremely restless. About 1,000 ml of blood was lost from mouth and nostrils. Physical examination revealed soft tissue laceration, bruises of the face, and ecchymosis of the left eyelid and both conjunctiva. Asymmetry of the pupillary size and restriction of adduction of the right eyeball were noted. X-ray of the skull showed fracture of the occipital bone with the fracture line extending to the base of the skull.

During the early resuscitation period the heart rate was kept at 120–140/min and blood pressure at 110/80 mmHg–120/100 mmHg. Fluid intake was restricted to 2,590 ml (700 ml blood, 540 ml physiologic saline, 550 ml 5% and 800 ml 25% mannitol) for the first 24 h postburn and 550 ml (400 ml blood, 150 ml 20% mannitol) for the second 24 h postburn. No salt-free water was supplied. Urinary output was 901 ml and 855 ml respectively. Sudden respiratory arrest was observed at the beginning of the 3rd postburn day. Emergency tracheotomy was performed and artificial respiration instituted. Under artificial hibernation and local anesthesia, a burr hole was made at the occiput fracture site, and a hematoma measuring 8 × 1.5 cm evacuated. The patient's respiration then became spontaneous, and 10 h after the operation he became conscious. Bleeding from the mouth and nostrils gradually ceased. On the 7th postburn day (4 days after the operation) the patient suffered from high fever, fretfulness, severe headache, psychoneurotic disturbances and meningism. CSF culture revealed positive growth of *Pseudomonas aeruginosa*, and intrathecal instillation of 1.5–2mg polymyxin B for each time was carried out five times. CSF culture became negative on the 28th postburn day. Upper gastrointestinal bleeding occurred on the 17th postburn day and stopped after conservative treatment. The patient survived. The final diagnosis was burn complicated by blast injury, contusion of the brain, fracture of the base of the skull, and hematoma of the posterior fossa.

2.3 Spinal Cord Injuries

Spinal cord injuries are usually accompanied by other compound traumas. In open spinal cord injury, debridement should be carried out as early as the patient's general condition permits. The purpose of the operation is to remove loose bone chips, foreign bodies, blood clots etc., which may exert pressure on the spinal cord or nerve roots. In closed spinal cord injury, the patient must be strictly immobilized and placed under close observation.

High cervical spinal trauma usually accompanies craniocerebral injuries. One of our patients had high tension electric burns of the head and concomitant spinal cord injury. The level of paralysis ascended gradually, resulting in dyspnea and finally leading to respiratory arrest. Immediate tracheotomy and artificial respiration were performed. Skeletal traction was performed by means of "tongs" through the part of the scalp affected by third degree burns. The patient's respiration again became spontaneous. The level of paralysis descended gradually. All of the lost neurologic functions were regained 1 month postburn. The patient survived.

3 Fractures

Fractures, along with soft tissue injuries, were the most frequently encountered traumatic complication accompanying burns in our series of 100 cases (Table X.2). The incidence is higher in the lower extremities than in the upper extremities (Table X.3).

Burn itself exerts no effect on the time of healing of the fractures. If deep burns overlay the fracture site and early excision and grafting have not been performed, osteomyelitis is likely to occur and may even lead to non-union of the fractures.

During resuscitation and transportation of the patient, simple and provisional immobilization of the fractures must be carried out. The concomitant nerve and vascular injuries must be properly treated in the early stage of management.

The blood loss caused by fracture of the femur, comminuted fractures of the ilium, fracture of the lumbar spines complicated by retroperitoneal hematoma, etc. should be taken into account and should be added to the regimen of shock resuscitation fluid replacement.

3.1 Closed Fractures of the Extremities:

All burn wounds are more or less infected; therefore the lymphatic drainage of a deep burn wound overlying a fractured bone is not sterile. In case of unstable fractures, before complete coverage of the wounds of the fracture site, open reduction and/or internal fixation are contraindicated, and pins and wires for skeletal traction are only permitted to pass through the cortical bones. In stable fractures, after closed reduction, immobilization is achieved by means of bivalved casts which are most convenient with regard to change of dressings.

Table X.3. The fracture sites in 41 cases of burns

Fracture site	No. of cases
Lower limb	24
Upper limb	13
Mandible	2
Ribs (multiple)	2

A turning frame further facilitates skeletal traction, wound exposure, and change of dressings.

3.2 Open Fractures of the Extremities

If open fractures are overlaid or surrounded by deep burns, the ideal treatment is excision of the burn wound with immediate coverage by grafts. After debridement the exposed fracture sites must be covered with healthy soft tissues. Sometimes a remote freeflap or local rotational flap is mandatory to achieve immediate closure of the wound. Skeletal tractions are usually better than casts for fractures of the lower extremities. Local and systemic sensitive antibiotics must be administered.

4 Soft Tissue Injuries

Thin partial-thickness skin graft is readily "taken" by almost any kind of recipient area devoid of necrotic tissue. We have successfully grafted the surfaces of exposed kidney, liver, brain, pleura, peritoneum, and omentum. Therefore, after soft tissue injuries we are used to closing the open wound by skin grafting; this is especially so in the cases of wounds which cannot be sutured for healing by first intention and areas with loss of large amounts of soft tissue.

If the wound is surrounded by burns, it is liable to be infected after debridement and suturing. Consequently the burn tissue must be excised before approximation is attempted; alternatively, the wound ought to be left open or properly drained. In some cases involving loss of large amounts of soft tissue, the wound may still be covered immediately by allo- or autografts (meshed or nonmeshed) if, after debridement, (a) all necrotic tissue is removed, (b) the repair of vessels, nerves, and tendons is satisfactory, and (c) the wound is not badly contaminated. Sometimes a large amount of soft tissue is crushed, lacerated, lost, necrotic, has deep penetrating wounds, or involves important nerves, vessels, and tendons; it is not suitable to treat such a complicated wound radically during the climax of the shock stage. Primary debridement, such as irrigation, hemostasis, and removal of dead tissue and foreign bodies, may be carried out. After the shock stage is over, removal of the rest of the dead tissues and covering of the exposed vessels, nerves, and tendons with adjacent healthy tissue may be performed. If there is no healthy surrounding tissue, skin grafts may be applied directly onto the sheaths of the nerves or vessels. Under certain circumstances, debridement may be divided into stages, and skin grafting is performed simultaneously, i.e., the wound is covered step by step while the necrotic tissues are being gradually removed.

Case Illustration. Male, aged 22. A red hot steel bar penetrated through the root of the patient's left thigh, perineum, buttock, external genitalia, and anus. Colostomy was carried out during the shock stage. The patient was transferred to Rui Jin Hospital 10 days after the burn. On the 12th postburn day, with the patient under general anesthesia, necrotic muscles of the medial and posterior aspects of the root of the thigh were excised together with the overlying eschar. After removing the dead tissues, 4 cm of femoral artery was exposed. Sartorius and adductor muscles were used to cover the exposed vessel. Subsequent operations were performed on the 18th, 28th, and 31th postburn days including excision of the necrotic lesser trochanter of the femur, drainage of the pus pockets, excision of the dead hip-joint capsule (lower portion), split-thickness autografting and closure of the colostomy. Bony ankylosis of the hip joint resulted. The patient survived.

5 Hot Roller Burns of the Hand (Hot Roller Hand)

Once a hand is caught in a hot roller, the thermal insult to the hand is complicated by crush injury. This is a serious trauma which may result in very poor functional recovery. Since the hand is caught in the roller with the forearm in full pronation, the dorsum of the hand and fingers are usually involved. A few such patients suffered superficial burns, but the majority were deeply burned. In some of the cases, no gross soft tissue injuries were seen. Some had manifestations of lacerations of the skin, exposure of the subcutaneous tissue and of the underlying bones and joints, and possible fractures of the metacarpals or phalangeal bones.

When burns to the hand are associated with crush injury, the latter will further damage the already deranged vascular linings, causing exceptionally severe edema and vascular thrombosis. A copious amount of exudation may weep from the wound, and the local swelling may extend far up to the elbow joint. Patient will suffer from intractable pain.

If a hot roller hand is not treated appropriately, the injured vessels will gradually become thrombosed. The clinical manifestations are coldness of the fingertips, impairment of capillary refilling of the nail beds, cyanosis, and blackening of the fingers and finally necrosis of the fingers and the palm.

Formerly, various conservative methods of treatment were used. Whenever a patient with hot roller hand was admitted, after blocking the brachial plexus, the involved hand was exposed to a warm environment. Vasodilators, such as phentolamine methane sulfonate and tolazoline hydrochloride, anticoagulant, such as heparin, and antisludging remedies, such as low-molecular dextran and injection of *Salvia miltiorrhiza*, were employed. In certain cases hyperbaric oxygen therapy was given. Such treatment was believed to be beneficial, yet no controlled studies had been carried out. Recently we have adopted a more aggressive and constructive method for the emergency care of hot roller hands. The primary debridement includes the radical excision of all the necrotic tissue. The fingers are sutured together to form a single block of tissue. An abdominal flap is prepared to cover the whole raw surface created. The fingers are separated in another operation after detachment of the pedicle. Five hot roller hands were treated according to the above method, and satisfactory functional results were achieved.

6 Trauma of the Chest and Abdomen

In chest trauma, not only the soft tissue of the chest wall but also the underlying bones, pleura, lungs, vessels, and heart may be involved. Usually the situation is very complicated, and sometimes there is coexisting intraabdominal contusion or rupture of viscera.

Fracture of the ribs is the most frequent complication. The fractured ends may penetrate the pleura, lungs, or vessels, causing pneumothorax (sometimes tension pneumothorax), hemothorax, or hemopneumothorax. This may disturb the normal respiratory and circulatory functions.

6.1 Rib Fractures

The ribs most commonly fractured are nos. 4–7. For simple fractures, only intercostal nerve block and analgesics are needed. In the case of double or multiple fractures in more than one rib, emergency measures must be taken to correct paradoxical chest wall movement and mediastinal flutter. Internal fixation of the fractured ribs or external traction is mandatory. Cuffed endotracheal tube insertion and assisted ventilation by use of a respirator are the best ways to secure optimal respiratory functions.

6.2 Pneumothorax

Pneumothorax may occur following laceration of the lung tissue. In very rare cases it may result from hyperinflation of the lung during burn injury. If the pneumothorax does not affect respiration, it may be left alone for the gradual spontaneous resorption of the air to take place. If the amount of leaked air is sufficient to cause collapse of the lung and shifting of the mediastinum, needle aspiration of the air is indicated.

Tension pneumothorax inevitably causes mediastinal temponade and seriously interferes with ventilation and cardiac function. A thoracostomy tube must be inserted for closed drainage. If the chest wall is burned, we usually first excise the burn eschar and graft the wound and then insert the thoracostomy tube and instill sensitive antibiotics into the pleural cavity.

6.3 Hemothorax

The pulmonary circulatory pressure is relatively low. If the bleeding is caused by laceration of the lung tissue, it may stop spontaneously. If there is massive intrapleural bleeding, rupture of the systemic (e.g., intercostal) vessels is likely to be the cause. A thoracostomy tube must be inserted for evacuation of blood and instillation of antibiotics. Aspiration by needle is usually inadequate. If active bleeding is suspected, emergency thoracotomy, hemostasis, insertion of a thoracostomy tube, and close drainage should be performed.

6.4 Abdominal Injuries

In the case of rupture of the viscera, the fluid replacement budget must include the estimated extra blood loss. If the laparotomy incision must pass through the burn wound, sensitive antibiotics should be instilled into the peritoneal cavity at the end of the operation.

Case Illustration. Male, aged 35. A red hot steel bar hit the patient's left flank, resulting in burns to 41% of the BSA, including third degree burns to 12.5%. A history of coma for 30 min–40 min was given. Chest roentgenography revealed fracture of the left 6th rib and 1–3 lumbar transverse processes. Gross hematuria was observed. During the first 2 days postburn the fluid needed to maintain an hourly urine output of 60 ml and 4 cm–18 cm H_2O CVP greatly exceeded the calculated budget. It included 9,200 ml colloids, 6,400 ml crystalloid, 5,300 ml water, and 600 ml mannitol and sorbitol. On the 3rd postburn day the patient became dyspneic. Rightward shifting of the mediastinum and left hemothorax were found by percussion and confirmed by X-ray film. Thoracocentesis was used to draw off 1,890 ml fresh blood. Under intravenous anesthesia, left thoracotomy was performed on the third degree burn eschar through the 6th intercostal space. Another 1,000 ml blood was evacuated from the pleural cavity. Rupture of the 6th intercostal artery caused by the fractured rib was found. After hemostasis, laparotomy was performed through the left diaphragm, and the subcapsular ruptured spleen was extracted. The external configuration of the left kidney appeared normal. The thoracic cage was closed by sutures. The thoracostomy tube was removed 24 h after the operation. Three additional operations involving excision and grafting of the third degree burns were performed. The fractures were treated by conservative measures. The patient recovered uneventfully.

Case Illustration. Male, aged 52. The patient sustained second degree burns to 50% of the BSA, complicated by chest injury, fracture of the lateral condyle of the left femur, and contusion of soft tissues. Chest roentgenography revealed multiple unstable fracture of the left ribs nos. 3–7, mediastinal emphysema, rightward shifting of the mediastinum, hemopneumothorax, and subcutaneous emphysema (Fig. X.1). The patient became dyspneic, and the dyspnea could not be relieved by tracheotomy. External rib traction was employed. Needle thoracocentesis was used to draw off 1,200 ml air and 30 ml blood. After traction and aspiration, paradoxical chest movement disappeared. For adequate drainage a thoracostomy tube was inserted at the 4th anterior intercostal space.

Whenever the external traction was stopped, the patient became dyspneic and cyanotic, with a thready pulse or absence of pulse. Consequently it was impossible to turn and to expose the burned back. Warm air treatment was instituted for the burned back, which was healed 16 days after the injury. Polymyxin B was instilled into the pleural cavity for the control of infection. Rib traction was discontinued on the 24th postburn day. The patient recovered uneventfully (Fig. X.2).

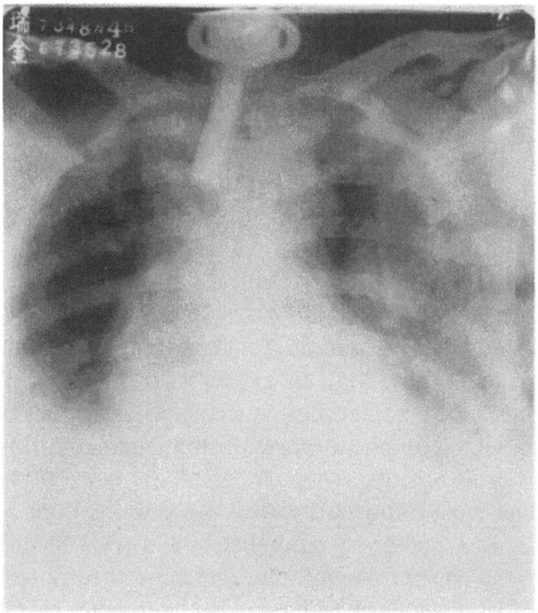

Fig. X.1. Multiple unstable fracture of the left ribs. Hemopneumothorax and subcutaneous and mediastinal emphysema are present. The mediastinum is shifted to the right

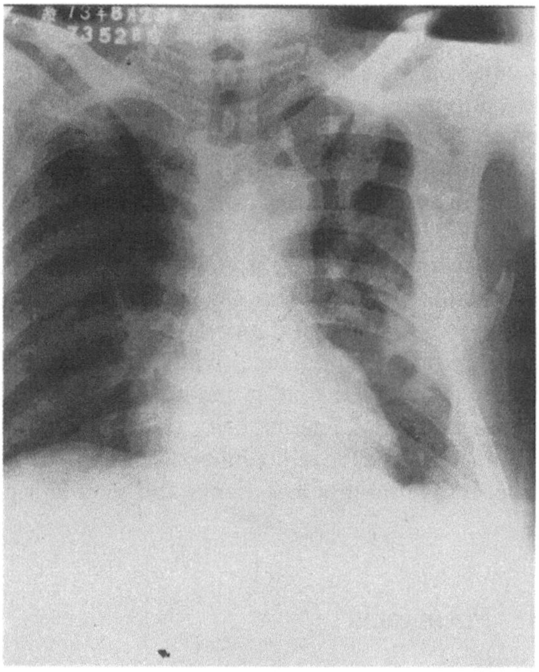

Fig. X.2. Same patient as in **Fig. X.1**, 27 days postburn. The left lung is fully inflated. The mediastinum has returned to its normal position

Chapter XI Systemic Complications of Burns

HSU WEI-SHIA, LIU YUE-LIANG, and YANG CHIH-CHUN

Translated by YANG CHIH-CHUN and LIU GUO-YU

Complications remain an important problem in burn management. Their incidence is quite high in extensive burns with prolonged uncovered third degree burns, and sometimes as many as six or seven complications occur in a single patient. Complications make management difficult, and may lead to death directly or indirectly.

The most important causes of complications are:

1. *Trauma:* stress diabetes, acute GI ulceration.
2. *Sepsis:* pneumonia, pyogenic thrombophlebitis, GU infection.
3. *Prolonged bed rest and metabolic disturbance:* GU stones, calcification or ossification of joints.
4. *Iatrogenic factors:* deep venous thrombosis from deep venous catheterization; overhydration, inappropriate fluid therapy during shock stage leading to lung and brain edema, acute renal failure.

Decreasing trauma stimulation, minimizing wound infection, covering the wound as soon as possible, early ambulation, and functional exercising are the important measures to minimize complications. Iatrogenic factors should be prevented.

The main complications encountered in the 4684 patients admitted from 1958 through 1978 are shown in Table XI.1.

In this chapter, pneumonia, cardia complications, deep venous thrombosis, GI bleeding, diarrhea, jaundice, stress diabetes, acute renal failure, and bone and joint complications are briefly introduced. These are the common and directly or indirectly fatal complications. Another common complication is fluid and electrolyte imbalance, which has been presented in Chap. VI. Edema of the brain and lung after inadequate fluid therapy during the shock stage is not so common. The majority of cases of brain edema were due to deep burns of the head in children, while pulmonary edema was seen after lower respiratory tract burns. Pulmonary edema and wound sepsis have been discussed in Chap. VII.

1 Pneumonia

Pneumonia is the most common pulmonary complication after burn (Table XI.2). Once it supervenes, not only does the patient's general condition become poor, but pulmonary infection per se is also difficult to control. Of the 109

Table XI.1. Complications in 4684 patients admitted from 1958 through 1978

Complications	No. of cases	%
Shock	319	6.81
Brain edema	31	0.66
Pulmonary edema	32	0.69
Acute renal failure	49	1.04
Septicemia	349	7.45
Burn wound sepsis[a]	225	4.80
Systemic mycosis[b]	25	0.53
Pneumonia	109	2.32
Deep venous thrombosis	33	0.70
Acute GI bleeding	78	1.66
Jaundice	68	1.44
Acute gastric dilatation	89	1.90
Diarrhea	296	6.31
Diabetes	17	0.36
Auricular chondritis	188	4.01

[a] 1967–1978 data
[b] 1970–1978 data

Table XI.2. Main pulmonary complications in 4,684 cases

Complications	No. of cases
Pneumonia	109
Pulmonary edema	37
Pulmonary atelectasis	14
Pulmonary embolism	10

patients whose condition was complicated by pneumonia, 47 died of pneumonia or of other causes but still with uncontrolled pneumonia (43.11%). In spite of healing of the wound, some patients still died of uncontrolled pneumonia.

After burns of the face and neck, the pulmonary toilet ability of the patient is impaired. If respiratory tract burn coexists, it will result in weakening or diminishing of the cilia function and will give rise to bronchopneumonia. Tracheotomy and anesthetic factors may increase the susceptibility of such patients to pneumonia. Of the 109 patients whose condition was complicated by pneumonia, 88 had burns of the face (80.73%). Tracheotomy and lung infection are closely related, for tracheotomy had been performed in almost 50% of the 109 patients. In our series, tracheotomy was performed in 337 patients, of whom 53 later developed pneumonia (15.7%).

In the early stage of respiratory burn, aspiration pneumonia is likely to develop owing to swelling of the epiglottis. So-called aerogenic pneumonia (bronchopneumonia) develops exclusively after lower respiratory burn.

Pneumonia may develop through hematogenous spread from septic foci of the wound with septic emboli. Generally it is preceded by septicemia or occurs secondary to other septic foci, such as pyogenic thrombophlebitis or abscess.

In our series, 74.11% of cases of pneumonia occurred within 2 weeks after burn; only 9.17% developed later than 1 month postburn. This shows that a high proportion of cases of pneumonia after burns may be secondary to septicemia and may be related to early semiconscious state, posture, epiglottic edema, and tracheotomy. Pneumonia may develop after the wounds has essentially healed. When the patient develops high fever, roentgenography should be performed even if auscultation of the chest gives negative results.

The majority of offending bacteria are gram-negative bacilli, with *P. aeruginosa* ranking first (Table XI.3). The bacteria yielded from the sputum usually corresponded with those on the wound: In the 52 cases with positive sputum and wound cultures, the same kind of bacteria were found in 45 cases (85.5%); only 7 were different (13.5%). This shows that pneumonia after burn often develops hematogenously, particularly secondary to septicemia.

Table XI.3. Distribution of 108 strains in 56 cases with positive sputum cultures

	P. aeruginosa	*Para. coli*[a]	*Aerobacter*	*Proteus*	*Klebsiella*	*B. anitratum*	*B. coli*	*Alkeligenes*	*Staphylococcus aureus*	*Streptococcus faecalis*	Others[b]
Strains	35	8	7	6	5	3	2	2	23	3	14

[a] Before 1973, Arizona, Citrobacter, Providencia, and late-lactose-fermenting *E. Coli* were reported as *Paracolobactrum*
[b] *Staphylococcus tetragenus, Staphylococcus albus, Streptococcus viridans, Neisseria,* and *Streptococcus pyogenes*

1.1 Clinical Manifestations

Burn patients may develop high fever, dyspnea, and leukocytosis suggestive of pneumonia. Owing to lack of positive findings on auscultation, the complicating pneumonia may be missed in some patients. Pneumonia most commonly develops during septicemia and after operation, so one has to pay special attention to the lungs during such periods. Besides dyspnea, patients usually develop flaring of the nostrils. Generally dry rales or wheezing manifest first and moist rales appear 2 or 3 days later. Sometimes coarseness of respiratory sound appears first; this warrants attention, and a chest roentgenogram may be necessary.

1.2 Management

General principles of management are the same as in ordinary pneumonia, but prognosis is poor owing (a) to the fact that in the majority of cases the pathogens are gram-negative bacilli and drug resistant staphylococci and (b) to the rather poor condition of the patients.

1. *Choice and use of antibiotics:* Antibiotics should not be chosen as in the routine management of ordinary pneumonia, but rather in accordance with the bacteria yielded from the wound when there is no sputum for culture. Repeated sputum culture is necessary because of constant change of bacteria. Generally, polymyxin B, gentamicin, isoxazolyl penicillines, and cephalosporins may be prescribed in combination.

The course of treatment should not be too short; withdrawal of antibiotics should be postponed until complete resolution of the foci is proved by chest roentgenography and by negative physical findings.

Besides systemic antibiotics, sensitive antibiotics may be administered 3–4 times a day as an aerosol for inhalation therapy.

2. *Promoting pulmonary toileting:*

a) Ultrasonic nebulization or humidified steam inhalation six times daily

b) Encouraging deep respiration and coughing

c) Postural drainage; increasing the number of times the body is turned

d) Tracheotomy

Tracheotomy is necessary if large amounts of tracheal secretion cannot be removed satisfactorily through the mouth. Irrigation, aspiration, and cough reflex stimulation are facilitated after tracheotomy. It is stressed that aspiration should be performed gently. Nebulization or steam inhalation is more effective through the tracheotomy opening than through the mouth. Nursing care is especially important. Once secretions have decreased, the tracheostomy tube should be removed promptly.

3. *Chinese herb medicine* (see Chap V).

4. Whenever *blood-borne infection* is suspected, foci should be sought for and eliminated.

2 Cardiac Complications

The etiologic factors of postburn cardiac complications include postburn hypermetabolism, systemic infection, toxemia etc. Other complications besides sinus tachycardia are arrhythmias, myocarditis, heart failure, and pericarditis.

Most extensively burned patients reveal sinus tachycardia, usually 120–140/min. In some patients the heart rate may reach 140–160/min and may further increase after minute stimulation. Tachycardia usually appears at the very beginning of the thermal insult and persists for quite a long period. In a few normothermic patients, tachycardia persists after the completion of the wound coverage. Generally speaking the increased heart rate cannot be lowered by tranquilizers or digitalis, and no specific treatment is necessary. If the heart rate suddenly increases to and persists at 180/min or more, it will evidently damage the myocardium. Corticosteroids, propranolol, and/or digitalis may be used in such cases. Extreme tachycardia is usually seen in patients with severe systemic infection or in the presence of bulky necrotic tissue. Searching and eradicating the infectious foci and active controlling of the wound infection must be carried out.

The incidence of cardiac arrhythmias is low, and they usually occur during the stage of infection. Arrhythmias usually encountered include supraventricular tachycardia, ventricular extrasystole, auricular fibrillation, and sinoatrial block with junctional escape. No treatment is necessary in the case of occasional ventricular extrasystole. Persistent or repeated ectopic rhythm which will further distress the involved heart must be controlled promptly. We have treated two cases of supraventricular tachycardia; one was controlled by digitalization, the other by electric conversion.

Case Illustration. Male, aged 25. The patient had burns to 75% of the BSA, including third degree burns to 31%. The burn wound was severely infected. On the 13th day postburn the patient had a high fever of 40 °C, and the heart rate suddenly increased to 214/min and could not be controlled by digitalis, practolol, Neo-Synephrine, and other measures. Supraventricular tachycardia proved by EKG persisted for 6 h. Under intravenous methohexitone anesthesia, DC synchronous electric shock, with energy discharge of 100 Watt-S was performed. Sinus rhythm was restored, and the heart rate decreased to 124/min. Despite oral administration of quinidine, the heart rate increased to 200/min 3 h later and fluctuated between 124 and 196/min during the next 24 h. Paroxysmal onset of supraventricular tachycardia continued for another 2 days. On the 17th day postburn a third electric conversion was attempted, followed by repeated autografting of the wound and oral administration of quinidine and practolol. Supraventricular tachycardia was thereby controlled. The patient's general condition improved and he was ultimately cured.

Toxic myocarditis is frequently seen in extensively burned patients and discovered in autopsy cases. The possible pathogenesis is the absorption of bacterial toxin and toxin liberated by the burned tissue. The clinical manifestations of toxic myocarditis are protodiastolic gallop rhythm and arrhythmias; EKG reveals low voltage and changing of the T wave. Oral prednisone and digitalization may produce some beneficial effect. Vitamins B_1 and B_6, ATP, coenzyme A, inositol, and hypertonic glucose are prescribed to "protect" the myocardium. But the ultimate aim of treatment must be the energetic eradication of dead tissues and effective control of wound infection. Although myocardial insults of various extent are frequently seen, heart failure is fortunately rare. Even if protodiastolic gallop rhythm appears, heart failure can be prevented by prompt treatment. In our cases, heart failure was usually the consequence of overhydration during the shock stage following lower respiratory tract burn.

Pericarditis occurred in only 0.2% of the patients admitted. Postburn pericarditis is usually formed secondarily to systemic infections. The most frequent microorganism encountered is *Staphylococcus aureus;* occasionally fungus may be isolated. We have had one case of systemic *Cephalosporium* infection with pericardial effusion. The diagnosis was made by chest roentgenography and cardiac blood pool scanning (Fig. XI.1). The purulent effusion drawn by pericardiocentesis revealed positive growth of *Cephalosporium.* The patient was cured by topical application of clotrimazole to the wound and systemic administration of amphotericin B.

The clinical manifestations of postburn pericarditis may be easily confused with those of wound sepsis. Even the important initial subjective symptom of precordial pain may not be manifested in postburn cases. Signs are also vague and atypical. For instance in certain cases there is no weakening of the apical beats observed, and sometimes an enlarged heart shadow on the chest film may coexist with a negative EKG tracing. Therefore cardiac blood pool scanning and/or pericardiocentesis is sometimes mandatory to make possible an exact diagnosis.

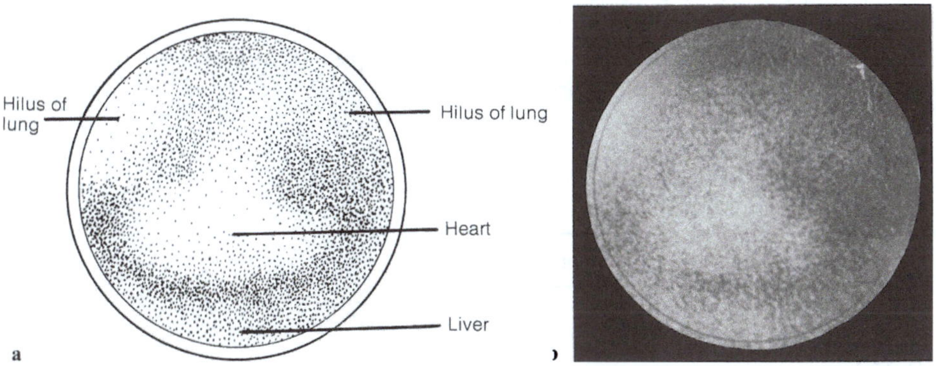

Fig. XI.1. Mycotic pericardial effusion. Cardiac blood pool scan showing normal heart image and radioactive defects between the heart and the liver and the heart and the bilateral pulmonary hili. These defects indicate the presence of pericardial effusion (proved by pericardiocentesis)

The principle of treatment is essentially the same as in ordinary purulent pericarditis. The antibiotics employed must be selected according to the result of sensitivity tests on the isolated microorganisms of the tapped effusion. In the case of fungi infection, amphotericin B remains the antibiotic of choice.

3 Deep Venous Thrombosis – Including Pulmonary Embolism

Being bedridden for a prolonged period, stagnation of blood flow, hemoconcentration, injury of the deep venous intimal lining due to catheterization or repeated venipuncture, and direct thermal injury of the veins can all lead to deep venous thrombosis. Of 4684 burn patients, 33 developed deep venous thrombosis. In deep venous thrombosis there is marked edema of the involved limbs. The pale and edematous granulation wounds result in a low rate of graft taking. Once infected venous thrombi will become septic foci. Dislodging of the deep venous thrombi will cause pulmonary embolism. Inferior vena caval thrombosis may increase the burden on the heart and cause heart failure. In fact, deep venous thrombosis involves a series of problems which complicate the burn treatment and influence the ultimate outcome.

Of 54 patients who received indwelling deep venous catheters in their lower extremities (femoral, iliac, or caval catheter via the great saphenous vein), 6 developed deep venous thrombosis (11%). During the same period, of 789 patients sustaining deep burns of their lower extremities but without catheterization, only four developed deep venous thrombosis (0.5%). It is evident that deep venous thrombosis is closely related to the indwelling catheters. Deep venous thrombosis of the upper extremities is exceedingly rare; of the 33 cases encountered, all the thrombi were located in the femoral vein, the iliac vein, or the inferior vena cava. In order to prevent this complication, central venous catheterization of the inferior vena cava should be avoided; superior vena caval catheter threading via the cephalic, jugular, or subclavian veins is advised.

If it is impossible to do this (e.g., the upper extremities, chest, and neck are deeply burned), and indwelling inferior vena caval catheter should be permitted for a very short period only, e.g., 3 days. Aseptic technique and meticulous nursing care are necessary to prevent infection.

Table XI.4. The onset[a] of catheter-induced deep venous thrombosis (24 cases)

Onset (days postburn)	No. of cases
<5 days	7
6–10 days	9
11–15 days	5
>21 days	3

[a] Date of onset according to patients' charts

Catheter-induced venous thrombosis may arise while the catheter is in situ or within several days after its removal. Of 24 catheter-induced venous thrombosis, 16 were formed within 10 days postburn (Table XI.4), at which time the deep wounds had not yet healed. The edematous and weeping wounds resulting from deep venous thrombosis rendered the wound treatment extremely difficult. On the other hand, in four cases of non-catheter-induced venous thrombosis, the onset was postponed until the 22nd, 32nd, 50th, and 116th postburn days. These cases were probably related to the long time for which the patients were bedridden: for such patients early ambulation is of paramount importance.

3.1 Clinical Manifestations

If the thrombus is located in the femoral, external, or common iliac veins, only one lower limb is affected, but if it is located in the inferior vena cava, both lower limbs are involved. Manifestations include:

1. Swelling and edema of the affected limb: If the proximal end of the thrombus extends beyond the external iliac vein, the perineum and lower abdominal wall may also appear swollen. The wounds are weeping and wet, the granulation tissue, pale and edematous.

2. Pain and tenderness along the course of the thrombosed deep veins.

3. Engorgement of the superficial veins. This sign may be concealed in the case of burns of the lower limbs.

Fever and leukocytosis usually occur in burn patients before the complete healing or coverage of their wounds; consequently they are not bound to reflect that the thrombus is infected. But in convalescents who are normothermic and who have a normal white blood cell count, the recurrence of hyperthermia and leukocytosis usually implies that the thrombus has been infected.

Pulmonary embolism is still a serious complication. Its symptoms and signs vary with the size and the number of the emboli. During the onset of massive emboli, the patient suddenly feels oppression of the chest, followed by dyspnea, fretfulness, paleness, profuse sweating, coldness of the limb, and weak pulse. Disseminated wet rales and lowering of the breathing sound are heard upon auscultation. A typical dense wedge-shaped shadow may be seen on the chest roentgenogram 3–5 days after the acute onset. Ten cases of pulmonary embolism were diagnosed on the basis of typical clinical manifestation, positive chest roentgenograms, or autopsy findings; of these ten patients, four had deep venous thrombosis (three thrombi were located in the inferior vena cava). Despite of ligation of the inferior vena cava, repeated attacks of pulmonary embolism occurred, leading to the death of three of the patients.

3.2 Management

The principles of treatment are to localize the thrombus, to control the infection, to eliminate the edema, and to prevent the occurrence of pulmonary emboli. Various points are listed below.

1. The affected limb(s) are *elevated*, even when the patient lies prone. If the condition of the wound permits, the limb(s) are dressed with elastic bandages.

2. *Systemic antibiotics* are used according to the result of sensitivity tests on the wound flora.

3. *Anticoagulants and fibrinolytic activators:* The newly formed venous thrombi are lysed and their extension prevented. Anticoagulants and fibrinolytic activators may be employed, and gratifying results can be achieved.

a) Heparin therapy should be started as soon as the diagnosis has been confirmed. The dose for adults is 50 mg q 6 h, i.v. The dosage must be constantly regulated according to the patient's whole blood clotting time (Lee and White). Ideally the clotting time should be adjusted to 1–2 times that of the normal control. In the case of hemorrhagic complications, 1 mg protamine sulfate is given for every milligram of heparin administered. The anticoagulant effect of heparin is immediate and it has no accumulation action after intermittent injection. Intramuscular administration should be avoided because of the danger of local hematoma at the injection site.

b) Coumarin derivatives: The onset of action occurs within 24 h–48 h of oral administration. A therapeutic level can only be reached 3–4 days after the institution of the drug. Therefore it must be used together with heparin. When coumarin derivative has reached its therapeutic level, heparin may be discontinued and the former used alone. The dosage is adjusted according to the prothrombin time, which ideally should be twice the normal control value. Its side effect is bleeding complications which can be antagonized by vitamin K_1 and the infusion of fresh blood. Between 5 and 6 days are needed to reduce the prothrombin time to normal after discontinuation of the drug. A smaller than average dose is advisable for patients with impaired hepatic or renal function.

4. *Fibrinolytic activators:* Both urokinase and streptokinase may be used. Because streptokinase is antigenic, it has recently been replaced by the nonantigenic urokinase. Whenever urokinase is used, heparin therapy is instituted at the termination of the fibrinolytic therapy to prevent rethrombosis.

5. *Operative treatment*

a) Thrombectomy is indicated in cases with a newly formed thrombus.

b) Ligation of the inferior vena cava may cause chronic venous insufficiency of the lower limbs. In some cases, wound edema and infection become a very serious or even an insoluble problem. Consequently ligation is only indicated in patients with repeated pulmonary emboli or pyogenic septic venous thrombi. After vena caval ligation, some patients still develop recurrent emboli, which seem to be either transported through the collateral veins or newly formed in the stump of the caval ligature.

Management of massive pulmonary emboli: Pulmonary embolism has a sudden onset. Massive emboli may block the pulmonary artery and cause fatal bronchial spasm and/or coronary arterial spasm. Emergency measures are intravenous administration of 1 mg atropine and infusion of 100 mg diluted papaverine. Patients suffering from pulmonary edema should be digitalized. Tracheal intubation and assisted respiration should be instituted for patients suffering from anoxia.

Active ambulation or passive moving may cause dislodging of the thrombi. Therefore it is advisable not to let the patient move around before the thrombi have been organized.

4 Acute Postburn Ulcerative Bleeding

In 1842 Curling first described acute postburn gastrointestinal ulceration in a scientific way; hence the term "Curling's ulcer." It is a common complication of burn, its reported incidence in the literature ranging from 0.1%–34%, with most authors reporting an incidence of 10%–30%. The incidence found on autopsy in Sevitt's series (1967) was 22%, the most common sites being the stomach and duodenum. Recently, the correct diagnosis of this complication has been considerably improved through the use of fibergastroscopy. Czaja et al. reported 32 patients (1974) in whom fibergastroscopy was performed after burn. Gastric erosions were present in 25 of 29 (86%) with extensive burns (35% of the BSA). Of 23 who had been studied within 72 h postburn, 17 (74%) had lesions. Nine patients developed duodenal ulcer, and eight had concomitant gastric disease. In the whole series, seven patients (22%) developed hemorrhage; in six cases ulcerative bleeding was involved.

The sudden onset of hematemesis and melena (usually without any prodromal symptoms) is one of the clinical characteristics of acute postburn ulcerative bleeding. Abdominal pain is very rare, even if the ulcer is perforated and results in peritonitis. Abdominal pain and gastrointestinal symptoms may be masked by the critical condition of the burn. Usually bleeding is intermittent. Sometimes ulcers are discovered only after autopsy (Table XI.5).

Generally, clinical diagnosis is based upon hematemesis, melena, stool occult blood determination, frank bloody stool, or shock. Therefore diagnosis is usually made only after bleeding has occurred, so that the true incidence was far higher than that indicated by clinical diagnosis. Of the 4684 burn patients admitted, 78 were diagnosed clinically as having acute ulcerative bleeding – an incidence of 1.66%. According to the classification of severity of burn set out by the

Table XI.5. Autopsy findings of acute ulceration in four burn patients.

Age	Sex	Autopsy findings
31	M	Four ulcers of various size on lesser curvature; acute necrosis of mid-portion of esophagus complicated by profuse bleeding
25	M	Giant bleeding ulcer on anterior gastric wall, adhering to liver and diaphragm, perforating into left lung, and eroding pulmonary artery; profuse bleeding
65	M	Lesser curvature ulcer
32	M	Superficial gastric ulcer

China National Burn Congress 1970, 1% of cases of acute ulcerative bleeding occurred in the "light" group, 8% in the "Medium" group, 20% in the "severe" group, and 71% in the "very severe" group. Thus it is clear that the incidence of acute ulcerative bleeding increases according to the severity of burn.

In this series of 78 patients, the ratio of male to female was 2.6:1 and their ages ranged from 5 months to 84 years, with an average of 27.3 years (see Table XI.6).

With respect to the period between burn and the onset of bleeding, the earliest occurrence was 6 h, and the latest, 63 days. The ratio of incidence before and after the 10th postburn day was 2:1 (55/23 cases), i.e., the majority of cases developed acute ulceration with bleeding within 10 days. This may be related to the severe burn stress and relatively pronounced homeostatic impairment during that period.

Of the 4684 patients, 319 developed burn shock, of whom 25 developed GI bleeding (7.8%). In the 4365 patients without shock, 53 developed bleeding (1.2%), i.e., there is a statistically significant lowered incidence in this group ($P<0.01$).

Of the 574 patients who developed burn wound sepsis and septicemia, 62 developed bleeding (10.8%), while of the 4110 without wound sepsis, only 6 developed bleeding (0.3%), revealing the close relationship between acute ulcerative bleeding and general sepsis.

The stomach and the duodenum are the most common sites of acute ulcers; the lower portion of the esophagus, the small bowel, and the colon may also be involved. Pathologically, the majority of duodenal lesions are solitary and ulcerating, while the majority of gastric lesions are multiple and manifest as hemorrhagic gastritis. Kissing ulcers may develop as well. The usual location of duodenal lesions is the posterior wall of the first portion, 1 cm–3 cm distal to the pylorus. Should multiple lesions occur, generally one is found there.

Table XI.6. Age distribution of patients with acute ulcerative bleeding

Age	<1	1–10	11–20	21–30	31–40	41–50	51–60	61–70	71–80	81–90
No. of cases	3	23	8	18	5	8	4	2	6	1

Acute duodenal ulcer is usually deeply seated, penetrating submucosa and muscularis right up to the pancreas. The calibre of penetrating duodenal ulcers is generally large (1 cm or more). The pancreaticoduodenal artery is the most common artery to be eroded, giving rise to hemorrhagic shock or even fatal bleeding. Gastric lesions are characterized as being superficial, multiple, and small. Usually they are diffusely distributed lesions of pinpoint size or slightly larger (diameter 3 mm) ulcers on the gastric fundus, the gastric body, and the pylorus with the intervening mucosa intact. The diameter of some ulcers may be as large as 4 mm–5 mm. As a rule, the entire gastric mucosa became swollen, congested, and pinkish with ecchymosis in the nonulcerated regions. Small erosion points without bleeding are not readily recognizable while those with bleeding are fairly distinct. This type of gastric erosion may heal within a few days, but it is also possible for it to develop into ulcers.

Erosion, congestion, necrosis, and sloughing of gastric mucosa are the main sources of GI bleeding during wound sepsis. Under such conditions, the shed blood is relatively scanty and small pieces of brownish-black necrotic sloughed mucosa may be seen in the gastric juice.

During bleeding, positive blood bacterial cultures were obtained in 21 out of 58 cases (36.2%) encountered from 1958 through 1973, 16 being gram-negative rods. Quite a number of patients with bleeding developed typical symptoms of wound sepsis, yet blood cultures were negative. This further shows the close relationship between acute ulcerative bleeding and general sepsis.

Recently, many investigators have used the method of neutralizing gastric acid, to lower the incidence of Curling's ulcer, especially in burn patients with impaired gastric mucosa barrier function. This has a significant effect in preventing acute ulceration, particularly in the duodenum. Joseph (1976) investigated two groups of patients with burns to similar areas of the body surface (in all cases more than 35%). He established a ratio of 1:7 with regard to the incidence of acute ulcerative bleeding in the two groups, the first with antacid therapy, the second, a control group ($P < 0.02$). The H_2 receptor blocker – cimetidine possesses the same prophylactic effect on acute ulceration after burn. In a double-blind study, McElwee (1979) reported the same prophylactic effect on acute ulceration with either cimetidine or antacid in patients with burned areas exceeding 30% of the BSA. Nearly all patients were free from duodenal lesion and the severity of gastric lesions was significantly reduced. Cimetidine is easy to administer and can be given as a stat dose intravenously.

After severe burn, an abrupt fall in the vitamin A level (even to zero) has been observed in 80% of cases. As Vitamin A is necessary for the metabolism of epithelium and mucosa, the repair of connective tissue, and the production of mucosa, Chernov advocated administration of 100,000 IU–400,000 IU (vitamin A) per day to reduce the incidence of acute ulcer. (In his data, the incidence in the treated group was 18%, that in the control group, 60%.)

In extensively burned patients, besides the routine prescription of large doses of vitamins A and D on admission, routine estimation of gastric pH through a gastric tube should be carried out and acidity maintained at around 7.0 with aluminum hydroxide, magnesium oxide, or/and cimetidine. This might have some benefit in preventing the occurrence of stress ulcer. In this series

Table XI.7. Data concerning the nine patients operated on for acute ulcerative bleeding

Sex	Age	Total BSA burned/III° (%)	Onset of bleeding postburn (days)	Amount of blood transfused preoperatively	Type of operation	Location and size of ulcer	Result	Ultimate outcome
M	25	31/28	17	1,200	B-II	Post. wall of first part of duodenum; 1.5 cm × 1.5 cm	No more bleeding	Survived
M	51	40/31.5	6	1,000	Jejunostomy	Negative	No more bleeding	Survived
M	51	40/0	4	900	B-I	Post. wall of first part of duodenum	No more bleeding	Survived
M	16	67/0	4	1,200	B-I	Post. wall of first part of duodenum Perforating to pancreas	No more bleeding	Survived
M	42	84.5/12	10	1,100	B-I	Prepyloric part of stomach; 1 cm × 1 cm		Died of sepsis
M	43	100/7	10	1,900	B-II	Post. wall of first part of duodenum Lesser curvature of stomach (multiple superficial ulcers)	Bleeding recurred; second op. performed	Died of sepsis
M	47	83/62.5	39	1,200	B-II	Post. wall of first part of duodenum; 2 cm × 2.5 cm Post. wall of perpendicular part of lesser curvature of stomach, 2 cm × 2.5 cm	No more bleeding	Died of sepsis
M	28	41/8	5	1,800	B-II	Post. wall of first part of duodenum; 2 cm × 2.5 cm Perforating to pancreas	No more bleeding	Survived
M	37	90/60	5	1,400	B-I	First part of duodenum (multiple ulcers) Lesser curvature of stomach (single ulcer)	No more bleeding	Survived

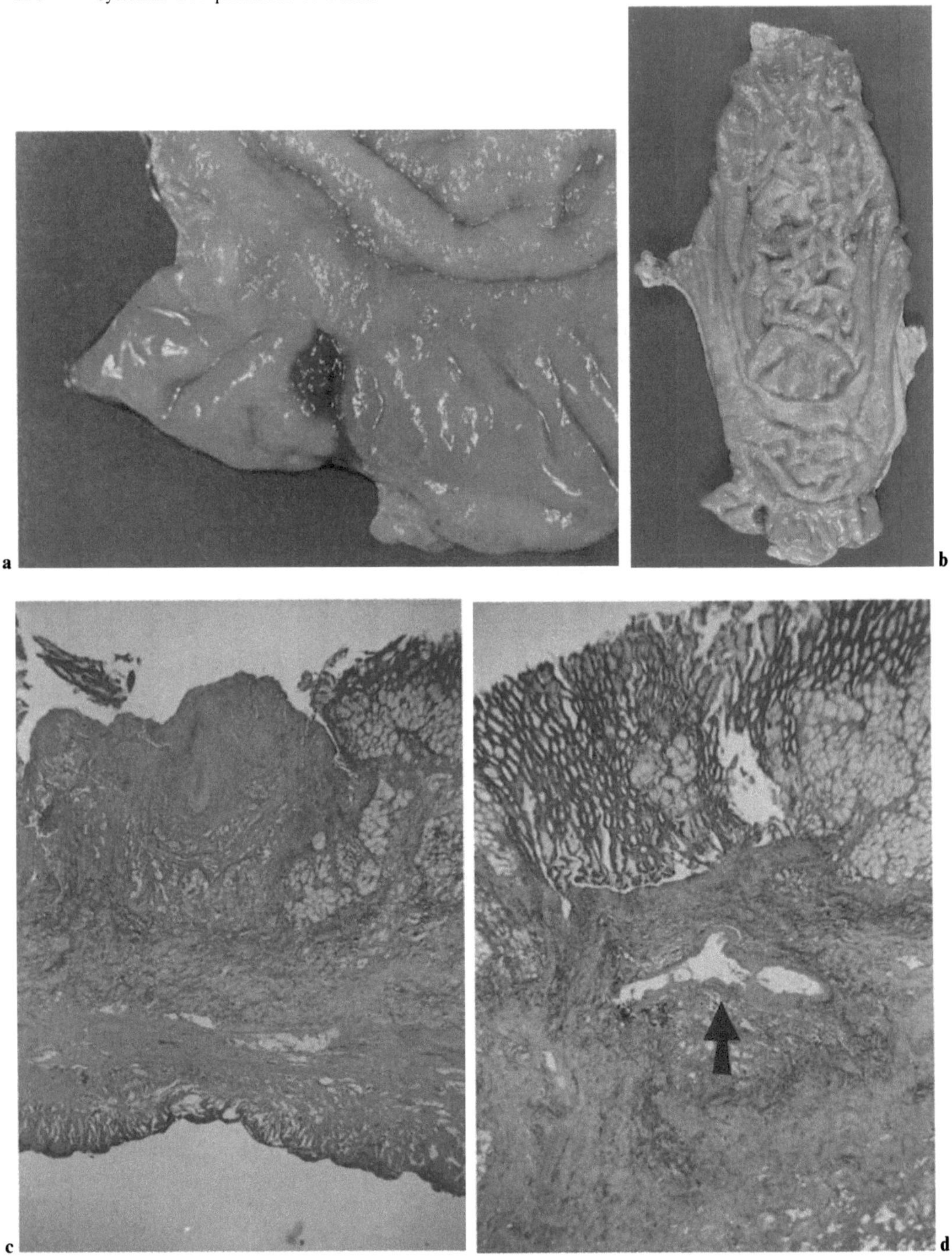

of 78 cases of acute bleeding ulcers, 69 developed either a moderate amount of occult blood, hematemesis, melena, or bloody stool. During the episode, the amount of blood transfused was less than 1,000 ml for each case and all patients gradually stopped bleeding after conservative treatment. As the majority

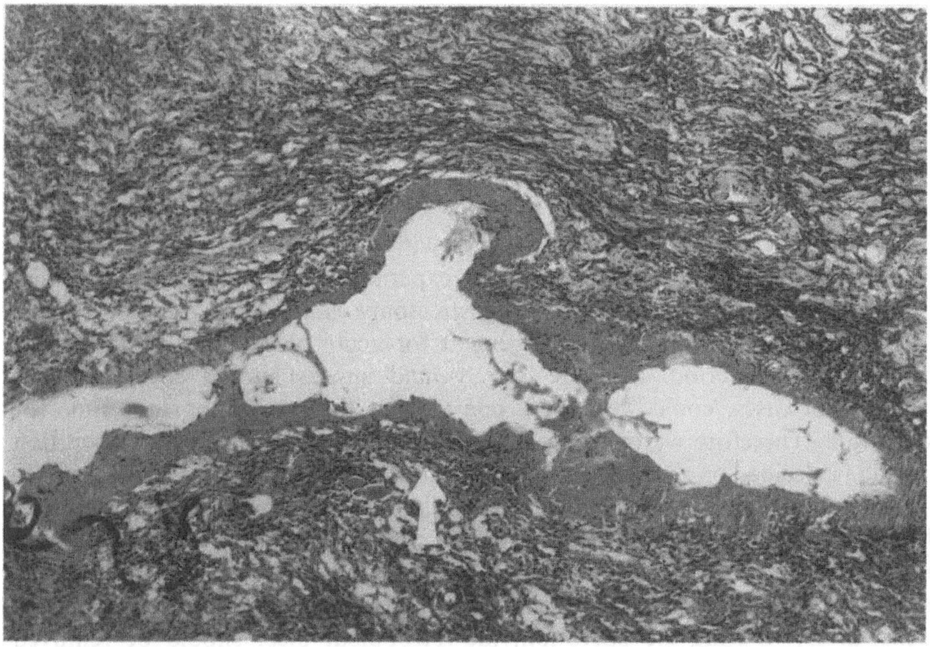

e

Fig. XI.2a–e. Acute postburn duodenal ulcerative bleeding in a 35-year-old male with burns to 91% of the BSA, including third degree burns to 15% (patient not included in Table XI.7). Melena and bloody stools were passed on the 28th day postburn. Laparotomy was performed 20 h later. Before and during the operation 2,600 ml blood was rapidly transfused. The patient survived, recovering uneventfully. Operative and pathologic findings: **a** Acute ulcer located at the posterior wall of the first part of the duodenum with ejective arterial bleeding at the center of the crater. **b** Congestion and petechial hemorrhage of the gastric mucosa. **c** Section through the center of the ulcer showing the eroded artery. H & E, ×10. **d** Section through the edge of the ulcer showing normal duodenal mucosa and necrotic arterial wall (*arrow*). H & E, ×10. **e** Magnified view of the necrotic arterial wall (*arrow*) H & E, ×25. Resection of the ulcer is necessary in cases such as this

of acute bleeding ulcers may be successfully managed conservatively, drugs including vitamin K, PAMBA, carbazochrome, and Pitressin as well as herbal medicines such as rhizoma *Bletillae* and radix *Sancki* (ground to powder, 50 mg three times daily p.o.) may be used. Another herb medicine, "Pai Yao" may also be used. In order to facilitate the hemostatic effect of the above-mentioned drugs, a relatively large dose of aluminium hydroxide is added to serve as an antacid.

Generally emergency exploration is warranted whenever conservative treatment fails and normal hemoglobin level and blood pressure can no longer be maintained in spite of transfusions. On this basis, 9 of the 78 cases were operated. The amount of blood transfused exceeded 1,000 ml in all but one case (900 ml) (Table XI.7).

According to our experience, indications for surgery in acute ulcerations are as follows:

1. Acute massive bleeding accompanied by shock
2. Recurrence of massive bleeding
3. Inability to maintain a normal hemoglobin level or progressive fall in blood pressure in spite of blood transfusions exceeding 1,000 ml within 24 h
4. Perforation

The procedure chosen in our series of nine cases was subtotal gastrectomy, with one jejunostomy upon negative findings. Except for the one case in which a second operation was needed, bleeding was checked by a single operation. The emergency operations were performed within 4–17 days postburn, excluding one on the 39th day. According to our experience, the foci can be identified and the results are good. Subtotal gastrectomy is the procedure of choice. Over prolonged conservative management for acute bleeding ulcer during the grave postburn period, with the burn wound unsatisfactorily covered in the majority of cases, could well cause one to miss the most opportune time for operation. Therefore we emphasize that after careful consideration, operation should be decided on promptly and opportunely. For those patients with transfusions of more than 1,000 ml, operation should be decided on as early as possible, because active bleeding ulcers are always present. Bleeding foci were found in eight out of nine cases in our series (88.9%), and in six they were located in the posterior wall of first portion of duodenum, eroding the pancreaticoduodenal artery. During the operation, the retrobulbar ulcer should be removed and the artery ligated in the normal tissue (Fig. XI.2). One operative failure was performed with simple suture ligature in situ, leaving the ulcer intact; this gave rise to rebleeding. Incision may be made through the burn wound if unavoidable, provided that the operative wound is sutured in layers. The peritoneum, muscle, fascia, and fat may all result in primary healing. During the operation any active bleeding points on the residual stomach or duodenum should be checked. The surgeon should carefully look for such points and choose his procedure scrupulously. As the main postoperative complications are wound disruption and stoma leak, nutritional support is very important. High caloric oral or total parenteral nutrition should be prescribed. Intravenous albumin may be necessary to maintain the plasma protein level above 5 g%.

Case Illustration. Male, aged 25. The patient had flame burns to 31% of the BSA, including third degree burns to 25%. He was transferred to our hospital on the 16th day postburn in 1959. On admission, the patient had pallor, cold sweating with a pulse rate of 156/min, and blood pressure of 84/40 mmHg. After rapid infusion of 300 ml physiologic saline and 500 ml plasma, his pulse rate decreased to 136/min and blood pressure was stabilized. On the 8th day after admission he developed shock. Four hundred milliliters of whole blood was transfused within 10 min, but, blood pressure fell further from 90/50 to 40/30 mmHg. Blood pressure was still unstable even after administration of 3,600 ml whole blood within 8 h. Therefore exploratory laparotomy was performed, disclosing an acute ulcer with a diameter of 1.5 cm on the posterior wall of the first portion of the duodenum. There was an active bleeder in its base. Suture ligature of the bleeder was carried out, and subtotal gastrectomy with gastrojejunostomy and jejunostomy were performed.

Nutrition was supplied through the jejunostomy beginning on the 3rd postoperative day. Two thousand five hundred calories a day were supplied through both intravenous and GI routes to maintain plasma protein level at 5.5 g% and albumin level at above 3 g%. The wound healed by first intention. The patient survived.

Before the diagnosis and decision with regard to operation are settled, it is necessary to rule out acute exacerbation of dysentery after burn, characteristic of which is diarrhea, later shifting to passing of fresh blood. Such patients were carriers before burn and the disease manifests itself once the host resistance is lowered, as it is after burns. Thus it is important to establish whether the patient had dysentery or chronic diarrhea before burn. Routine examination and culture of the stool may help in the differentiation. Two cases of burn complicated by dysentery with massive GI bleeding were encountered; in both cases the pathogenic bacteria were Flexner's dysentery bacillus. One of the patients had been operated for uncontrollable bleeding.

Case Illustration. Male, aged 19. There were soda lime burns to 100% of the BSA, including third degree burns to 33%. The patient developed diarrhea 8 days after burn, with three passages a day and 400 ml in quantity. Routine stool examination revealed occult blood+, RBC++, WBC+++, phagocyte 0–1/HP. In spite of treatment with chloromycetin and polymyxin B, passages increased day by day, reaching eight a day with an amount of 1,000 ml. He began passing fresh blood on the 11th day postburn, as frequently as 25 times a day. Even though the amount of a single motion was not large, the total amount reached 1,800 ml. The bleeding became more profuse the next day, so laparotomy was performed. On exploration, there was small amount of bloody fluid in the free peritoneal cavity, and the ascending and transverse colon were prominently swollen. There was a little blood in the ileum and no blood was seen in the jejunum, duodenum, or stomach. Stool culture revealed Flexner's dysentery bacillus. Neomycin and furazolidone were administered orally, and bleeding stopped 2 days afterward. The patient survived.

---

5 Diarrhea

Surgeons who are experienced in handling patients with extensive burns may have the impression that those patients who retain a good appetite will ultimately be cured. But unfortunately, not a few patients suffer from postburn anorexia or diarrhea. Anorexia can be compensated by tube feeding or parenteral nutrition, but if diarrhea cannot be promptly controlled, malnutrition, water and electrolyte disturbances, and disturbance of the intestinal flora will ensue and will increase the difficulties in treatment.

Table XI.8. Time of onset of 74 cases of postburn diarrhea

Time of onset (days postburn)	No. of cases
5	22
6–10	23
11–15	8
16–20	8
>21	13

The most frequent cause of postburn diarrhea is wound sepsis (or septicemia). In 74 cases of diarrhea, 19 revealed positive blood cultures. Some of the patients had clinical signs and symptoms of septicemia, although their blood cultures were negative. In most of the patients the onset of diarrhea was within 10 days after the injury, which coincided with the peak onset of wound sepsis or septicemia. Only about 20% of the cases had their onset later than 3 weeks postburn (Table XI.8). Another common causal factor is improper oral dietary. During the late 1950s and early 1960s our patients were overenthusiastically fed with chocolate and homogenized milk. The incidence of diarrhea rose to 10% of burn inpatients; this figure soon dropped to 3% after this lopsided practice was corrected.

With regard to pathogenic factors, special attention should be paid to disturbances of the normal intestinal flora. After long-term administration of broad-spectrum antibiotics, drug-resistant Clostridium difficile pseudomembranous enterocolitis or mycotic enteritis is liable to occur. Owing to lowering of general resistance, acute flare-up of bacillary dysentery may take place in dysentery carriers. In rare cases diarrhea may be induced by oral administration of amphotericin B or potassium chloride.

The consistency of the diarrheal stool varies from pasty mucoid to watery. Mucin, foam, or undigested food may appear in the stool. The frequency varies from 7–8/day to over 10 passages per day. The amount of watery diarrhea

Table XI.9. Results of routine examination of 46 specimens (stool of diarrheal patients)

Routine changes of stools	No. change	WBC	RBC, WBC	RBC, WBC, phagocytes
No. of cases	10	13	19	4

Table XI.10. Results of bacterial culture of 31 specimens (stool of diarrheal patients)

Bacteria	Normal intestinal flora	*Shigella dysenteriae*	Other pathogenic[a] bacteria
No. of cases	16	5	10

[a] Twenty strains were isolated from ten specimens

may reach 1,000 ml–2,000 ml/day. Leukocytes are found in 80% of the specimens (Table XI.9).

Except for *Shigella dysenteriae*, positive findings of pathogenic microorganisms are not common (Table XI.10). Five of ten other pathogenic bacteria isolated were *Streptococcus faecalis; Pseudomonas aeruginosa* took second place. It is difficult to determine the cause of diarrhea by routine examination of the feces only. Microscopic examination of stained fecal smears and differential count of cocci and bacilli may provide some useful information. Although yeastlike fungi may be present in normal feces, if there are repeated positive findings a provisional diagnosis of mycotic enteritis can be made, especially if the amount of fungi is large and hyphae are present. The final diagnosis can only be made after identification of the cultured pathogens of the stool.

For intractable cases, besides "etiologic treatment," special attention should be paid to dietary regulation. If the condition can be mitigated by proper dietary regulation, a certain portion of nutritional supplements may be given via the gastrointestinal route. Etiologic treatment includes controlling wound sepsis, suppression of *Shigellae dysenteriae*, and oral administration of sensitive antibiotics. Mycotic enteritis can be readily controlled by oral administration of nystatin, amphotericin B, and/or 5-fluorocytosine. Dietary regulation includes discontinuation of chocolate and homogenized milk intake and substitution with rice soup, powder of rhizoma *Diascoreae*, apple sauce, skimmed sour milk, and casein. The amount must be increased gradually by dripping or by use of a peristaltic pump. Some cases of idiopathic intractable diarrhea can be mitigated by dietary regulation. "Antidiarrheal compound" may be administered three times a day for patients with "functional diarrhea." This compound contains 0.25 g tannalbin, 0.2 g biofermin, 0.3 g bismuth subcarbonate, and 0.5 g calcium lactate. After the infection factor has been ruled out in cases of copious amounts of watery diarrhea, tincture camphor compound may be prescribed. Supplement of potassium salt is of paramount importance; water, electrolyte, and acid-base disturbances should be promptly adjusted.

6 Jaundice

Of the 4,684 patients, 68 developed jaundice. The main causes were wound sepsis (septicemia) and serum hepatitis; hemolytic jaundice was the third most common cause (Table XI.11).

6.1 Hemolytic Jaundice

Red cell destruction after burn may cause jaundice. In hemolytic jaundice, serum bilirubin rarely exceeds 3 mg%, and liver function tests are usually normal (Table XI.12). The concentration of plasma unconjugated bilirubin is increased; little or no bilirubin is excreted in the urine. Tests of urinary urobilinogen yield a positive reaction. Hemolytic jaundice usually appears within 2 weeks after burn; it lasts for about 1 week and then subsides. In a few cases jaundice may not subside until 3 weeks after its onset. Hepatic parenchymal damage

Table XI.11. Etiology of jaundice in 68 burned patients

Cause of jaundice	No. of cases
Wound sepsis (or septicemia)	24
Serum hepatitis B	15
Hemolytic jaundice	11
Infectious hepatitis A	5
Phosphorus and copper poisoning	3
Chlorpromazine-induced jaundice (cholangiolitis)	3
Idiopathic factors	6
Hepatorenal failure	1
Total	68

Table XI.12. The results of serum total bilirubin, SGPT, and flocculation liver function tests in cases of homologous serum hepatitis, jaundice caused by sepsis, and hemolytic jaundice

<table>
<tr><th></th><th colspan="2">Serum total bilirubin, SGPT and flocculation tests</th><th>Homologous serumhepatitis (n)</th><th>Jaundice caused by sepsis (n)</th><th>Hemolytic jaundice (n)</th></tr>
<tr><td>Serum total bilirubin (mg%)</td><td></td><td><2</td><td>2</td><td>7</td><td>1</td></tr>
<tr><td></td><td></td><td>2–3</td><td>1</td><td>5</td><td>7</td></tr>
<tr><td></td><td></td><td>3–5</td><td>3</td><td>5</td><td>3</td></tr>
<tr><td></td><td></td><td>5–10</td><td>6</td><td>1</td><td>0</td></tr>
<tr><td></td><td></td><td>>10</td><td>2</td><td>3</td><td>0</td></tr>
<tr><td>SGPT (U)</td><td></td><td>Normal</td><td>0</td><td>6</td><td>8</td></tr>
<tr><td></td><td></td><td>40–400</td><td>7</td><td>12</td><td>3</td></tr>
<tr><td></td><td></td><td>>400</td><td>6</td><td></td><td>0</td></tr>
<tr><td>Serum flocculation tests</td><td>CCFT</td><td>Negative</td><td>0</td><td rowspan="2">15</td><td rowspan="2">10</td></tr>
<tr><td></td><td></td><td>+</td><td>2</td></tr>
<tr><td></td><td></td><td>++</td><td>6</td><td>1</td><td>1</td></tr>
<tr><td></td><td></td><td>+++</td><td>6</td><td>4</td><td>0</td></tr>
<tr><td></td><td></td><td>++++</td><td>1</td><td>0</td><td>0</td></tr>
<tr><td></td><td>TTT (U)</td><td>0–6</td><td>2</td><td>16</td><td>11</td></tr>
<tr><td></td><td></td><td>>6</td><td>13</td><td>3</td><td>0</td></tr>
<tr><td></td><td>ZnTT (U)</td><td>2–12</td><td>2</td><td>13</td><td>11</td></tr>
<tr><td></td><td></td><td>>12</td><td>10</td><td>6</td><td>0</td></tr>
</table>

Abbreviations: CCFT, cephalin-cholesterol flocculation test; TTT, thymol turbidity test; ZnTT, zinc sulphate turbidity test

in hemolytic jaundice is much milder than in toxic hepatitis; therefore no special treatment is necessary. Both anesthesia and surgery can be undertaken during its onset. Since chlorpromazine or other phenothiazine derivatives and topical antimicrobial agents have been extensively used in our practice, chlorpromazine-induced jaundice and other drug-induced hepatitis must be differentiated from hemolytic jaundice. Chlorpromazine-induced jaundice is caused by intrahepatic biliary obstruction and cholestasis. Besides discontinuation of the offending drug, chloropromazine-induced jaundice can be treated by oral administration of 2 g cholestyramine q 4 h to relieve pruritus. If there is prolongation of prothrombin time, vitamin K should be administered. Jaundice caused by topical agents is always accompanied by impairment of hepatic function.

Jaundice is characterized by yellow discoloration of the sclerae and skin. In case of nonobstructive jaundice, the patient may also have black tea-hued urine, which is caused by increased concentration of urinary urobilinogen. In burn patients, the increased serum bilirubin not only stains the skin and sclerae but also tinctures the wound exudate yellow. If the wound dressing is stained yellow, jaundice should be strongly suspected.

6.2 Serum Hepatitis

Formerly so-called serum hepatitis was considered to be transmitted solely by the parenteral route. However, it was later proved by pathogenic and epidemiologic studies that the pathogen of serum hepatitis is hepatitis B virus, which can be transmitted both enterally and parenterally. Since hepatitis B has a long incubation period (60–160 days), all the cases listed under this item in Table XI.11 had their onset at least 2 months after burn, the latest case occurring on the 118th day postburn. Jaundice caused by hepatitis B lasts a long time, usually subsiding 3 weeks after the onset; the longest duration in the present series was 45 days. The jaundice may be very severe. In 8 of 14 cases the serum bilirubin value exceeded 5 mg%, and in 3 cases it exceeded 9 mg%, the highest being 13 mg%. All the patients had suffered from severe liver damage, with a high serum GPT value and positive serum flocculation tests (Table XI.12). Tenderness over the region of the liver, anorexia, nausea, and vomiting are the usual clinical symptoms.

Prognosis is mainly depend upon the condition of wound coverage. If the burn wounds have been covered or have healed before the onset of serum hepatitis, prognosis is good. If this has not occurred, hepatitis will aggravate the burn, and infection of the burn wounds, anesthesia, and surgery will in turn further damage the diseased liver. Since we adopted the energetic policy of radical excision and immediate coverage, 13 of 14 patients recovered uneventfully. The exception was a patient with fulminating hepatitis who quickly developed hepatic coma and died within 24 h after the onset of jaundice.

The treatment is the same as that for acute viral hepatitis A. Large doses of the vitamin B complex and C should be prescribed. Intravenous supplementation of 2,000 ml–3,000 ml GIK solution (1,000 ml 10% glucose, 30 ml 10% KCL, and 20 IU regular insulin) may be added to the ordinary diet. The recommended dose of prednisone for an average adult is 10 mg–20 mg. In cases of fulminating viral hepatitis B, 200 mg–300 mg hydrocortisone or 5 mg–10 mg dexamethasone may be given daily.

6.3 Wound Sepsis (or Septicemia)–Induced Jaundice

Jaundice is a bad omen which implies the aggravation of the course of sepsis. Only 6 of 24 cases survived wound sepsis-induced jaundice. Jaundice cannot

Table XI.13. Blood culture of 15 cases of burn septicemia complicated by jaundice

Bacteria	No. of cases[a]
Staphylococcus tetragenus	1
Staphylcoccus aureus	8
Pseudomonas aeruginosa	7
Aerobacter aerogenes	1
Bacterium anitratum	1
Bacillus alcaligenes	1
Citrobacter	1

[a] Three cases revealed two kinds of bacteria in one culture
One case revealed three kinds of bacteria in one culture

serve as a criterion for differentiating gram-positive coccal septicemia from gram-negative bacillary septicemia (Table XI.13).

In most cases the onset of wound sepsis (or septicemia)-induced jaundice was within 3 weeks postburn. In nearly half of the cases the onset occurred within 10 days postburn. The jaundice is mild, and serum bilirubin level rarely exceeds 5 mg% (Table XI.12). The jaundice may subside spontaneously after the sepsis is controlled, but persisted in those cases which succumbed to sepsis. With regard to the laboratory findings, most cases revealed an elevated SGPT value, but in none of the them did it exceed 400 U. Serum flocculation tests showed negative results in most cases (Table XI.12), whereas in hepatitis B the SGPT value is increased and the serum flocculation tests reveal positive reactions. Half of the patients who suffered from hepatitis B had an SGPT value exceeding 400 U. Therefore it is possible to differentiate septicemia-induced jaundice from hepatitis B jaundice with the help of laboratory findings. We had two cases of septicemia-induced jaundice which occurred 2 months after the burn. Both patients had a relatively low SGPT value and negative flocculation tests, which are different from the laboratory findings in serum hepatitis B with a long incubation period.

7 Stress Diabetes

Besides stress diabetes, postburn hyperglycemia may occur after high-caloric tube feeding, rapid infusion of hypertonic glucose solution, or deficiency of endogenous insulin. In the present section only stress diabetes is discussed. The incidence of postburn stress diabetes is low – about 0.36% in our inpatients.

7.1 Clinical Characteristics

Postburn stress diabetes is characterized by glucosuria, hyperglycemia, and absence of ketonuria. In our patients its onset was within 15 days postburn, and most of those affected had received high-caloric nasal tube feeding. In grave cases the fasting blood sugar may exceed 300 mg%, and in one case it exceeded 700 mg%. Most cases of stress diabetes can be controlled by 2 weeks of regular insulin therapy and prompt coverage of the wound, thus having no serious ill-effect on the course and prognosis of the injury. In extensive third degree burns, especially in cases with bulky muscle destruction, stress diabetes may aggravate the wound infection and may also cause gangrene of the necrotic muscles. As mutually interacting cause and effect, diabetes and infection may form a vicious circle. Uncontrollable diabetes and infection will eventually lead to sepsis and death.

Case Illustration. Male, aged 23. The patient had flame burns to 95% of the BSA, including third degree burns to 85%. No glycosuria was found immediately after admission. On the 3rd day postburn urinary sugar fluctuated between + + and + + +. GIK solution was given, with 1 IU regular insulin (RI) for each 5 g glucose. On the 12th postburn day dehydration and hyperosmolarity occurred. The serum sodium level increased to 150 mEq/liter, and the serum chloride level, to 135 mEq/liter. Despite RI therapy (96–120 IU/day), the blood sugar level still fluctuated between 319 mg and 700 mg %. The 24-h urinary sugar value amounted to 32 g–144 g; no ketonuria was found. Although 60% of the wound had been excised in stages and immediately covered with allo- and autografts, the wound became badly infected, together with progressive wet gangrene of the left upper limb and systemic mycosis. The patient died on the 22nd postburn day with uncontrolled diabetes.

The average total BSA burned and the average BSA affected by third degree burns in eight fatal cases complicated by stress diabetes were 88.6% and 54% respectively. Of the survivors, the most severe case involved burns to 85% of the BSA, including third degree burns to 52%.

With regard to the clinical symptoms, the three "polys" do not usually have diagnostic value in postburn stress diabetes: Polydipsia is usually present in ordinary burn patients, excessive catabolism and antibiotic-induced renal tubular damage may evoke polyuria, but polyphagia is rarely seen in burn patients. In extensive burn patients glycosuria may be due to rapid infusion of hypertonic glucose solution, so the criteria for diagnosis of stress diabetes must be the fasting blood sugar level and the glucose tolerance test. If the daily urinary output exceeds 4,000 ml and glycosuria, + +, the fasting blood sugar level should be determined.

7.2 Management

The principles of management are the same as for cases of diabetes in patients who have undergone surgery. No dietary control is necessary. With regular insulin treatment (dosage is monitored according to quantification of glucosuria), excisional operations and grafting can be carried out as usual. The level of fasting blood sugar concentration must be determined on the morning of the operative day; it must be brought to normal by RI before the operation and repeated checks should be made postoperatively. GIK in physiologic saline solution must be infused during the operation. If hypertonic glucose solution is given the glucose–insulin ratio should be set at 3:1 (g/IU) – 4:1 (g/IU).

Since postburn stress diabetes is evoked by the systemic response to the burn insult, it will subside spontaneously following the healing or coverage of the burn wound.

8 Acute Renal Failure (ARF)

In postburn ARF, the patient's blood volume is adequate and shock is relatively stabilized, but daily urinary output is less than 400 ml or, although the daily urine exceeds 400 ml, the blood urea nitrogen level shows a steep rise, the blood and urine urea nitrogen ratio is less than 1:15, and urine specific gravity is low and fixed at around 1.010–1.020. After extensive burn, the ability of the body to retain sodium means that the urinary sodium concentration can no longer be relied upon as a diagnostic index.

Postburn ARF may occur during the shock stage or may be a terminal symptom of fatal wound sepsis. Only shock stage ARF is discussed here.

8.1 General Considerations

Twenty-three guinea pigs were scalded in 70 °C water for 1 min. A burn of 50% of the BSA was thus created. The animals were killed 2 and 4 h postburn. The kidneys were extracted, and routine fixation, embedding, sectioning, and staining of the specimens were performed. Some of the sections were stained with benzidine. Microscopic examinations revealed congestion of the glomeruli and marked cloudy swelling of the renal tubules. Protein and granular casts were seen in 14 animals, hemoglobin casts in 7, and tubular necrosis in 2. The above findings implied that one type of postburn kidney damage is plugging of the renal tubules by casts (especially hemoglobin casts).

We have encountered 35 cases of shock stage ARF, of which seven were caused by chemical intoxication. The other 28 patients sustained extensive third degree burns, their average total burn area being 73.88% of the BSA, including third degree burns to 51.1%. Nine patients were either over 60 or below 6 years of age. Within 6 h postburn, antishock treatment was inadequate in seven patients who manifested anuria at the time of their admission. The above figures denote that the aged, infants, and those whose early antishock treatment was inadequate are liable to suffer from ARF. Another factor which influences the occurrence of ARF is the depth of burn. In the young and middle-age group, the average total BSA burned was 80% including third degree burns to 66.9%; all the patients had muscle involvement. Extensive muscle involvement may lead to intense hemoglobinuria and myohemoglobinuria. Hemoglobin and myohemoglobin casts, plugging the renal tubules, are stained blue by benzidine.

Case Illustration. Male, aged 47. There were flame burns to 96% of the BSA, including third degree burns to 94%. The patient was admitted 1 h postburn. The bladder was found to be empty. After rapid fluid administration (including 250 ml of 20% mannitol) dark soya sauce-colored urine flowed out from the indwelling catheter. The cardiovascular system was stable during the first 24 h. The amount of fluid administered during this period was 9,600 ml. The urinary output was 2,330 ml of hemo- and myohemoglobinuria. Starting from the second 24 h, urinary output suddenly dropped and abruptly turned clear; anuria ensued despite energetic treatment with various diuretics. At that time CVP was 10 cm water column. After 48 h postburn blood urea nitrogen increased to 48.4 mg%, and peritoneal dialysis was started. Due to massive destruction of the muscles of the legs and left forearm, debridement, bilateral disarticulation at the knees, and amputation of the left forearm were performed on the 3rd and 5th days postburn. The patient died on the 6th postburn day, leaving large amounts of necrotic muscle of the chest and amputation stumps still untreated. Despite adequate fluid replacement, prompt blood volume restoration, and early employment of various diuretics, ARF still could not be avoided.

Case Illustration. Male, aged 34. The patient had high tension electric burns to 21% of the BSA, including third degree burns to 16.5%. The patient was admitted in a state of shock after 3 h of long-distance transportation, during which time no intravenous fluid therapy was given. Fluid administered during the first 24 h amounted to 8,155 ml (including 500 ml of 20% mannitol, 250 ml of 5% sodium bicarbonate, and 700 ml of 1.25% sodium bicarbonate), urinary output (hemoglobinuria), 1,862 ml. At the beginning of the second 24 h the urine suddenly turned clear with a fixed specific gravity of 1.018. Oliguria and anuria quickly followed and did not respond to any diuretics employed. At that time CVP was 20 cm water column. On the 4th postburn day the patient's blood urea nitrogen increased to 55 mg%, creatinine to 6.1 mg%, and serum potassium to 6 mEq/liter. Peritoneal dialysis was started and retained for 11 days. By the 22nd day postburn the patient entered the polyuric phase, with a maximum daily urinary output of 5,000 ml. Renal function gradually recovered during the next 2 months, and the patient finally survived.

Owing to the destruction of large amounts of muscle, excisional and grafting operations were performed on days 2, 4, 7, and 11 postburn. All the deep burn eschar together with the necrotic muscle bellies were radically excised and immediate coverage was achieved.

The key to the successful management of this patient was early diagnosis, radical excision, and immediate coverage before the onset of invasive infection. The fact which contributed considerably to the successful management was that although the patient's burn was deep, it was not very extensive.

The absorption of toxic chemicals, such as phenol, α or β-sodium naphthol, chromic acid, mercury, bismuth, carbon tetrachloride, etc., from the wound may result in ARF. Seven of the present series of ARFs were caused by chemical intoxications; six received peritoneal dialysis and one hemodialysis. Three patients survived. We are convinced that further improvement of the techniques of dialysis and of excision and grafting will further lower the mortality.

8.2 Prevention and Early Diagnosis of ARF of the Shock Stage

In cases of extensive third degree burns, high tension electric injury, or burns complicated by chemical intoxication, besides the usual resuscitation measures, two intravenous lifelines must be established, one for fluid replacement and one for rapid infusion of 20% mannitol and 5% or 2.5% sodium bicarbonate. 20% mannitol 1,000 ml in separate doses (usually four or six) may be given in 24 h. If hemoglobinuria and myohemoglobinuria still exist after the first 24 h postburn, another one or two doses of 250 ml of 20% mannitol should be given. The total amount of daily sodium bicarbonate infused to alkalinize the urine may reach 24 g. After rapid infusion of 20% mannitol, the total urinary output within the next 3 h should exceed the amount of mannitol infused. If it does not, impairment of renal function is to be strongly suspected. Infusion of 300 ml–500 ml of 5% glucose within 30 min or injection of ethacrynic acid or furosemide may give some beneficial effects in such circumstances (see Chap. II). If, after the above-mentioned treatment, blood pressure and CVP are normal, oliguria still exists, and the urine is water-clear with a fixed specific gravity of 1.010–1.020, the diagnosis of ARF can be ascertained.

Owing to the large amount of water loss from the wound, the daily water intake should not be restricted to 500 ml in postburn ARF.

8.3 Peritoneal Dialysis in Postburn ARF

8.3.1 Timing

Peritoneal dialysis should be started as soon as possible for two reasons:

1. A large amount of fluid is administered during the shock stage so that the complications of heart failure and pulmonary edema, which may precipitate fulminating septicemia during the resorption period, are likely to occur.

2. Since catabolism is greatly enhanced after burn, hyperkalemia and azotemia will progress with extreme rapidity. After ARF, 48–72 h are enough to raise the serum potassium concentration to a dangerous level. Therefore in our opinion peritoneal dialysis should be started within 48 h after the diagnosis of ARF is made.

Case Illustration. The diagnosis of ARF was established 18 h after a burned child was admitted. At that time the blood urea nitrogen (BUN) was 22.8 mg%; during the next 12 h it increased to 63 mg%. Peritoneal dialysis was started 32 h postburn. Forty-eight hours after dialysis BUN decreased to 48 mg%. Ten grams of urea nitrogen was dialyzed, and 1,100 ml water were drawn via the peritoneal cavity during this 48-h period, with significant subsidence of the patient's edema.

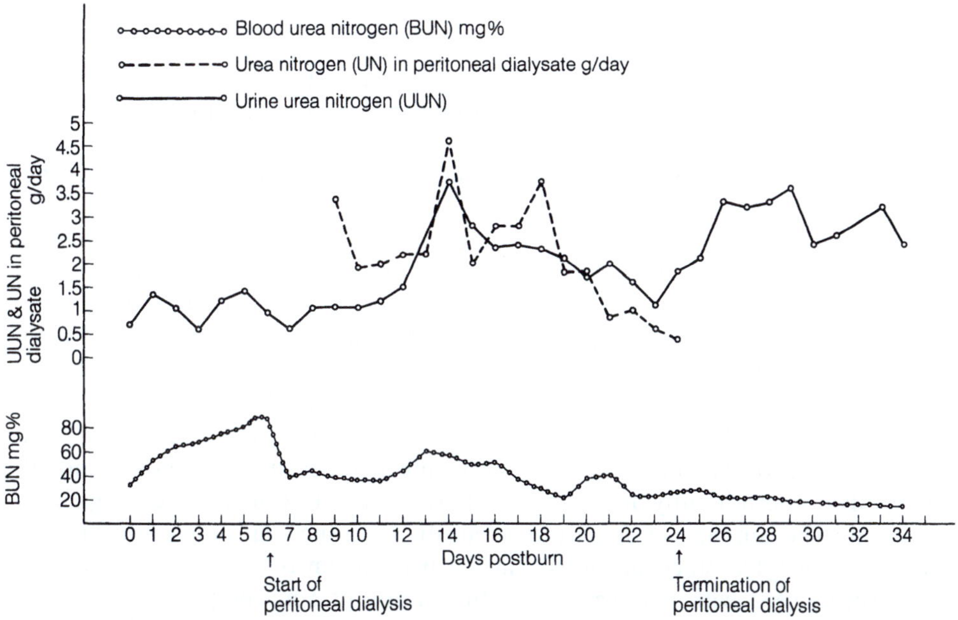

Fig. XI.3. Illustration of the course of polyuric ARF in a 6-year-old girl with burns to 49.5% of the BSA, including third degree burns to 29%

In the polyuric type of ARF, azotemia increases steeply although there is no menace of fluid overloading. Early dialysis without hesitation will lead to a rapid recovery.

Case Illustration. Female, aged 6. The patient had burns to 49.5% of the BSA, including third degree burns to 29%. She was admitted 5.5 h postburn, after long-distance transportation without fluid therapy. The patient sustained polyuric ARF. Despite a satisfactory urinary output, BUN increased to 85 mg% and creatinine to 10.3 mg% on the 5th postburn day. Peritoneal dialysis was started on the 6th day and continued for 19 days. After excision and graftings, the patient survived with normal renal function (Fig. XI.3).

In order to expel the toxic chemicals in ARF with chemical intoxication, dialysis may be started even earlier: the earlier it is started, the sooner will normal renal function return.

8.3.2 Preparation and Instructions

1. To each liter of peritoneal dialyzing fluid, 3 mg–5 mg heparin and 25 mg tetracycline (or 100 mg cephalothin) are added. Since tetracycline and cephalothin are detrimental to the liver and the kidney and are readily absorbed via the peritoneum, we usually employ the intermittent instillation method (instilled q 4 or 6 h).

2. If the skin of the abdomen is not burned, a peritoneal dialysis tube may be inserted via a median incision below the umbilicus. Alternatively some other nonburned or relatively shallow burned area may be chosen. The important point is that the tube must be inserted into the rectovesical fossa or the Douglas cul-de-sac.

3. During daily changing of the inlet and outlet tubing, strictly aseptic technique should be used.

4. It is advisable to prewarm the dialyzing fluid to 37 °C. One liter of dialyzing fluid is allowed to run into the peritoneal cavity within 15 min and is drained out 45 min later. If the drainage is not free, the dialysis tube may be readjusted, the posture changed, or gentle massage performed. The tube may be flushed aseptically with heparin–physiologic saline solution (1 mg heparin in 100 ml physiologic saline) to release the fibrinous plugs.

5. If the fluid let out from the peritoneum is turbid, as is frequently seen in extensive burn patients, it is likely to be infected. Sensitive antibiotics should be instilled intermittently according to the sensitivity test of the microorganism revealed. The amount of nephrotoxic antibiotics, such as polymyxin B and various aminoglycosides, absorbed via the peritoneum is very small; therefore they can be used with relative safety. (Instillation of 5 mg polymyxin per liter, 10 mg gentamicin per liter, 50 mg kanamycin per liter, 50 mg amikacin per liter, or 50 mg vancomycin per liter may be carried out intermittently.)

6. If the serum potassium concentration drops below 4 mEq/liter during dialysis, 3 ml of 10% KCl must be added to each liter of dialyzing fluid.

7. Urea nitrogen and protein content in the dialyzing fluid should be determined daily in order to appraise the effectiveness of the dialysis and the amount of protein loss. The dietary protein intake may not be restricted if the serum urea nitrogen concentration is not high. The amount of protein loss must be supplemented by plasma or human albumin.

8. High caloric dietary intake, parenteral nutritive support, and intravenous administration of antibiotics all need water as solvent. Twenty grams of glucose, which can extract 300 ml of excessive water, may be added to each liter of dialyzing fluid to prevent dilutional hyponatremia.

9. The usual complication of postburn peritoneal dialysis is infection. Peritoneal dialysis ought to be abandoned if the infection is uncontrollable. The alternative is hemodialysis. Complications such as abdominal pain, diarrhea, intestinal distension, and intraperitoneal hemorrhage can be mitigated by symptomatic treatment.

8.4 Other Managements of Postburn ARF

8.4.1 Nutrition

Energetic nutritional support must be given to meet the needs of massive evaporative heat loss, extremely enhanced catabolism, wound infection, tissue repair etc. The concrete requirements are as follows:

1. Daily caloric intake for adult must be kept over 2,000 cal.

2. Ordinarily protein intake in ARF must be restricted according to the

Table XI.14. High caloric liquid diet cases of ARF (1500 ml)

Constituents (g)	Protein (g)	Fat (g)	Carbo-hydrate (g)	Caloric supply
Rice soup (1,250)	5	0	40	180
Chocolate (150)	18	72	45	916
Cane sugar (100)	0	0	100	400
Peanut oil (10)	0	10	0	90
Total	23	82	185	1,586

creatinine clearance. The amount of protein can be increased greatly if the patient's BUN is below 100 mg% and under effective dialysis.

3. In polyuric ARF, sodium and potassium loss is tremendous, and they must be supplied according to urinary loss. Intravenous and intramuscular supplementation of vitamins is undertaken for patients who are under total parenteral nutritive support.

4. High caloric ARF liquid diet: each liter supplies 1,000 cal (Table XI.14). With regard to parenteral nutrition, see Chap. XII.

5. Protein loss via the peritoneum must be replaced in the form of plasma or human albumin.

6. Anuric or oliguric patients are advised not to eat edible mushroom, pickled vegetable root, potato, or fruit juice, all of which are rich in potassium.

8.4.2 Fluid Intake

In oliguric patients, overhydration will cause hyponatremia, pulmonary edema, or heart failure. The daily schedule of water intake should be strictly calculated on the basis of the sensible and insensible water loss minus the water of oxidation. The daily insensible loss from the normal skin and respiratory tract is 12 ml/kg; from the burn wound it is 300 ml–500 ml per 10% of the BSA burned. Edema, hyponatremia, and increase of body weight imply that the patient is overhydrated.

8.4.3 Management of Hyperkalemia

In postburn ARF, there is always a steep rise in the serum potassium level. If its concentration exceeds 5.6 mEq/liter, the following emergency measures should be carried out together with dialysis:

1. Intravenous infusion of 250 ml of 5% sodium bicarbonate.

2. Hyperkalemia, hypermagnesemia, and hypocalcemia usually coexist, thus enhancing their individual toxic effects upon the myocardium. In order to mitigate their detrimental effects, 10 ml–20 ml of 10% calcium gluconate may be given intravenously. The daily dose may reach 50 ml–100 ml.

3. Intravenous infusion of 250 ml of 50% glucose mixed with 30 IU RI.

4. Gastric lavage with hypotonic saline solution may wash out a considerable amount of potassium.

Table XI.15. Bone and joint complications in 58 burn patients

Complications	No. of cases
Osteomyelitis	31
Purulent arthritis	22
Ectopic calcification and ossification	5

8.4.4 Management of Dilutional Hyponatremia

Restriction of fluid intake and prompt dialysis is the only way to combat dilutional hyponatremia.

8.4.5 Management of Metabolic Acidosis

It is unjustifiable to treat metabolic acidosis in ARF by administration of sodium bicarbonate or sodium lactate. A low carbon dioxide combining power is a strong indication for immediate dialysis.

9 Bone and Joint Complications

Postburn bone and joint complications are usually related to local or systemic infection and prolonged immobilization. The early changes include osteomyelitis and purulent arthritis. Late changes are osteoporosis, ectopic calcification, ectopic ossification, and osteophyte formation. Of 973 burn patients admitted over a 6-year period, 58 developed destructive or hyperplastic bone and joint changes (Table XI.15). This figure cannot reflect the true extent of this complication since a general bone survey has not been carried out in all of the patients admitted. Roentgenologic examination was performed only in cases which revealed clinically significant bone and joint involvement. Some were discovered during the follow-up studies or when the patients were readmitted for reconstructive surgery.

9.1 **Bone Destruction** (Fig. XI.4)

Most cases of bone destruction are elicited by direct thermal injuries. A few are caused by infection of the adjacent soft tissues. Sites where soft tissues are scanty, such as the anterior tibial region, the ankle, the dorsum of the hand, the head, etc., are liable to be affected.

9.2 **Joint Destruction** (Fig. XI.5)

Joint destruction can be caused by either direct thermal insults or hematogenous purulent arthritis. Loss of a certain degree of articular motion will inevitably result in most cases, and in some it will eventually lead to ankylosis of the

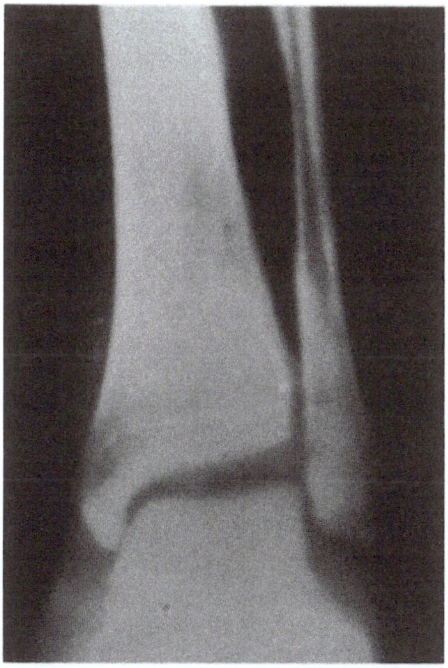

Fig. XI.4. Bony destruction of the lower end of the fibula and of the ankle joint. Linear ossification of the soft tissue is seen at the lower inner aspect of the tibia. (83 days postburn)

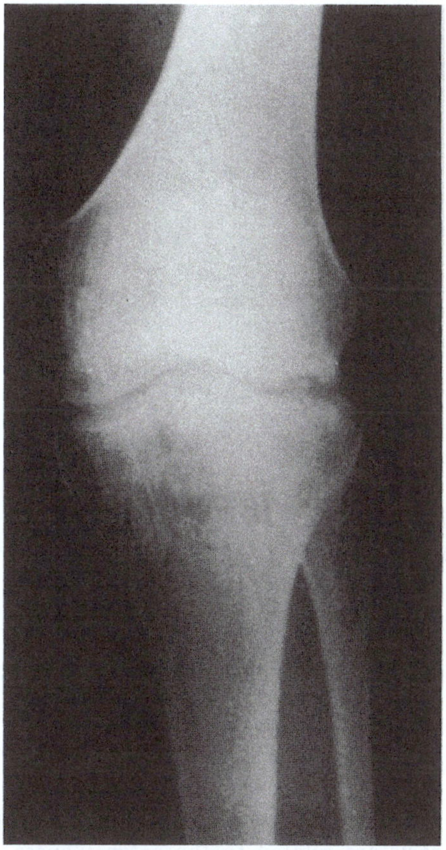

Fig. XI.5. Extensive destruction of the knee joint and osteoporosis. (212 days postburn)

joint. Purulent arthritis of the superficial joints, such as the interphalangeal joints, the elbow joint, and the ankle joint is usually due to direct extension of infection from the adjacent burn wounds, whereas the purulent arthritis of hematogenous dissemination usually affects deep-seated joints such as the hip. The principle of treatment is the same as in ordinary purulent arthritis.

9.3 Hyperplastic Periostitis

If the periostitis is caused by infection of adjacent soft tissue of a long bone shaft, the hyperplastic change will be linear and extensive, whereas the lesion is localized if it is caused by periarticular infection.

9.4 Osteoporosis

Osteoporosis is frequently seen in postburn bony changes. It has not been listed in Table XI.13. In mild cases, only punctating translucent areas of one to several millimeters breadth are seen on the X-ray film. They are scattered in the cancellous ends of the long bones, and may also be seen in the cortex and the medullary cavity in severe cases. Translucent belts may be demonstrated

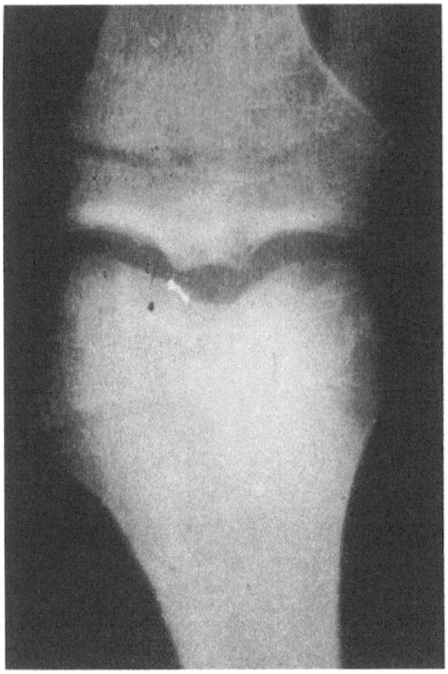

Fig. XI.6. Osteoporosis of the ends of the long bones. Translucent belts are seen at the epiphyseal region. (190 days postburn)

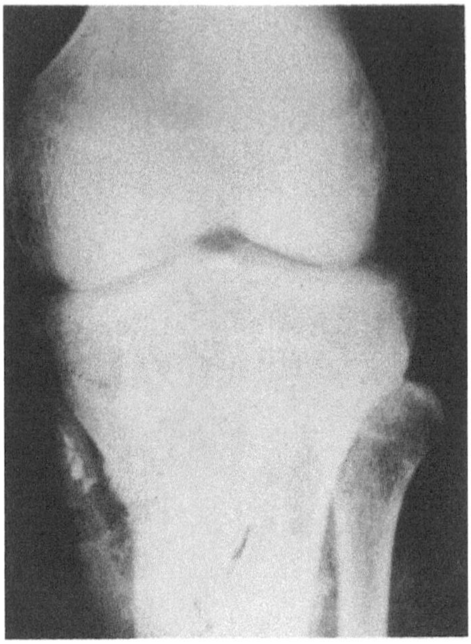

Fig. XI.7. An area of ossification shadow is seen at the inner aspect of the tibia. Osteophyte formation, narrowing of the knee joint space, and subluxation are also present. (63 days postburn)

near the epiphyseal region (Fig. XI.6). The extensiveness and severity of osteoporosis are related to the extensiveness and the duration of the course of burn. In patients with extensive burns, osteoporosis can usually be detected 1 month postburn. Generally speaking, after 1–2 years of convalescence, generalized osteoporosis will no longer be apparent or at least will be greatly improved. But localized osteoporosis may exist for a long time in patients who suffer from functional derangement of the limbs.

Osteoporosis in senile patients may precipitate pathologic fractures.

The most important and effective measures in the prevention and treatment of postburn osteoporosis are early ambulation and functional drilling.

9.5 Ectopic Calcification and Ossification

Infection and immobilization are possible causes of postburn ectopic calcification and ossification. The characteristic changes usually manifest later than 2 months postburn. The clinical sign is the restriction of motion of the involved joint. Calcification may progress to ossification. The process can be revealed by growth in the density and formation of the bony trabeculae of the calcification spots in serial roentgenographic follow-up studies. Calcification and ossification may coexist. According to site of occurrence, they can be further classified into paraosteal and paraarticular types, of which the latter is more frequently seen.

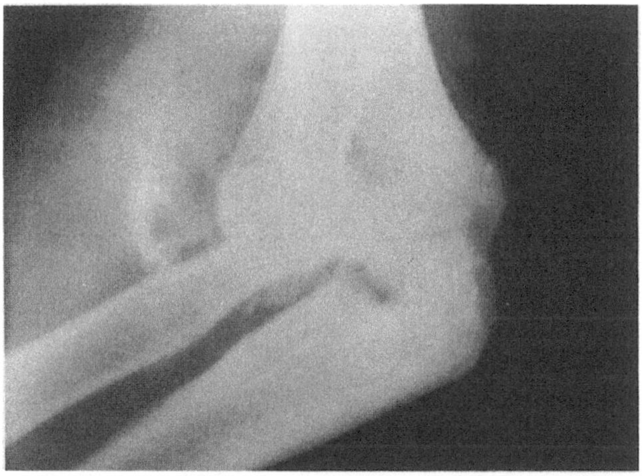

Fig. XI.8. Irregular linear ossification of the elbow joint, which has been destroyed. (96 days postburn)

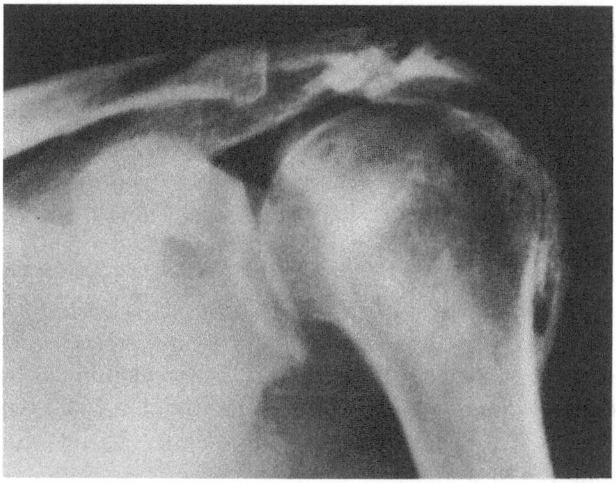

Fig. XI.9. Ossification, osteoporosis, and bony ankylosis shoulder joint. (301 days postburn)

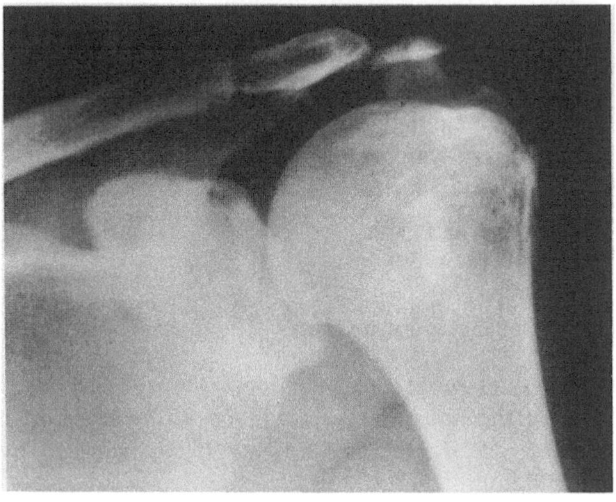

Fig. XI.10. Ossification and bony ankylosis of area of the shoulder joint

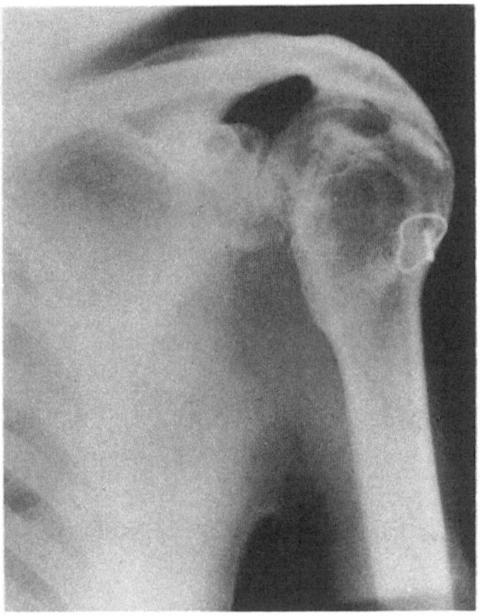

Fig. XI.11. Same patient as in **Fig. XI.9**, 16 years postburn. A rotational osteotomy of the humerus was performed 1 year postburn. Functional recovery is excellent

Roentgenographically the paraosteal type is characterized by linear or ossification shadows in paraskeletal tissues. They are usually solitary, not connected with the skeleton, and deeply situated underneath full-thickness burn wounds (Fig. XI.7). Paraarticular calcification or ossification usually involves the elbow joints, and may be single or multiple. The lesions are usually seen around the joint capsule where tendons and ligments are attached, and finally the whole joint capsule may be completely surrounded by ossification tissue. Whenever the joint is involved, limitation of articular motion ensues (Figs. XI.8–XI.10). The ossification and calcification lesions may be formed both in burn and nonburn areas.

Early coverage of the wound, avoiding forced passive movement of the joint, and early joint motion are the main steps in the prevention of calcification and ossification. The restricted joint motion due to calcification may be improved by physical therapy. In a few patients, painstaking exercises may result in resolution of the calcified spots and restoration of full range motion of the joint. Various conservative measures usually end in failure in cases of ossification. Operative intervention is considered in patients with functional disturbances. Radical excision together with orthopaedic corrections are usually rewarding (Fig. XI.11).

9.6 Osteophytes Formation

Osteophytes often protrude from the bony ends. If bony bridges are finally formed, the adjacent joint will be ultimately ankylosed. If the joint motion is greatly restricted or completely lost, surgical excision of the osteophytes is mandatory.

Chapter XII Nursing Care in Burns

TAO XIANG-LING and XU WEI-ZHEN

Translated by LING LI-LI

1 Sources of Infection, Disinfection, and Isolation

There are two routes through which the burn wound may be contaminated by microorganisms: firstly, autoinfection, and secondly, cross infection. The infection of burn wounds due to cross infection is more liable to cause invasive infection, and the cross infection may also cause the spread of drug-resistant bacterial strains.

1.1 Sources of Cross Infection

The main routes by which cross infection takes place are pollution of the air, contamination by utensils, and contamination by medical personnel.

The main causes of airborne pollution are related to the frequent entrance and exit of the medical personnel, changing of dressings, general cleaning of the wards, and poor ventilation (Tables XII.1–XII.4). The most serious airborne pollution of the wards occurs during changing of dressings; therefore, changing of dressings should not be carried out for two patients simultaneously in the same ward. Changing of bed sheets should be done gently. Soiled bedding and clothes and soiled dressings should be placed in containers. The number of persons going in and out of the ward should be strictly limited.

The air pipes of an air conditioner of the circulating type might be the source of spreading of microorganisms (Table XII.5). Unidirectional cold and warm air passage pipes should be used (see Table XII.6).

The dressings, bedding, clothing, medical instruments, furniture, and mattress which had been in contact with burn patients were proved to carry pathogenic

Table XII.1. Number of bacterial colonies in the air before, during, and after changing of dressings

Time	No. of bacterial colonies per m^3
Before changing of dressings	930
During changing of dressings	6,890
After changing of dressings	1,310

Table XII.2. Comparison of the number of bacterial colonies in the air before and after general cleaning

No. of bacterial colonies per m^3 before general cleaning	No. of bacterial colonies per m^3 within 15 min after general cleaning
936	10,240

Table XII.3. Effect of frequency of passage of personnel on the number of bacterial colonies in the air

No. of persons moving about the same ward	No. of bacterial colonies per m^3
8	21
20	144
23	158

Table XII.5. Number of colonies after formalin fumigation (15 ml/m^3) performed three times

Site	No. of colonies of fungi
Entrance of air pipe No. 1	3
Exit of air pipe No. 1	147
Entrance of air pipe No. 2	48
Exit of air pipe No. 2	218

Table XII.4. Number of bacterial colonies in the air when the room is tightly closed or ventilated

	No. of bacterial colonies per m^3
Air in tightly closed room	20–35
Air in ventilated room	0– 6

Table XII.6. The results of investigation 575 days after installation of unidirectional cold and warm air pipes

Site	No. of colonies[a]
Entrance of air pipe No. 1	0
Exit of air pipe No. 1	0
Entrance of air pipe No. 2	1
Exit of air pipe No. 2	0

[a] 15 min after opening Petri's dish

organisms. Using the bacteriophagic typing method, the strains of *Staphylococcus aureus* isolated from the burn wound were found to be identical to the strains isolated from the air and various utensils used in the burn wards. (Table XII.7a, b). We are of the opinion that emphasis should be put on the final disinfection after transfer to another ward, discharge, or death of the patients. All the materials pertaining to the bed must be sterilized with ethylene oxide before they can be used again (Fig. XII.1).

Table XII.7a. Bacteriophagic typing of 182 strains of *Staphylococcus aureus* isolated from burned patients. (Courtesy of Dr. Lan Hong-tai)

Group number	Phage type	No. of strains	Total	Percentage
I	79	1	3	1.64
	52/80	1		
	52/52A/80	1		
II	55/71	11	20	10.9
	55/71$^+$	1		
	71	6		
	71$^+$	1		
	3A	1		
III	54	20	81	44.5
	53/83A	8		
	53	6		
	53$^+$	2		
	75	6		
	53/75/77	6		

Group number	Phage type	No. of strains	Total	Percentage
	7	4		
	7/47/53/54/75/83A	4		
	75/77	4		
	42E	2		
	47/53	3		
	7/47/54/75+	2		
	6/7/47/53/54/73+	2		
	47	1		
	77	1		
	77+	1		
	7/75	1		
	53/77	1		
	7/47/54	1		
	7/47/57	1		
	47/53/54/77	1		
	47/54/75/77+	1		
	7/47/53/54	1		
	6/7/47/53/54/75	1		
	47/53/54/75/77	1		
Undetermined	81	11	16	8.78
	187	5		
Mixed group	52/52A/80/81	24	62	34.0
	52/52A/80/81+	7		
	52/81	3		
	80/71	2		
	52/52A/80/71	2		
	29/53	1		
	29/81	1		
	52/81	1		
	80/81	1		
	80/7+	1		
	42E/81	1		
	80/71	1		
	52A/79/77	1		
	80/53/81	1		
	29/79/83A	1		
	29/52/81+	1		
	52/80/81	1		
	80/53/81	1		
	71/7/47	1		
	52A/79/75+	1		
	54/75/81+	1		
	52/6/47/53	1		
	80/71/53/75	1		
	52/6/7/47/53/54	1		
	52/52A/80/54/75/81+	1		
	42E/47/53/54/75/81	1		
	6/7/42E/47/53/54/75/81	1		
	52/52A/79/80/7/47/55/77/83A+	1		
	6/7/42E/47/53/54/75/77/81/83A	1		

The above table shows that the most frequent type of *S. aureus* isolated was type 52/52A/80/81. The most frequent group was group III; the second most frequent group was the mixed group

Table XII.7b. Bacteriophagic survey of carriers (59 strains of "typable" *Staphylococcus aureus*). (Courtesy of Dr. Lan Hong-tai)

Group number	Carrier	Phage type	No. of strains	Total	Percentage	Total
I	Medical personnel	29^+	1	6	10.17	10.17
		29/52	1			
		79	1			
		80	1			
		52/52A/80	1			
		29/52/52A/80	1			
	Air and utensils		0		0	
II	Medical personnel	55^+	3	10	11.8	15.95
		55/71	3			
		$55/71^+$	1			
	Air and utensils	71	3		4.15	
III	Medical personnel	53	1	16	10.17	27.12
		54	1			
		53/75/77	1			
		$47/53/75/77^+$	1			
		7/47/54/75/77	1			
		$6/7/42E/47/53/54^+$	1			
	Air and utensils	53/75/77	3		16.95	
		47/53/75/77	2			
		7	1			
		7^+	1			
		42E	1			
		54	1			
		77	1			
Undetermined	Medical personnel	81	2	11	6.78	18.64
		187	2			
	Air and utensils	81	2		11.86	
		187	5			
Mixed group	Medical personnel	52/52A/80/81	2	16	11.8	27.12
		53/187	1			
		52/80/81	1			
		$52/52A/80/81^+$	1			
		29/79/42E/47/53/75	1			
		29/52/52A/80/7/42E/81	1			
	Air and utensils	$52/52A/80/81^+$	3		15.32	
		52/52A/80/81	2			
		80/81	1			
		80/42E	1			
		$52/80/81^+$	1			
		$29/52/52A/80/71/6/7/53^+$	1			

The above table shows that the most frequent type of *S. aureus* isolated from the carriers was also type 52/52A/80/81. The most frequent groups were group III and the mixed group

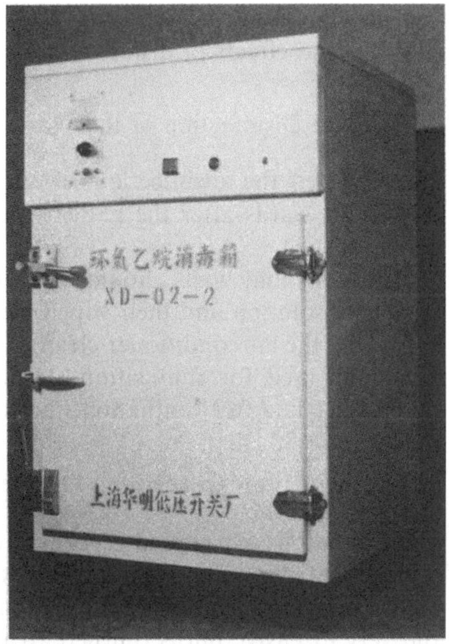

Fig. XII.1. Ethylene oxide sterilizer

The incidence of bacterial contamination of the hands is highest after changing or adjusting dressings, and is also high after basic nursing of patients (Table XII.8). After contact with the patients or soiled dressings, the hands of the attending personnel must be washed with soap and running water.

Formerly the incidence of carrier state in the nasopharynx of medical personnel in our burn wards was 100%. One of the common sites is the nasal cavity, and several sites may be involved at the same time. The chief microorganisms revealed are gram-positive cocci. Local application of antibiotics cannot eradicate the carrier state of the nasopharynx. Nowadays medical personnel are allowed periodic temporary leave from the burn wards for a few months; this will cause a natural decline in the incidence of carriers.

Table XII.8. Bacteriologic investigation of both hands of attending personnel before disinfection

No. of cultures	Positive (*n*)	Nonpathogenic bacterial (*n*)	*Staphylococcus aureus* (*n*)	Fungi (*n*)
12	0	2	9	1

1.2 Measures of Disinfection and Isolation

Maximum effort should be made to prevent cross infection, especially before the formation of scab of the wound surface in the early stage of burns. Owing to the varying opinions regarding asepsis and isolation, the measures taken in different institutes also vary. The following is a simple account of the disinfection and isolation measures in our institute, based on investigation of cross infection and effects of disinfection in the past.

1.2.1 Final Disinfection of the Wards

This denotes the disinfection of air and all the utensils which have been used in the wards after the patients have been discharged, transferred to other wards, or died.

The floor and walls should be brushed with 5% lysol mixed with sodium carbonate solution and then wiped clean with water. Attention should be paid to keeping the air conditioner clean. Formaldehyde and bleaching powder (3:2) should be used for fumigation sterilization, and the room should be tightly closed for 6 h. After ventilation, the room is again ready for use.

1.2.2 Regulations Concerning Disinfection and Isolation in the Wards

The regulations are graded according to the severity of burns.

1. Disinfection and isolation for extensively burned patients are carried out in the early stage of burns to more than 50% of the BSA (before scab formation) and very extensive burns (burned area exceeding 80% of the BSA).

a) After debridement, the patient should be moved into a clean single room. It is desirable to have two single rooms for alternative used for patients with very extensive burns.

b) The attending personnel should wear a clean working suit, masks, caps, and shoes, and if necessary, a sterilized suit.

c) The attending personnel should wash their hands with soap and running water before and after entering or leaving the ward, after contact with patients, and after changing dressings.

2. The procedures regarding disinfection and isolation for ordinary burn patients are also applicable when dealing with patients with burns to medium or minor body surface areas.

a) The patient should be moved into a clean ward after debridement.

b) The attending personnel should be wearing caps and working suits on entering the room. Masks should be put on prior to changing dressings, turning over the patient, or carrying out treatment. Hands must be washed after coming into contact with the wound surface or soiled materials and after helping the patient in defecation or urination.

1.3 Problems and Prospect of Improvement

The incidence of cross infection between the wards in medical units with a large number of burn patients is still very high in spite of investigation of the sources of cross infection and repeated modifications of the measures of disinfection and isolation. The measures which we now take to reduce the incidence of cross infection are still far from adequate, and they are rather tedious. If the attending personnel does not have a good understanding of

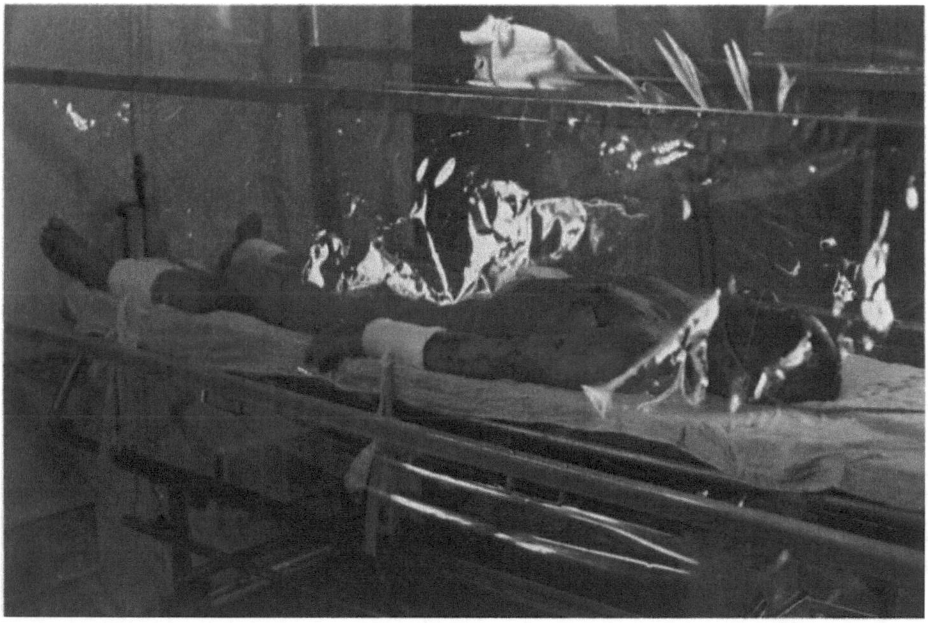

Fig. XII.2. Laminar flow cabinet, introduced by Boston Shriner's Institute. It has recently been tried out in the People's Republic of China with respect to its effectiveness in controlling cross infections

the dangers of cross infection, the above measures are even more difficult to implement. It is therefore necessary to investigate further effective measures of disinfection and isolation to reduce the incidence of cross infection as far as is possible (Fig. XII.2).

2 Nutrition

The increase in metabolism and constant exhaustion of tissues of body are characteristic features of severe burn reactions. The hypermetabolic state starts from the 2nd day postburn and remains until the wounds have healed. The calorie requirement in patients with extensive burns exceeds that in any other diseases, and if such requirements are not fulfilled, there will be a loss of body weight directly proportional to the severity of the burn. It is difficult to satisfy the nutritional demand even in patients without complications because the amount of calories required is great, whereas factors such as neuroendocrine changes, gastrointestinal dysfunction, and sepsis will cause even more difficulties in achieving nutritional balance in burn patients.

Malnutrition and hypoproteinemia cause delay in healing of the wound, lower resistance to infection, render control of infection difficult, and produce liability to various kinds of complications. Nutritional deficiency is one of the causes of death in patients with extensive and deep burns.

2.1 Nutrient Requirements

Owing to high fever, exudation from the wound surface, repeated operations, and anesthesia, the amount of water evaporated daily and the exhaustion of heat are great. The daily loss of water and nitrogen may reach 3,000 ml–5,000 ml and 30 g–50 g, and the reduction of body weight may be 1 kg per day in severe cases. Generally, our patients have their wounds largely covered by the 30th–40th day postburn, therefore, the positive nitrogen balance may be achieved 1 month postburn. Before healing of the wounds the protein loss via the wound surfaces may exceed the catabolic loss. Within this period the plasma protein is usually very low in burn patients in spite of transfusion of large amounts of blood, plasma, and albumin during the course of treatment. In most cases, the plasma protein is only 4 g%–5 g% (occasionally only 3 g%–4 g%), and plasma albumin, 1.5 g%–2 g%; in addition there may be reversal of the albumin–globulin ratio. The patients are markedly emaciated. One of our cases had burns to 95% of the BSA, including third degree burns to 10%. The body weight was 75 kg on admission, but only 55 kg 1 month later (a 27% reduction). It is evident, therefore, that the requirements of calories, protein, and vitamins in burn patients are much greater than in normal persons.

2.2 The Nitrogen–Calorie Ratio

It is important to pay attention to the proportion of carbohydrates, proteins, and fats in the supply of calories and the proportion of nitrogen and non-nitrogen caloric content in order to achieve satisfactory nourishment. Generally speaking, protein supplies 15% of the total caloric intake; fat, 35%; and carbohydrates, 50%. The ideal non-nitrogen caloric intake for each gram of nitrogen is 150–200 cal.

In a patient who requires 4,500 cal/day, the amount of protein is 4,500 cal × 15% = 675 cal (about 170 g); the amount of fat, 4,500 cal × 35% = 1,757 cal (175 g); and the amount of carbohydrate, 4,500 cal × 50% = 2,250 cal (560 g).

2.3 Routes of Administration of Nutrients

2.3.1 Enteral Administration

2.3.1.1 Oral Feeding

In patients with medium or minor burns, food can be given soon after the burn. In patients with extensive burns, diet can be started with the restoration of normal intestinal peristalsis, generally 48 h postburn. Sugar water, rice soup, and fruit juice may be tried first, 25 ml–50 ml at a time. If these can be taken without ill-effect, the amount of food can be increased gradually.

2.3.1.2 Nasal Feeding

When a peristaltic pump is employed in nasal feeding, a soft silicone gastric tube of 0.15 cm–0.2 cm in diameter may be used.

Preparation of nutrient liquids: Nutrient liquids for nasal feeding consist of rice soup, 10%–15% concentrated bean milk and cow milk. Cow milk may be used as the chief constituent, supplemented by chocolate, sugar, glucose, and eggs to make up the "nutrient milk." Alternatively, concentrated bean milk may be used as the chief constituent, supplemented by sugar and bean oil to make up "whole bean milk nutrient liquids." Casein and amino acids can also be made into nutrient liquids for nasal feeding. In diarrheal patients, casein is used instead of cow milk. Our clinical practice indicates that casein possesses some antidiarrheal property and that it may even cause constipation in patients with normal gastrointestinal function. These nutrient liquids may be selected or supplemented according to the functioning of absorption and digestion.

*2.3.1.3 "Element Diet"**

"Element diet" is composed of the most elemental nutrients and is prepared according to the nutritional requirements of the body. In the element diet, nitrogen can be supplied by crystalline amino acids and the proportion of essential amino acids and nonessential amino acids is 35% : 65%. It also contains fat and carbohydrate compounds, such as glucose, fructose, or sucrose. Various kinds of vitamins may be added. By means of the element diet one can supply large amounts of calories and amino acids. It may be made into liquids by the addition of water just before use. Utilization of the full amount of this kind of diet will supply 3,000 cal and 20 g amino acids (equivalent to 120 g protein) per day.

The element diet may be administered by either oral feeding or nasal feeding. Spices may be added in oral feeding, and the food should be taken in small amounts but with greater frequency. The concentration of the preparations may be adjusted into four kinds (5%, 10%, 20%, and 24%), or three kinds (5%, 12%, and 24%). Generally, each milliliter of the 24% element diet furnishes 1 cal. In patients with extensive burns, nasal feeding of 5% or 12% element diet may be started on the 3rd day postburn: 25 ml–50 ml may be administered per hour. If there are no side effects, such as gastric retention, diarrhea, and glucosuria, the concentration and rate of administration may be increased gradually.

There are plenty of carbohydrates in the element diet and they may cause osmotic diuresis. The rate of instillation should be constant; it should be readjusted if the rate is so high as to cause glucosuria. The amount of feeding should be reduced gradually until it is completely withdrawn.

Case Illustration. Male, aged 25. The patient sustained flame burns to 73.5% of the BSA, including third degree burns to 40.3%. The allograft transplanted after excision of the eschar underwent lysis and sloughed off around the 30th

* Supplied by "East Sea" Pharmaceutical Factory, Shanghai.

day postburn. The granulation tissue was exposed, the wound surface was heavily infected by *Pseudomonas aeruginosa*, and there was disturbance of electrolytes balance. The patient was extremely emaciated. Administration of element diet was commenced, and at the same time high protein diet including casein and eggs was given orally. About 200 g protein and 4,000 cal–5,000 cal were supplied per day for 34 days. The wound surface was covered after several operations. The body weight increased from 44.3 kg to 52.8 kg, the plasma protein level from 5.5 g% to 6.3 g%, and the hemoglobin level from 9.7 g to 11.5 g. The patient survived.

2.3.2 Intravenous Alimentation

2.3.2.1 Composition of Intravenous Aliments

The nutriments administered intravenously are chiefly glucose and amino-acids. In order to prevent the severely injured body from mobilizing proteins and for the utilization of administered glucose, insulin should be given together with glucose in the proportion of 5:1 or 4:1 (e.g., 1 unit of insulin for every 5 g glucose).

Amino acid solutions are given chiefly for the synthesis of proteins. Generally, a mixture composed of 5% protein hydrolysate, or 9% or 12% amino acid may be used. Protein hydrolysate is not as effective as amino acid solutions owing to its high content of short peptides which cannot be fully utilized by the body. Furthermore, patients who are allergic to proteins are liable to suffer from the side effects of hypersensitivity. The mixture of amino acids used at present is composed of L-amino acids.

2.3.2.2 Preparations of Intravenous Aliments

1. One unit comprises 300 ml of 50% glucose solution and 500 ml of 5% protein hydrolysate in 5% glucose solution. Each milliliter of the mixture will supply 1 cal.

2. One unit comprises 500 ml of 25% glucose solution and 200 ml of amino acid solution. Each milliliter of the mixture will supply 1 cal.

To enhance utilization of the intravenous nutrient liquids, for every unit the following constituents may be added: 2 g potassium chloride, 40 mg adenosine triphosphate (ATP), 100 units coenzyme A, 100 mg inosine, 100 mg vitamin B_1, and 100 mg vitamin B_6. Insulin is added in the ratio of 5:1 or 4:1 according to the amount of glucose in each unit. Two or three units may be given per day. Various kinds of vitamins (including fat soluble ones) and trace elements should be supplemented to total parenteral nutrition.

In our treatment of severely burned patients, besides the daily 2–3 units of parenteral nutriment, 2,000 ml of a solution composed of glucose, insulin, potassium chloride, and vitamin C (or GIKC) should be supplemented. Each 1,000 ml of 10% glucose solution contains 20 units of insulin, 30 ml of 10% potassium chloride, and 1 g vitamin C.

Table XII.9. Parenteral aliments administered 4–45 days postburn in a 37-year-old male with burns to 90% of the BSA, including third degree burns to 60%

Human albumin	500 ml of 25% glucose solution and 200 ml of 9% amino acid	Glucose
550 g (25% 2,200 ml)	95 units	5,000 g (10% 50,000 ml)

Case Illustration. Male, aged 37. The patient sustained burns to 90% of the BSA, including third degree burns to 60%. He developed acute gastric dilatation and gastrointestinal hemorrhage on the 5th day postburn. Subtotal gastrectomy and gastrojejunostomy were performed on the 10th day, after which he had complications of toxic myocarditis, gastrointestinal disturbances, etc. Parenteral nutrition were given from the 4th day onward. Three units which contained 3,000 cal and 80 g–100 g protein were given per day. Peristaltic pump nasal feeding was started on the 10th day, and gradually substituted the intravenous nutriment. On the 43rd day postburn, the whole amount of nutrients was supplied through the gastrointestinal pathway and parenteral hyperalimentation was discontinued (Table XII.9). The patient underwent 11 operations in all. His general condition was good by the 55th day, and the patient was discharged.

Case Illustration. Male, aged 24. The patient sustained burns to 60% of the BSA, including third degree burns to 3%. Starting from the 5th day postburn, 12% amino acids and 25% glucose were used for intravenous nourishment. Two to three units were administered per day, with 2,000 cal–2,300 cal supplied by the intravenous route and 1,000 cal–1,500 cal by mouth. The amount of nitrogen given intravenously was 8 g–11 g, while the amount given orally was 6 g–10 g. Positive nitrogen balance was achieved from 11th day postburn (not including the loss of nitrogen from the wound surface). The third degree wound surface was completely covered by autografts on the 18th day postburn. The body weight increased from 56.5 kg (on admission) to 63.6 kg (15th day postburn). The plasma protein level increased from 4.6% (on admission) to 5.3 g% (17th day postburn) (Fig. XII.3).

2.3.2.3 *Administration of Parenteral Nutriments*

The choice of routes of administration needs special attention. In patients with extensive burns, the incidence of infection is very high in central venous catheterization. Culture of intravenous catheters which have been retained for more than 3 days often shows growth of pathogenic bacteria. According to our experience, it is better, if possible, to use peripheral venous puncture instead of central venous catheterization. Although dripping of hypertonic solution into the peripheral veins may easily cause swelling due to exudation and cannot

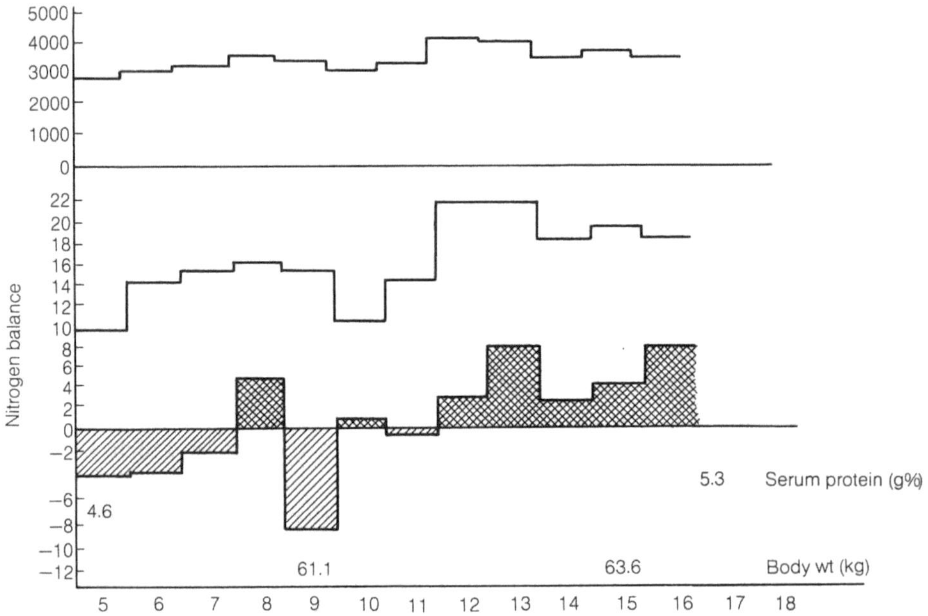

Fig. XII.3. Caloric intake and nitrogen balance in a 24-year-old male with burns to 60% of the BSA, including third degree burns to 3%. A positive nitrogen balance was achieved after the 11th day postburn

be retained for more than 24 h–48 h, the daily requirement to meet clinical demands can be given if the technique of puncturing the small veins and selection of the peripheral small veins are well mastered.

During the supply of parenteral nutriments, the two bottles (one bottle of glucose and one bottle of amino acid solution) of 1-unit solutions can either be given separately through two peripheral veins at the same time or be given after mixing the two bottles of solutions beforehand. The rate of dripping should be properly adjusted.

2.3.2.4 Important Points in Parenteral Nutrition

1. Appetite and gastrointestinal function might be affected during parenteral nutrition; therefore dripping is usually done at night to supplement any deficiency in nutritional intake during the daytime.

2. If total parenteral nutrition is instilled, it is important to calculate meticulously the amount of water intake.

3. Intravenous alimentation solutions should be prepared fresh under strict, aseptic conditions. Urinary sugar should be determined every 6 h; if the urinary sugar is over + +, the rate of infusion should be reduced.

We usually use the combined routes of oral, nasal, and intravenous administration of nutrients simultaneously in severely burned patients. Total parenteral

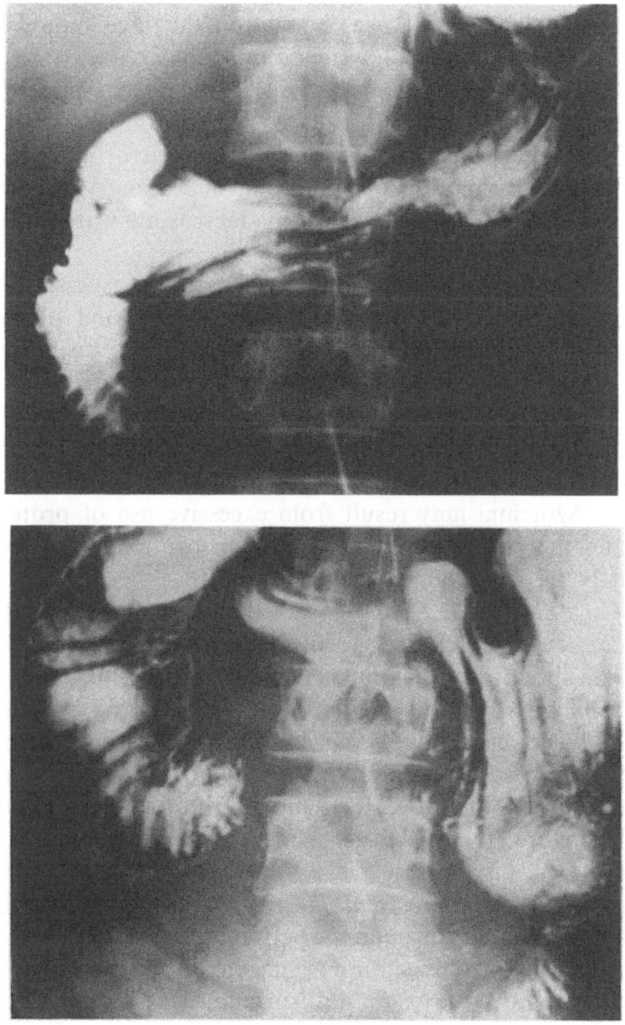

a

b

Fig. XII.4a, b. Superior mesenteric artery syndrome in a 30-year-old male with burns to 69.5% of the BSA, including third degree burns to 17%. **a** Roentgenogram showing dilation of the proximal part of the duodenum and a sharp cut-off at the root of the superior mesenteric vessels. No contrast material is seen beyond the obstruction. **b** Same patient in prone position. A small amount of contrast medium is seen in the intestine, which implies that the obstruction is slightly relieved when the patient is prone. Total parenteral nutrition was given before and after surgical intervention. The patient survived

nutrition is seldom used except in patients with severe gastrointestinal disturbances (e.g., in patients suffering from superior mesenteric artery syndrome) (Fig. XII.4).

2.3.2.5 Complications and Their Prevention

The incidence of complications is related to the duration of application: it rises markedly in patients with administration for more than 3 weeks. Most of the complications can be prevented if special attention is paid and preventive measures are taken during intravenous hyperalimentation.

1. *Systemic infection and thrombotic suppurative phlebitis:* These are life-threatening complications caused by bacterial or fungal contamination. Aseptic technique should be strictly followed during preparation and administration,

and peripheral venous puncture should be employed as often as possible. In cases which necessitate catherization, the tubes should be withdrawn immediately if there is any hint of systemic infection.

2. *Metabolic complications:* The chief complications are hypertonicity and dehydration due to hyperglycemia and osmotic diuresis. They can be regulated by gradual increase of the total amount of calories and nitrogen intake and frequent estimation of the blood and urinary sugar and urea nitrogen level, and they can be corrected by increasing water intake or additional use of GIKC.

Metabolic acidosis may be caused by excessive intake of amino acids or dysfunction of the liver or kidney. The blood pH and standard bicarbonate value should be monitored frequently, and an adequate amount of alkaline salts may be given for prevention.

Hypoglycemia may result from sudden stoppage after prolonged intravenous hyperalimentation; therefore, the dosage should be reduced gradually before complete withdrawal.

Azotemia may result from excessive use of protein hydrolysate in patients and the latter should be used with caution in patients with liver diseases. It is better to use amino acid solution.

3. *Electrolyte Disturbances:* Hypokalemia, hyponatremia, and hypernatremia are the chief electrolyte disturbances. We routinely add potassium chloride into the intravenous nutrient fluid, and hypokalemia seldom occurs. The level of blood sodium is related to the amount of water intake. The concentration of blood electrolytes and output of urinary electrolytes are measured daily in our cases, and the electrolytes are supplied or adjusted according to the output. Furthermore, the daily intake of water is as much as 5,000 ml–6,000 ml. Therefore, there is little chance of development of serious electrolyte disturbances.

4. *Tissue necrosis at the site of puncture:* Administration of intravenous nutrient liquids through the peripheral superficial veins is liable to cause ischemic necrosis due to exudation at the site of puncture. The needle should be immediately removed if exudation is found.

3 Intravenous Fluid Administration

3.1 Venipuncture of Veins of Unusual Sites

3.1.1 Superficial Veins of the Trunk

Superficial veins are distributed on the anterior and lateral aspects of the trunk. The largest and most superficial are those of the lower abdomen (above the inguinal regions) and axilla, followed by those of the lateral aspects of the trunk (Fig. XII. 5). The superficial veins of the trunk empty into the femoral, great saphenous, and axillary veins. Therefore puncture must be carried out centrifugally (umbilicus as the center). The index finger is used to press the proximal end of the vein to block the venous return. The thumb of the same

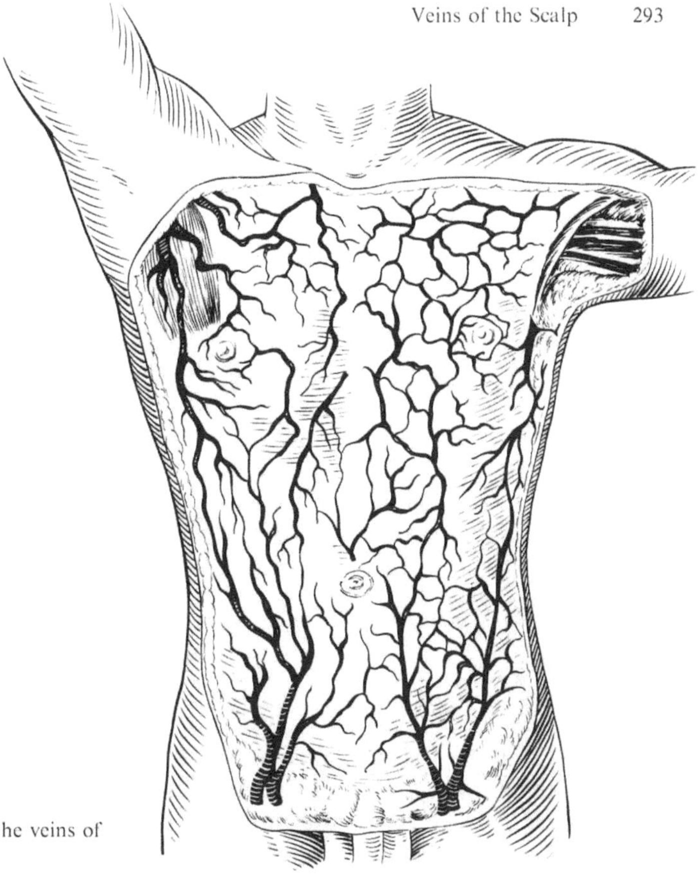

Fig. XII.5. Distribution of the veins of the trunk

hand is used to push the blood from the distal end upward to distend the vein to be punctured. They are superficially situated; therefore direct puncture is employed with the needle almost parallel to the skin. The skin is slightly lifted by the needle and the needle is gradually moved toward the lumen of the veins. During inspiration, the chest wall is expanded and veins become well exposed; this is the best time to introduce the needle. If backflow of the blood is seen the needle should be introduced 0.5 cm–1 cm further.

3.1.2 Veins of the Scalp

The veins which can be seen easily are the superficial temporal, frontal, posterior auricular, and occipital veins and their tributaries (Fig. XII.6). The superficial temporal vein has two to three branches which are superficial and better exposed; they are long, straight, and can be easily fixed. The frontal vein lies in the midforehead, and divides into Y-shaped branches near the hairline. These veins are large, short, straight, and deep, and can hardly be seen in fat patients. They can be punctured by inserting the needle from the hairline along the sagittal plane, with the needle directed toward the tip of the nose. The posterior auricular and occipital veins can be exposed only after shaving of the hair. They are large, long, straight, and superficial, are easily seen, and are easy

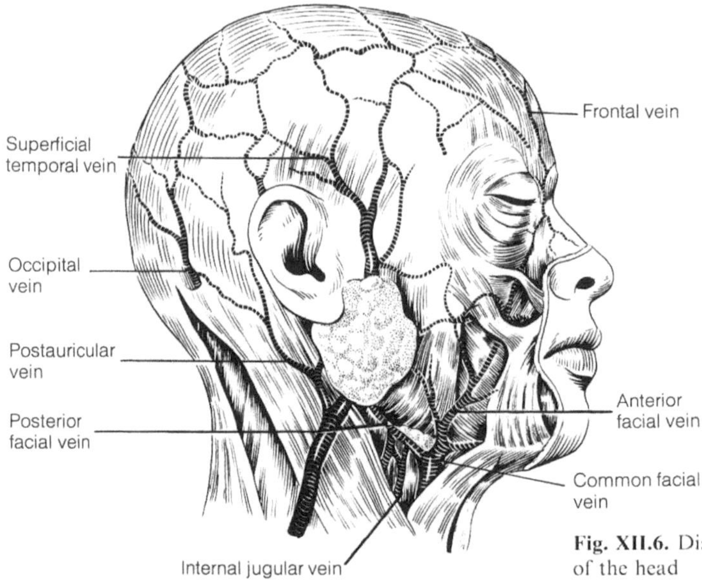

Fig. XII.6. Distribution of the veins of the head

to puncture and fix. The scalp veins should be palpated before puncture in order to differentiate the veins from arteries. Hair on the forehead and scalp should be shaved before puncture to ensure cleanliness of the site of puncture. The head should be placed in medium position when the frontal veins are punctured. It should be turned toward the contralateral side and slightly elevated when the superficial temporal veins are punctured. Owing to their rich distribution, the scalp veins are regarded as the chief avenues for blood transfusion and fluid replacement in patients with extensive burns. The veins can be made to distend by pushing lightly to and fro along the sagittal and coronal sutures with the finger or with the aid of a hot compress locally; the hidden veins can then be easily detected. Adhesive plaster cannot keep the injection needle in place because of the sebaceous secretions and hair. A paste can be made from 10 g plaster powder and 5 ml water (2:1) to fix the injection needle (Fig. XII.7). The nurse must be alert to the veins of unusual sites. For instance, the scalp veins are usually visible when the patient has a high fever or experiences pain during changing of dressings, or during crying in children. The nurses should keep in mind the position and direction of the distended veins which will be useful for later puncture.

3.1.3 Veins of the Fingers and Toes

For veins of the fingers and toes, a short needle should be used. Backflow of blood cannot be seen easily during puncture of the veins of fingers and toes; therefore a small amount of fluid may be injected to detect the result of puncture. The injection needle may be fixed with a tongue depressor and adhesive plaster.

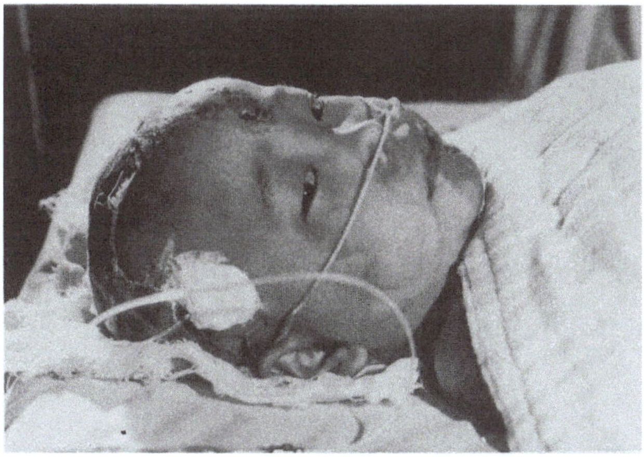

Fig. XII.7. Use of plaster of Paris to fix the injection needle. The method of fixing the nosogastric tube is also shown

3.1.4 External Jugular Vein

The external jugular vein not only can be easily punctured but can also be easily fixed after puncture. The head of the patient should be turned to the contralateral side, and the assistant stands by the contralateral shoulder with the left hand holding the head and the right index finger pressing the proximal part of the external jugular vein to make it distend. If the distension is not sufficient, the patient may be asked to perform a Valsalva maneuver. The person making the puncture will stand behind the patient's head on the side of puncture with the right hand holding the needle and the left thumb pressing the vein toward the distal end. The needle is then punctured into the vein after passing through the skin, and it should be introduced further (0.5 cm–1 cm) after backflow of blood is seen.

3.1.5 Internal Jugular Vein

The internal jugular vein arises from the base of skull and terminates at the inner margin of the first rib behind the clavicle. It joins with the subclavian vein to form the innominate vein. The internal jugular vein lies behind the upper margin of the clavicle and deep to the inner margin of the clavicular head of the sternocleidomastoid muscle. It is situated behind the internal carotid artery and then runs to the lateral side of the common carotid artery; finally, it courses to the anterolateral aspect of the common carotid artery and is enclosed in the carotid sheath. The superficial surface of the vein is covered by the sternocleidomastoid muscle throughout its whole course.

Generally, venipuncture is performed on the right side (the right internal jugular vein follows the same direction as the right innominate vein) with the patient in a supine position with his head turned to the contralateral side. The head is lowered by 20°–30° or the shoulder and occipital region are placed in a position of hyperextension to increase the distention of the vein and prevent

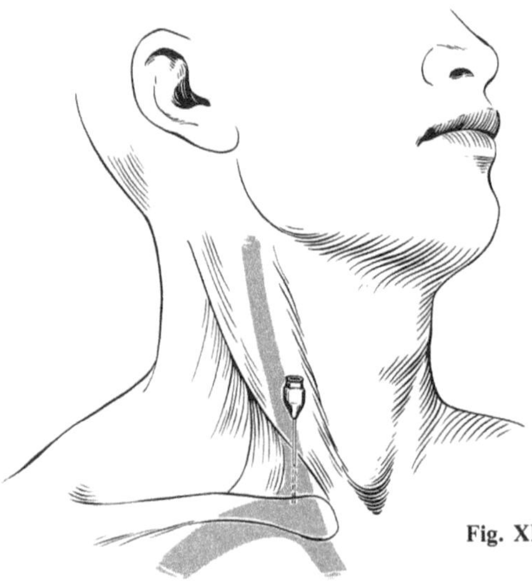

Fig. XII.8. Puncture of the internal jugular vein

the occurrence of air embolism. The clavicular head and sternal head of the sternocleidomastoid muscle and the triangular area formed should be identified. The top of the triangle is the site to be punctured (Fig. XII.8). In fat patients, the head should be elevated in order to expose the contour of the sternocleidomastoid muscle after they have been lying in supine position. Trial puncture may be performed under local infiltrative anesthesia before the acutal puncture is made. The needle is inserted at an angle of 30° to the sagittal and coronal planes; it is then introduced downward, backward, and slightly outward, pointing to the inner margin of the clavicular head of the sternocleidomastoid muscle and the posterior aspect of the upper margin of the clavicle. Generally a distance of 2 cm–4 cm is sufficient for puncture into the vein. Intravenous catheterization usually involves puncturing of the internal jugular vein.

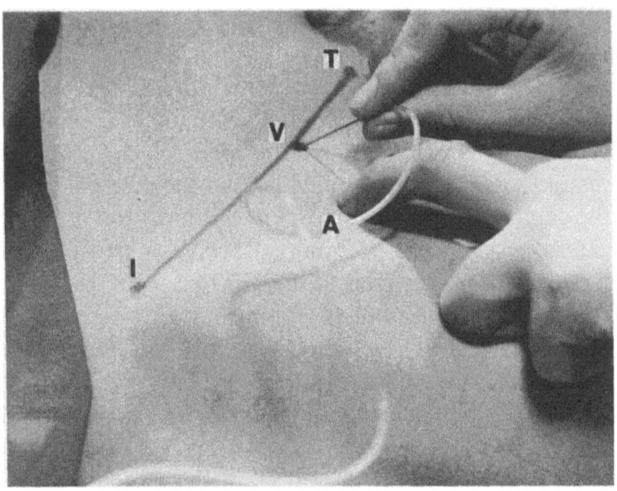

Fig. XII.9. Puncture of the femoral vein. *T*, pubic tubercle; *V*, femoral vein; *A*, pulsation of femoral artery; *I*, anterior superior iliac spine

3.1.6 Femoral Vein

The person performing the puncture should stand on the ipsilateral side of the site of puncture. After feeling the pulsation of the femoral artery with the index finger, puncture may be carried out at its medial side. The skin is first made taut with the left index finger and middle finger, and the right hand holds the needle, which should be directed toward the umbilicus, forming an angle of 30°–40° or being perpendicular to the skin (Fig. XI.9).

3.1.7 Superficial Veins Beneath the Healed Wound Surface

Bluish, superficial, small veins are usually seen beneath the healed wound surface of the trunk, palms, and soles. They are very superficial and may be punctured for fluid administration. Thin plaster paste may be used for fixation.

3.1.8 Popliteal Vein

The popliteal vein may be punctured for collection of blood when the patient is in the prone position. The knee joint is hyperextended before puncture, and the puncture is performed at the midpoint of the transverse skin fold of the popliteal fossa with the needle perpendicular to the skin. Aspiration is done at the same time until backflow of blood is seen.

3.1.9 Subclavian Vein

The subclavian vein has a large lumen and a good blood flow. It is distended during expiration. The third portion of the subclavian vein is to be punctured through the supraclavicular route. This portion of the subclavian vein starts from the midpoint of the clavicle and ends at the sternoclavicular joint, where it enters the innominate vein. The anterior surface of this portion of the vein is adjacent to the clavicle, and the anterior scalene muscle lies behind it.

The apexes of the lungs and pleurae are situated posterior to the artery. Only subcutaneous tissue and superficial fascia are present between the subclavian vein and the skin above the clavicle. The highest point of the subclavian vein is generally at the lateral margin of the sternocleidomastoid muscle. This portion of the vein is fixed between the clavicle and anterior scalene muscle and is supported laterally by the first rib at its lower part; therefore its position is fairly constant. The patient should lie supine and in a slight Trendelenburg position to avoid air embolism. If the infraclavicular route is to be taken, the patient's head is turned to the opposite side. The point of puncture is 1 cm below the midportion of the clavicle. The needle is directed toward the suprasternal notch. As the needle is advanced, slight negative pressure is applied to the syringe. When the subclavian vein is entered, blood will flow back freely. The position of the first rib prevents the needle from entering the pleural cavity, thus making the infraclavicular approach safer than the supraclavicular route (Fig. XII.10).

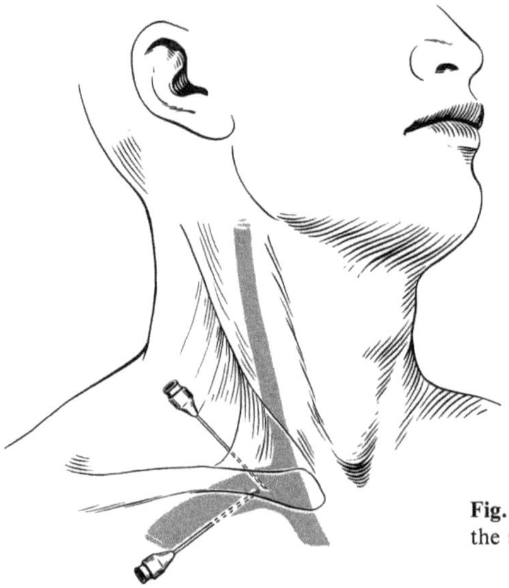

Fig. XII.10. Supra- and infraclavicular puncture of the subclavian vein

3.1.10 Axillary Vein

This vein is located at the apex of the axilla, anteromedial to the axillary artery. During puncturing, the arm should be fully abducted and supinated to make the axillary vein more superficial. The procedure of puncture is similar to that in puncturing the external jugular vein. It can be used for collection of blood or for percutaneous catheterization.

3.2 Intravenous Catheterization Through Puncture

The methods of performing intravenous catheterization through puncture consist of "closed fluid-drive" (Fig. XII.11), "water jet puncture" (Fig. XII.12), and "open puncture." The intubation may be carried out on the external jugular, internal jugular, cephalic, femoral, or subclavian veins.

4 Basic Nursing Care

4.1 Turning Over the Patient by Means of the Turning Bed

4.1.1 Advantages

The turning bed (Fig. XII.13) helps in the alternate exposure of the anterior, posterior, and lateral parts of the wound surface and prevents the aggravation of infection due to prolonged pressure and formation of bed sores. The height of the turning bed is adjustable, and the patient may be sent to the operating room and operated upon while lying on it. By restricting movement of the patient, this will cause less suffering, and it will also make the nursing care of defecation and urination easier.

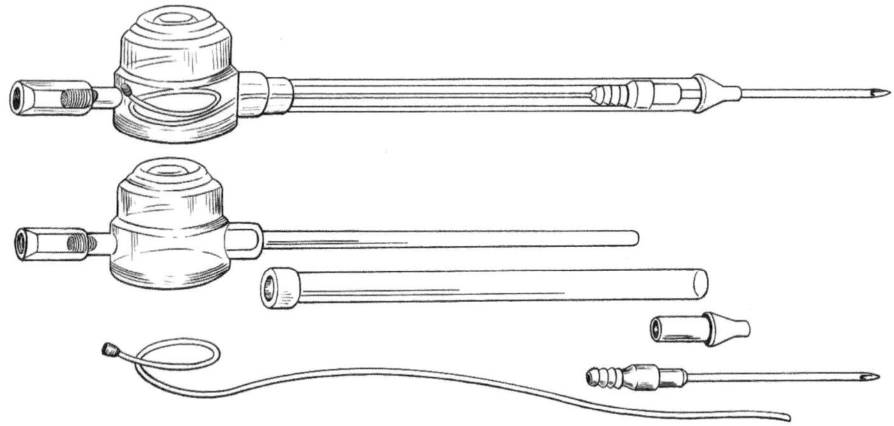

Fig. XII.11. Equipment for "closed fluid drive" intravenous catheterization

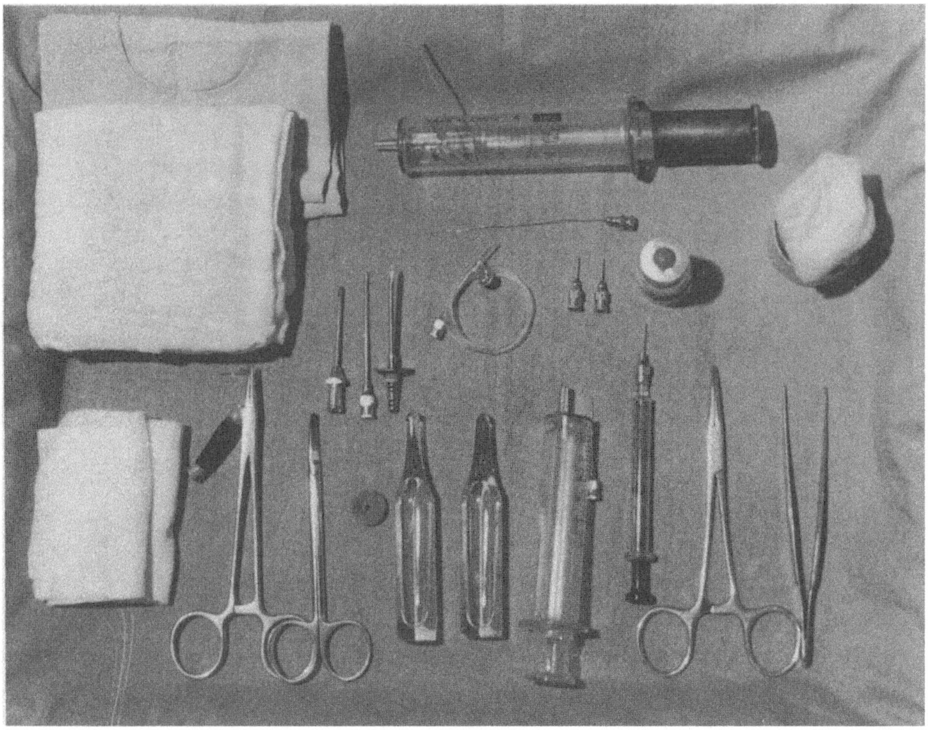

a

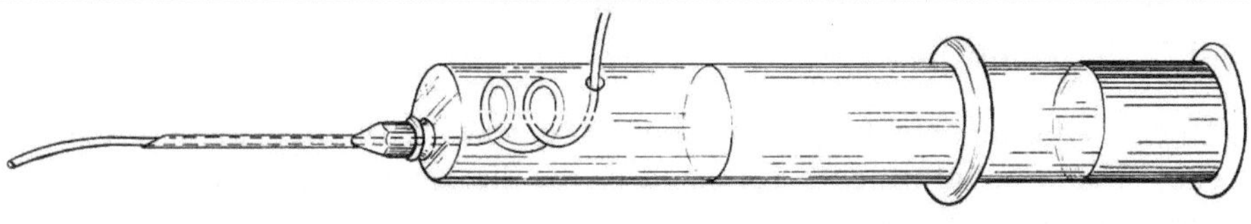

b

Fig. XII.12. a Equipment for "water jet puncture" intravenous catheterization. **b** The side-hole is sealed using the index finger. The syringe is then filled with physiologic saline. After the needle is introduced into the veins, the plunger is pressed to send the catheter into the vein

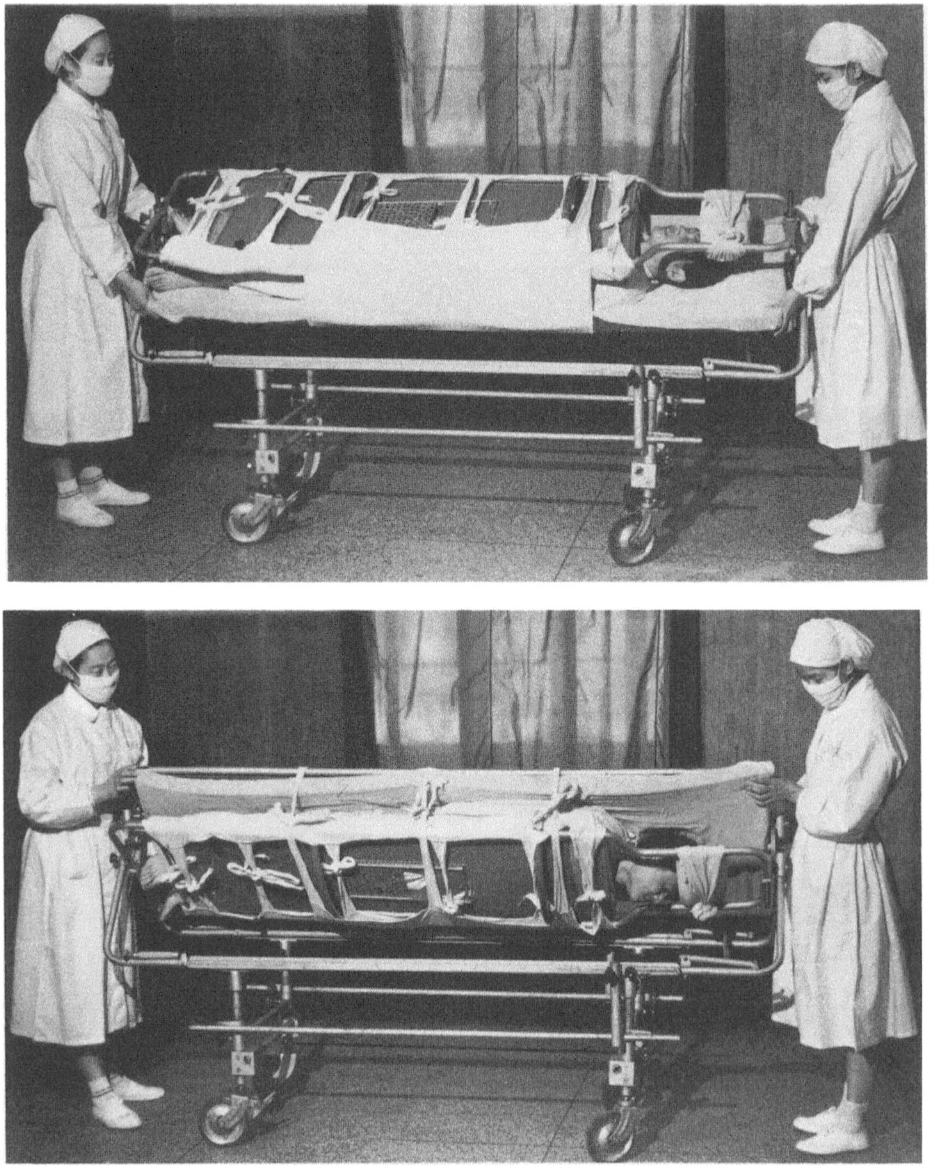

a

b

Fig. XII.13a, b. A turning bed. **a** The patient is supine, with protection straps in place. **b** Patient turned prone

4.1.2 Procedure

Patients who are mentally clear should be relieved of their anxiety and fear. They should be informed beforehand of the therapeutic significance and procedure in order to make them cooperative.

The upper and lower bed frames should be locked with adequate pressure between the frames, and soft pillows should be placed between the frames to serve as cushions in those parts (such as the lower extremities) where the frames cannot be closed up tightly. Protection straps should be fixed between the shoulder joints and the middle of the thigh to protect the patient from slipping between the bed frames on turning over (Fig. XII.13).

Two persons are needed to turn over the patient in bed. The screws of the frames should be examined first and then the leg support can be removed. The protection straps are fixed and the safety spring on the revolving plate is then removed. The patient may now be turned over, but not too rapidly. After turning over the patient, the safety spring is immediately replaced, leg support is fixed, and the protection straps and the upper bed frame can be removed (Fig. XII.13b).

4.1.3 Important Points to Note

Turning over the patient in bed is contraindicated in patients with respiratory tract burn, heart failure, or severe generalized anasarca or within the first 2–3 days of the shock phase (especially when the patient is under artificial hibernation).

The time for which the patient is allowed to lie in the prone position should generally be restricted to 1 h at first; this may gradually be increased according to the state of adaptation of the patient.

When an extensively burned patient is turned over into the prone position for the first time, respiration, pulse, and symptoms of anoxia should be carefully watched for. Instruments and medicine for emergency treatment should be prepared beforehand. Attention should be paid particularly to patients with burns of the head, face, and neck.

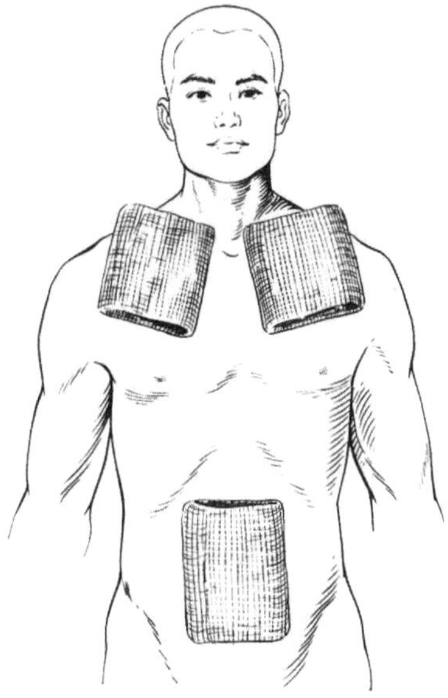

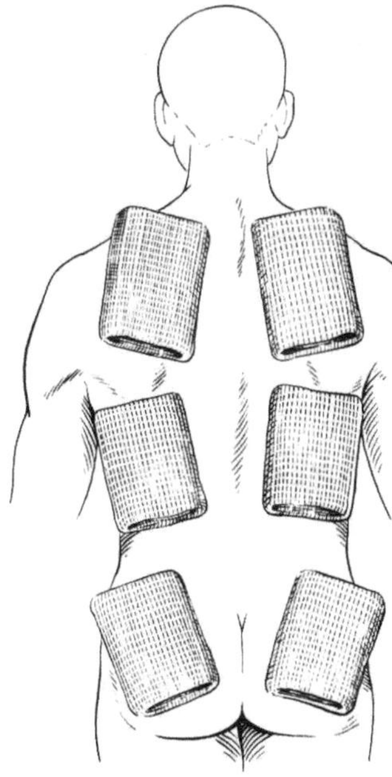

Fig. XII.14. Sites for placing pads for the prevention of bed sores

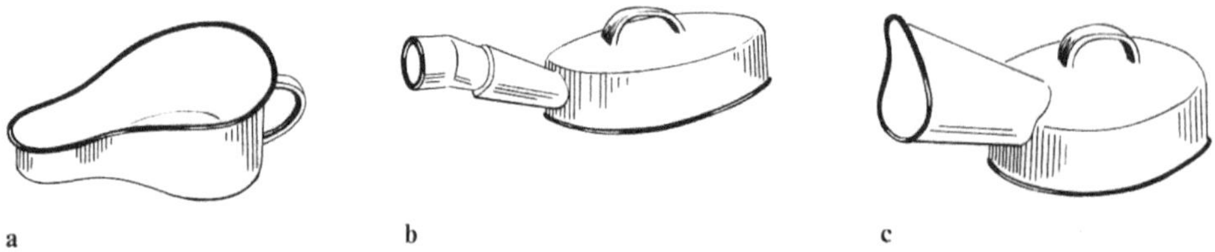

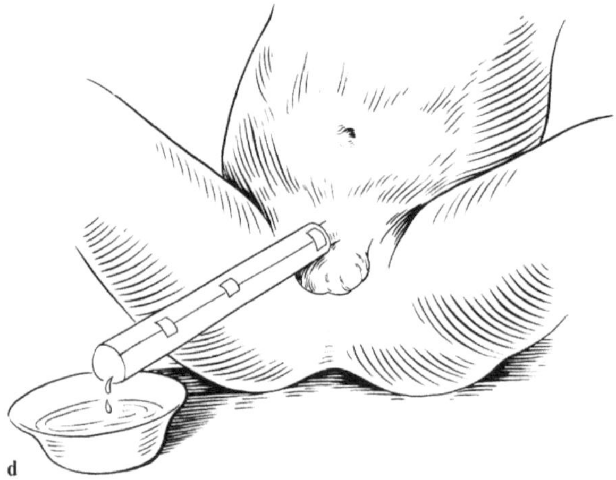

Fig. XII.15a–d. Specially designed bed pan and urinals

The turning bed is usually narrow in width, and patients who have psychic symptoms or who are not cooperative should be carefully fixed, especially around the extremities. The hand and foot supports may also be used as protection frames to prevent the patient from falling.

Bed sores may be prevented by the use of sponge pads (Fig. XII.14).

4.2 Nursing Care of Defecation and Urination in Extensively Burned Patients

The object of nursing care of defecation and urination in extensively burned patients is to prevent contamination of the wound surfaces by urine or feces. Bed pans and urinals of various kinds should be used (Fig. XII.15).

4.2.1 Defecation

When patients with burns of the buttocks or lower extremities defecate in the supine position, the bed pan cannot be set easily and cleaning is difficult owing to the close approximation of the anus to the bed sheet. The patient should be trained to form the habit of defecating in the prone position.

When the patient defecates in the prone position, both lower extremities should be abducted and inner aspects of the upper parts of both thighs should be wrapped with sterilized paper to avoid contamination of the dressings by the feces. The dustpan type of bed pan should be placed in the middle of the perineum, and the part above the anus should be covered with layers of sterilized toilet paper. The anus and perianal region should be cleaned after removing the bed pan.

When the patient lies in the supine position, both lower extremities should be abducted and the inner aspects of the upper parts of both thighs should be wrapped with sterilized paper. A shallow pan may be placed under the anus, and cleaning should be done after defecation.

In patients with severe diarrhea or loss of control of defecation and urination, pads or towels may be used if the patient lies on an ordinary bed and has no wound surface on the buttocks or on either thigh. If the patient lies on a turning bed, sterilized oily paper or gauze should be padded under the buttocks before the patient is turned over. The feces will flow into the bed pan through the opening during defecation. The inner aspects of the upper parts of both thighs may be protected by sterilized paper.

4.2.2 Urination

The long neck urinal is narrow and, as the name suggests, long. It will not touch the wound surface on the inner parts of the thigh and its volume is not less than that of the ordinary urinal. In children or in patients with loss of control of urination, a condom may be used. The terminal end of the condom may be cut with scissors, and it is put on the penis reversely and fixed with adhesive plaster. It is important to watch for any edema of the penis due to tightness of the condom. In patients with atrophy or deformity of the penis due to burns, thick sterilized paper may be rolled up into a tube to direct the urine into a container (see Fig. XII.15d).

Chapter XIII Pathologic Anatomy of Burns

CHEN ZHI-RANG

Translated by WANG PAO-MEI

1 Local Pathologic Changes

1.1 Cutaneous Burns

Cutaneous burns may be divided into three degrees according to the depth of injury.

First degree burns: Such burns are manifested by erythema and edema. Microscopically the stratum corneum of the epidermis is loosened and clefts may appear in this layer. The stratum corneum is separated from the stratum granulosum and superficial vesicles may be formed. The stratum lucidum and the superficial part of the stratum spinosum are degenerated and necrotic. The nuclei of the cells are lightly stained and the cytoplasm is fused into eosinophilic patches. The cells in the deeper part of the stratum spinosum show pyknosis and distortion with paranuclear and perinuclear vacuoles. Some of the basal cells are disintegrated, showing liquefaction. The blood vessels in the dermis are congested and the dermal papillae are edematous and infiltrated with a few neutrophilic leukocytes.

Since in first degree burns only the superficial layers of the epidermis are involved and some of the degenerated cells are not necrotic, the function of the epidermis can be restored. After the absorption of the exudate, the destroyed epidermal cells can be repaired by proliferation of the cells in the deeper part of the epidermis.

Second degree burns: In superficial second degree burns the epidermal cells are necrotic. The nuclei are pyknotic, fragmented, or totally disappear. Sometimes the necrotic epidermis is very thin with only a few layers of cells. The cells are distorted and closely packed. The nuclei are small and dense and the cytoplasm is fused into a mass of amorphous necrotic tissue. The most characteristic finding is separation of the epidermis from the dermis with exudate accumulating between them, forming subepidermal vesicles.

Generally, the thinner the injured skin (for example, the skin of the abdominal wall or the inner side of the limbs), the larger the vesicles. The superficial part of the dermis is edematous. The fibrous tissue may show mild degeneration or necrosis. The endothelial cells of the blood vessels are swollen and there are deposition of fibrin and agglutination of erythrocytes forming hyaline thrombi in the vascular lumen. The dermal appendages in the deep dermis are intact. Pathologically in superficial second degree burns the epidermis is affected chiefly by vesicle formation. The dermis underlying the vesicles is also affected, but only to a rather mild extent.

Deep second degree burns: Both the epidermis and superficial part of the dermis undergo coagulative necrosis. The necrotic tissue on the surface is the eschar. Underneath the eschar is an inflammatory zone, and granulation tissue forms at a later stage. The blood vessels are congested, and some of them contain agglutinated red blood cells with perivascular infiltration of inflammatory cells. If the necrotic tissue sloughs off, granulation tissue is exposed. The deeper part of the dermis is also damaged, but some dermal appendages still remain. When necrotic tissue and exudate are removed, deep second degree burns are actually composed of granulation tissue with some remaining epithelial cells. After healing, the deep second degree burn wound is a layer of granulation tissue (scar) covered with epithelial cells.

Third degree burns: Microscopically, the epidermis and dermis, including all the skin appendages, are destroyed, with disappearance of the nuclei of the cells and coagulation of the cytoplasm, forming a homogeneous hyaline band. Clinically this is called an eschar. Sometimes the cutaneous fat is also affected, showing karyolysis and eosinophilia of the cytoplasm. Inflammatory reaction is located in the subcutaneous tissue. In burns involving the subcutaneous fat and muscles, H & E staining gives the necrotic fibroadipose tissue a blue striated appearance. If muscles are burned the striations disappear, the cytoplasm is coagulated, and spaces are formed between the cell membrane

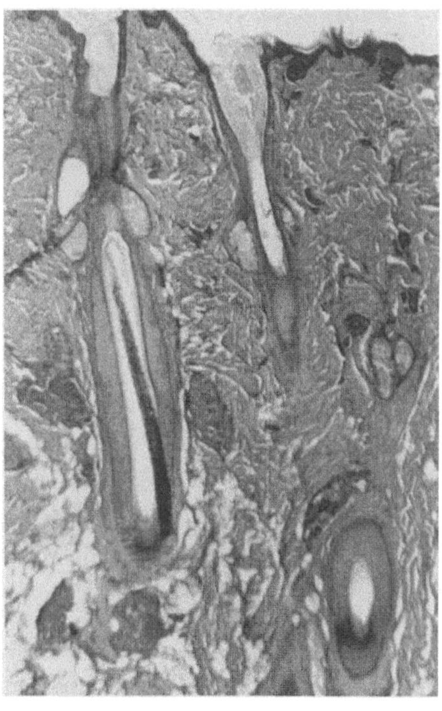

Fig. XIII.1. Section of the human scalp. The hair follicles are deeply seated in the subcutaneous adipose tissue

and the cytoplasm. The nuclei are pyknotic or completely disappear. The necrotic fibrous tissue between the muscle cells is basophilic.

Secondary infection often develops in second and third degree burns. Severe infection may transform second degree burns into third degree burns. Microscopically, bacterial colonies are seen on the surface of the necrotic tissue and pus cells and neutrophils are present under the necrotic tissue. Sometimes hemorrhage, caused by injury of the superficial veins and capillaries, is very prominent. Sometimes infection of the wound surface is very severe, large numbers of bacteria multiply rapidly in the deeper tissue, and clinical manifestations of pyemia appear. By this time, regardless of whether the blood culture is positive or not, we refer to wound sepsis. Severe infection and tissue necrosis may interfere with granulation formation and delay wound healing, Generally in infection with gram-positive cocci there are numerous neutrophils in the exudate, while the major lesions caused by gram-negative bacilli are tissue necrosis and hemorrhage, neutrophils being rarely seen.

The thickness of human skin varies and the distribution of the skin appendages varies also. The epidermis and dermis of the scalp are thicker with numerous hair follicles in the subcutaneous tissue, the blood supply is rich, and the regenerative power is strong (Fig. XIII.1). The scalp is as an important donor area for skin grafting. The stratum corneum of the skin of the palms and soles are very thick and the sweat glands are often located in the subcutaneous tissue, which favors the regeneration of the epithelial cells of these appendages. When the donor area for skin grafting is insufficient, the skin of the soles may be used.

1.2 Burns of the Respiratory Tract

After death caused by burns of the respiratory tract, postmortem examination of the larynx, pharynx, vocal cord, trachea, and bronchi reveals tissue congestion, necrosis, and sometimes superficial ulcers. Microscopically most of the epithelial cells of the trachea and bronchi are seen to be desquamated. The remaining epithelial cells are small and the nuclei are deeply stained. The basement membrane is necrotic and stained homogeneously. The soft tissue under the basement membrane is edematous, congested, and infiltrated with many inflammatory cells. Lung abscess may be present in some burned patients. In one case in which the burn lesion extended deep into the lung tissue, histologic examination revealed bronchioles and alveoli to be covered with hyaline membrane.

2 Systemic Disturbances Caused by Cutaneous Burns

Forty-two autopsies after deaths caused by burns showed the most common cause of death to be septicemia or wound sepsis (26 cases). The second most frequent cause was respiratory tract infection, including, bronchopneumonia, interstitial pneumonia, lung abscess, and pleuritis (11 cases). Two patients died of acute heart failure, two died from hemorrhage caused by gastrointestinal ulcers, and one died of acute renal insufficiency 1 day postburn.

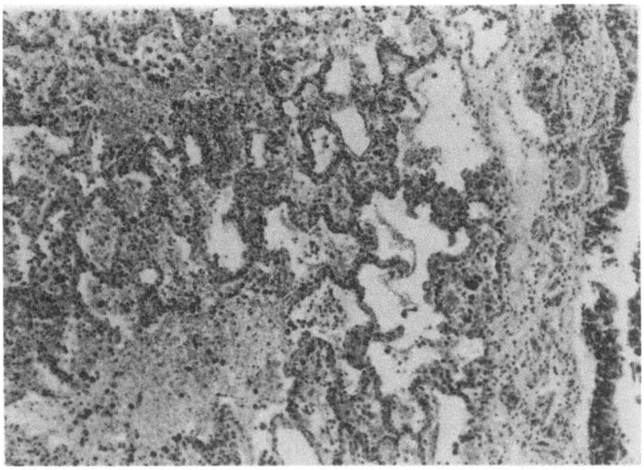

Fig. XIII.2. Passive congestion and edema of the lung. H & E, ×125

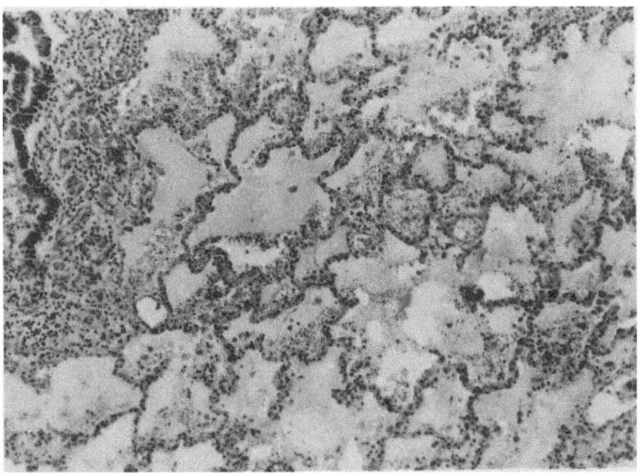

Fig. XIII.3. Pulmonary edema. The alveolar spaces are filled with serous fluid. H & E, ×125

Tissue sections of all thoracic and abdominal viscera, brain, and skin were examined. Besides H & E stain, PAS and stains for myelin sheath were used, with the following results.

2.1 Lung, Trachea, and Bronchi

Pulmonary congestion and edema were frequently seen in patients who died soon after burn (Figs. XIII.2, XIII.3) (19 cases). Clinically, cough, dyspnea, and copious sputum were present. In patients who died of septicemia or wound sepsis, pulmonary congestion often coexisted with congestion of liver and kidney and a tendency to bleeding. After the shock stage, bronchopneumonia (Figs. XIII.4, XIII.5) and interstitial pneumonia were frequent (23 cases: bronchopneumonia 18, interstitial pneumonia 5), especially in the aged and children because their body resistance was low. The morphological changes of pneumonia were

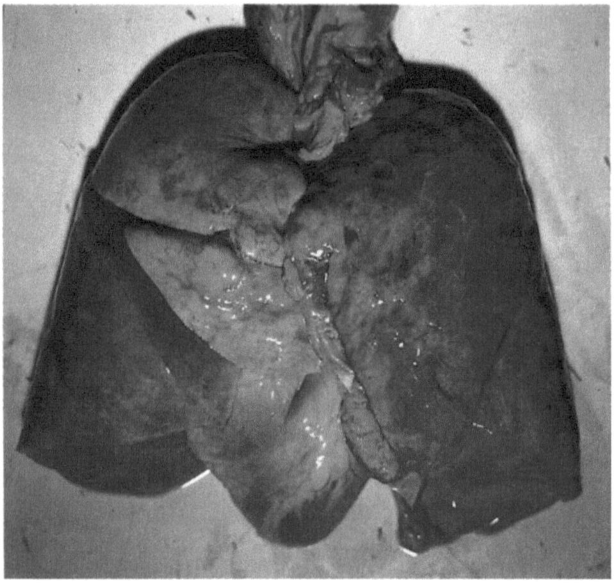

Fig. XIII.4. Numerous irregular purplish-red areas, which represent foci of bronchopneumonia, are seen on the surface of the lungs. (Patient died of postburn bronchopneumonia)

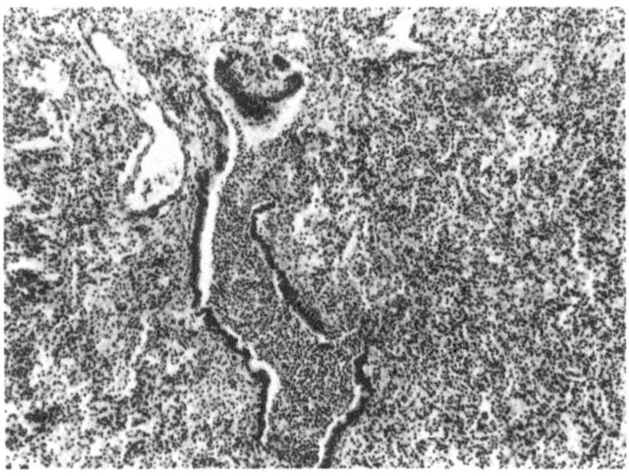

Fig. XIII.5. Bronchopneumonia. The alveolar spaces and the lumina of bronchioles are filled with polymorphonuclear leukocytes. H & E, ×125

related to the pathogenic organism and the general condition of the patient. Pneumonia caused by gram-negative bacilli was characterized by congestion, hemorrhage, and necrosis of bronchi and alveoli. Bacterial colonies were found in the center of the necrotic area (Fig. XIII.6). The infiltrating cells were mainly large mononuclear cells and lymphocytes. Fibrin and large mononuclear cells were found in the adjacent alveoli. In pneumonia caused by *Staphylococcus aureus,* the bronchi were filled with purulent exudate and the alveoli were filled with polymorphonuclear neutrophils. Generally the consolidated foci are lobular in distribution. Sometimes they may be confluent and form large patches and may even involve the entire lobe; in such cases we refer to confluent pneumonia.

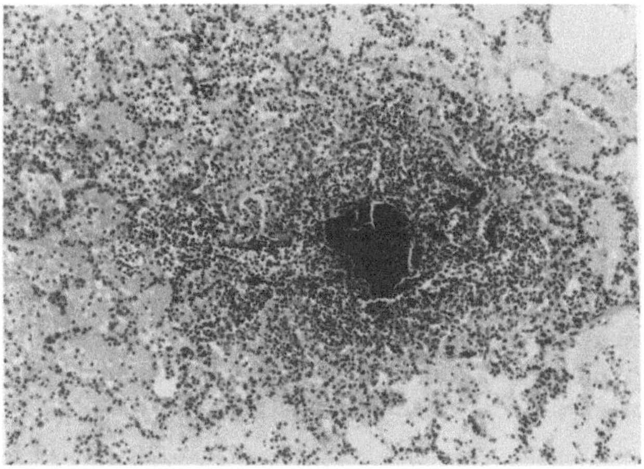

Fig. XIII.6. Lung abscess. Bacterial colonies are seen in the center of the abscess. H & E, ×125

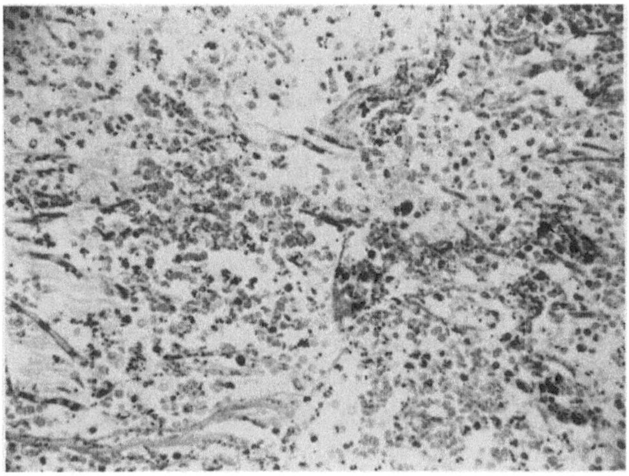

Fig. XIII.7. Fungal infection of the lung. Numerous mycelia and inflammatory cells are present in the alveoli. H & E, ×250

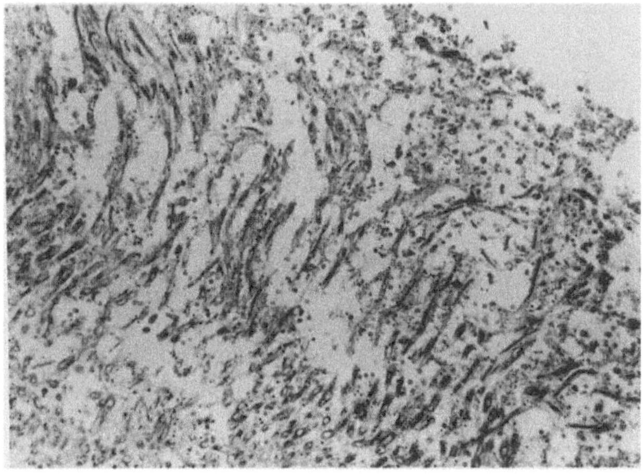

Fig. XIII.8. Fungal infection of the pleura. Numerous mycelia are seen arranged parallel to each other in the visceral layer of the pleura over the surface of the lung. H & E, ×150

Occasional cases were complicated by empyema. In eight cases there was thrombosis of the femoral vein, and two cases were complicated with multiple hemorrhagic infarcts of the lung. Among the cases involving septicemia and wound sepsis there were 12 complicated by multiple abscesses of the lung. A few patients had fungal infection (Figs. XIII.7, XIII.8).

Case Illustration. Female, aged 3. The patient had burns to 35% of the BSA, including third degree burns to 25%. The wound was infected early with *Pseudomonas aeruginosa*, and the child had persistent high fever. Fourteen days postburn the child became comatose and dyspneic, and rales appeared on both lungs. Generalized edema and anuria were present. Finally the child died of general failure. Bilateral confluent bronchopneumonia with pleural and peritoneal effusion were found at autopsy.

Case Illustration. Male, aged 31. The patient had burns to 90% of the BSA, including third degree burns to 80%. Both forearms were amputated because the muscles were completely destroyed, and allografting was performed. Twenty-eight days postburn the condition of the patient deteriorated. He was dyspneic, and rales appeared over the lungs. Tracheotomy was performed and strips of necrotic tissue were aspirated. The patient died of massive hamatemesis.

Autopsy findings revealed multiple infarcts and abscesses in both lungs, acute necrosis and hemorrhage of the esophageal mucosa, minute necrotic foci of all the organs, and multiple ulcers of the gastric mucosa. The cause of death were lung abscesses and gastrointestinal hemorrhage.

2.2 Wound Sepsis and Septicemia

Case Illustration. Female, aged 4. There were superficial second to deep second degree burns to 99% of the BSA. Bloody stools appeared 3 days postburn, followed by high fever, dyspnea, anuria, and hemorrhage and necrosis of the wound all over the body. The patient died on the 7th day postburn.

Autopsy revealed severe infection of the wound and edema, degeneration, necrosis, and hemorrhage of the viscera. The spleen was soft in consistency; the cut surface resembled mud, and could be scraped off easily with a knife. Microscopically, neutrophilic infiltration and hemolysis were seen. The pathologic diagnosis was wound sepsis.

Case Illustration. Female, aged 27. There were burns to 99% of the BSA, including third degree burns to 96%. The shock period passed smoothly. The eschars of the two lower limbs were excised 6 days postburn, and allografts with holes were transplanted. The eschars of the two arms were excised 9 days postburn and allografts transplanted. At the same time split-thickness grafts from the scalp were inserted into the holes of the allografts of the lower limbs. Both transplants had taken. Thirteen days postburn the eschar of the

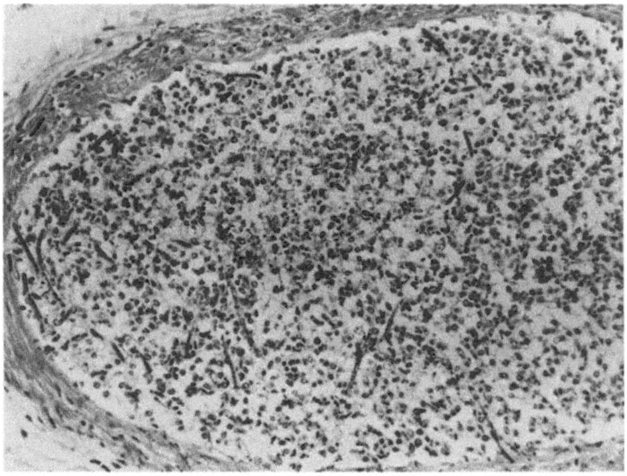

Fig. XIII.9. Fungal thrombus in the lumen of a blood vessel. H & E, × 150

chest was excised, allografts were transplanted, and autografts were inserted into the holes of the allografts of the upper limbs. The condition of the allografts of the chest was unsatisfactory. Diabetes appeared 8 days postburn. Three weeks postburn the unexcised eschar was severely infected. Twenty-eight days postburn necrotic patches appeared over the wound surface and the patient died. Blood culture was negative at the time of death.

Autopsy revealed severe infection of the wound and edema and congestion of the lungs, liver, kidneys, and spleen. Except for mild interstitial pneumonia, no evidence of infection of the other organs was found. Pathologic diagnosis was wound sepsis.

Case Illustration. Male, aged 39. There were burns to 75% of the BSA, including third degree burns to 40%. He was transferred to our hospital 3 days postburn. The wound was infected with *Pseudomonas aeruginosa,* and blood culture was positive with respect to this species. The two lower limbs were amputated because of severe necrosis. Eleven days postburn the patient died of complicating bronchopneumonia.

Autopsy revealed *P. aeruginosa* infection of the wound associated with fungal infection. Numerous mycelia were found in the lungs, heart, kidneys, liver, and meninges. Colonies of fungus were also seen in the lumen of the blood vessels (Fig. XIII.9).

2.3 Kidneys

Lesions of the kidneys mainly occur in the renal tubules. Of the 42 autopsy cases. 35 had cloudy swelling of the epithelial cells of the tubules. Microscopically the epithelial cells of the tubules are swollen and crowded together. The cyto-

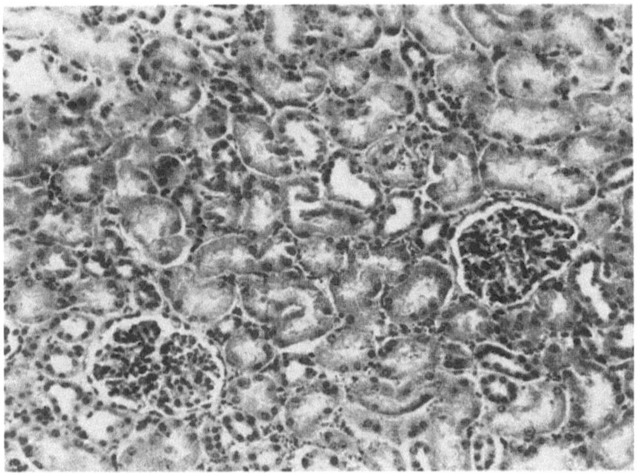

Fig. XIII.10. Granular degeneration (cloudy swelling) of the epithelial cells of the convoluted renal tubules. H & E, ×150

plasm is fine granular and the nuclei are pyknotic or vesicular. Sometimes the nuclei disappear and the cell membrane ruptures, with the surface of the epithelial cells protruding irregularly into the lumen of the renal tubules (Fig. XIII.10). In some patients with septicemia or wound sepsis, besides degenerative changes of the renal tubules there are also necrosis, calcification, and desquamation of the tubular epithelial cells into the lumen, causing obstruction of the renal tubules. At the same time since there is congestion and edema of the interstitial tissue the collecting tubules are compressed and make the obstruction more severe. Clinically, there are symptoms of uremia such as oliguria and anuria. Sometimes granular, hyaline casts and RBC casts are found in the lumen of the renal tubules. In patients with massive hemorrhage, pigment casts may be seen. The light yellowish crystals seen are the degradation products of hemoglobin. Large amounts of pigmented casts obstructing the tubules may

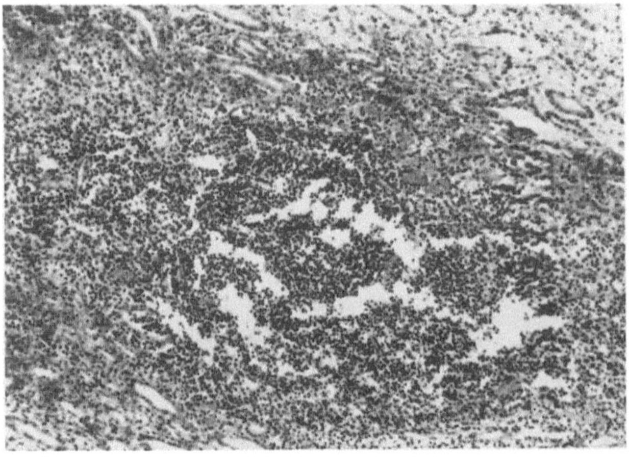

Fig. XIII.11. Acute renal abscess. H & E, ×125

induce acute renal failure. When there is obstruction of the renal tubules and the collecting tubules, the renal glomeruli are congested and the Bowman's capsules are dilated and filled with serous fluid. Erythrocytes may also be seen in the Bowman's capsule. In patients with pyemia, multiple abscesses may be seen scattered over the renal surface and the renal parenchyma (Fig. XIII.11).

Case Illustration. Male, aged 63. There were burns to 95% of the BSA, including third degree burns to 94%. Despite antishock treatment after admission, there was oliguria and even anuria. The patient died of circulatory failure 24 h postburn.

Autopsy findings revealed the size of kidney to be markedly increased. Microscopically, there was granular degeneration of the renal tubules and protrusion of the cytoplasm into the lumen of the tubules. There were many protein and granular casts. The epithelial cells of some of the renal tubules were necrotic. These changes were compatible with acute renal failure.

2.4 Heart

Ventricular dilatation was present in about one-third of the autopsy cases (often both the left and right ventricles are dilated), but was rarely accompanied by hypertrophy of the left ventricle. Microscopic examination disclosed hydropic degeneration of cardiac muscles, disappearance of striations, interstitial edema, and proliferation of interstitial cells. The pathologic changes of the heart were frequently seen in the middle and late stages of burns. Fragmentation of cardiac muscles may be found in patients who have died during the early stage. Hemorrhage in the myocardium was found in some cases. There was one case of interstitial myocarditis. One patient had multiple abscesses of the myocardium and myocardial infarction. These were the causes of myocardial failure and ventricular dilatation.

Case Illustration. Male, aged 29. There were burns to 64.5% of the BSA, including third degree burns to 31.5%. The left leg was amputated because of thrombosis of the femoral vein leading to wet gangrene of the left lower limb. The patients general postoperative progress was uneventful, but 1 month postburn the patient suddenly developed precordial pain, dyspnea, and pinkish frothy sputum. The clinical diagnosis was acute pulmonary edema. The patient's condition improved after emergency treatment. One week later the patient suddenly became dyspneic again. Respiration and heart beat stopped. Resuscitation was ineffective, and the patient died.

The major findings at autopsy were enlargement of the heart (378 g) and dilatation of both left and right ventricles. The dilatation and hypertrophy of the left ventricle were especially prominent (the papillary muscles were also hypertrophied). Microscopically there was degeneration of the cardiac muscles.

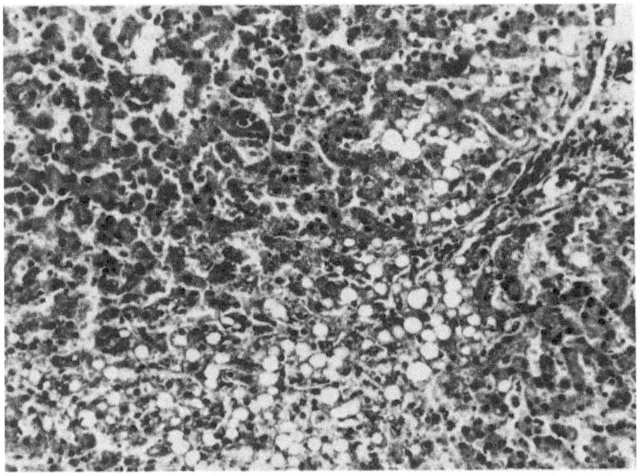

Fig. XIII.12. Fatty degeneration of the liver; fat droplets are seen in the hepatic cells. H & E, ×150

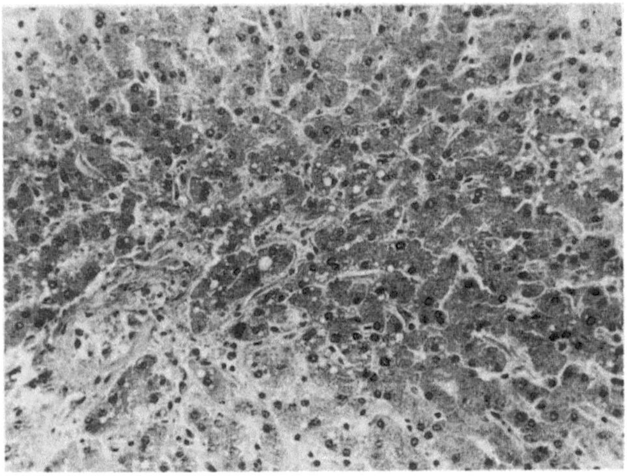

Fig. XIII.13. Cloudy swelling of the hepatic cells, some of which show fatty degeneration

The myocardial fibers varied in thickness, with vacuoles and lipochrome in the cytoplasm. The pathologic diagnosis was compatible with acute cardiac failure.

2.5 Liver

Passive congestion of the liver is frequently seen in patients who have died of burns it occurred in over 50% of the autopsy cases. The parts surrounding the central vein were often congested. Sometimes the liver was diffusely congested. The sinusoids were dilated and filled with red blood cells. Cloudy swelling of the hepatic cells was common, but fatty degeneration was not frequently seen and, when present at all, was mild (Figs. XIII.12, XIII.13). Focal necrosis of the liver was seen occasionally. Multiple abscesses of the liver were found in only three cases.

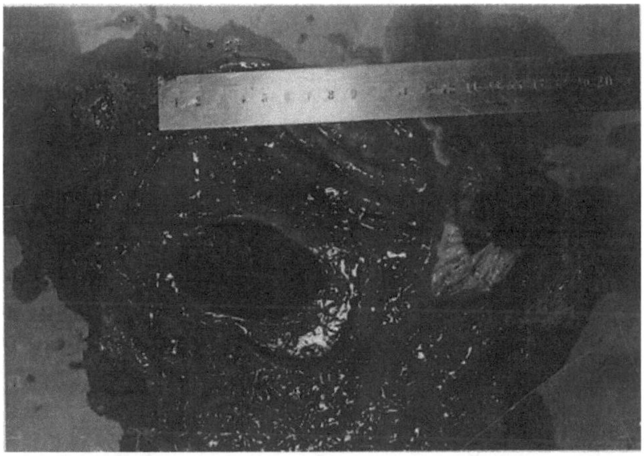

Fig. XIII.14. Huge penetrating ulcer located at the anterior wall of the lesser curvature. Its edge is not elevated; its base penetrates into the lower left lobe of the liver

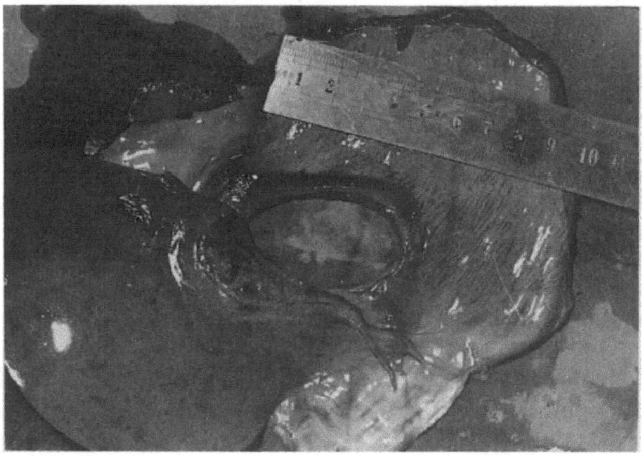

Fig. XIII.15. Huge gastric ulcer in the center of the serosal surface of the stomach. On the left is the liver, the left lobe of which has been penetrated

2.6 Spleen

Splenomegaly (200 g–500 g) was seen in some of the burned patients. In cases of septicemia and wound sepsis the spleen was enlarged and soft. The cut surface was purplish-red, resembling mud, and could be scraped off with a knife. Microscopic examination disclosed hemolyzed red blood cells in the sinusoids, deposition of hemosiderin, proliferation of reticuloendothelial cells and lymphocytes, active phagocytosis, and hyaline change of the walls of central arteries. Multinucleated giant cells were also to be found.

2.7 Stomach and Duodenum

Ulceration or erosions may develop in the fundus of the stomach. Acute ulcers, varying in number, are situated predominantly on the anterior and posterior wall of the fundus. The ulcers are shallow, extending to the submucosa only.

In one case in this series the gastric ulcer was as large as 6 cm in diameter. This ulcer penetrated the diaphragm and invaded the lung (Figs. XIII.14, XIII.15). Gastric erosions are often multiple in number and limited to the superficial part of the mucosa. Stress ulcers may develop in the duodenal bulb also. The lesions of the stomach and duodenal bulb described above may lead to gastrointestinal hemorrhage.

Case Illustration. Male, aged 25. There were burns to 76.5% of the BSA, including third degree burns to 40%. The patient was transferred to our hospital 3 days postburn suffering from high fever, delirium, restlessness, and severe wound infection. The condition of the patient improved after treatment. Jaundice, gastrointestinal hemorrhage, and rales on the left lung base appeared 21 days postburn. X-ray film showed patchy opacities in the base of the left lung. The diagnosis of lung abscess and pneumonia was made, and the patient was treated accordingly. Twenty-two days postburn the patient suddenly developed bloody stool, hemoptysis, palor, and shock. Emergency treatment was ineffective, and the patient died.

At autopsy, a giant ulcer 6 cm in diameter was found in the fundus of the stomach. The edge of the ulcer was slightly elevated. The base of the ulcer perforated through the left lobe of the liver and the left diaphragm and eroded into the left lower lobe of the lung. The left pulmonary artery was ruptured, leading to massive hemorrhage.

2.8 Adrenal Glands

Atrophy of adrenal glands was observed in 31 of the 42 autopsy cases. The atrophic lesions involved the glomerular, fascicular, and reticular zones of the adrenal cortex (where they were most prominent) (Fig. XIII.16). There were 12 cases of hemorrhage in the adrenal cortex. Microscopically the cortical cells were small, and the lipoid content in the cytoplasm of the cells of the fascicular-zone, decreased. The cells of the adrenal cortex were grouped into nests of different sizes. Red blood cells could be seen infiltrating into the interstitium and individual interstitial cells were separated by the red blood cells. Clinically, eosinophilia was observed in patients with hypofunction of the adrenal cortex.

2.9 Central Nervous System

Edema of the brain was frequently seen at autopsy. The pathologic manifestations are congestion of the meninges, widening of the gyri, and shallowness of the sulci. Clinically, high fever, convulsions, vomiting, and oliguria are present. In patients with mycotic septicemia there may be mycotic meningitis and brain abscesses (Figs. XIII.17, XIII.18). Microscopically, degeneration of the nerve cells is commonly seen. The nerve cells are lightly stained and the Nissl's bodies have disappeared. Neuronophagia occurs, glial cells proliferating and entering into the nerve cells. Some nerve fibers are demyelinated. There were

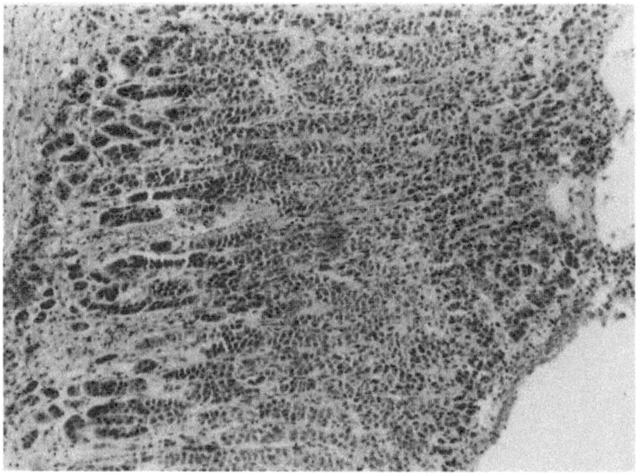

Fig. XIII.16. Cortical atrophy of the adrenal gland. The cells are small, the cytoplasm is condensed, and the lipoid content is decreased or has disappeared completely. H & E, ×125

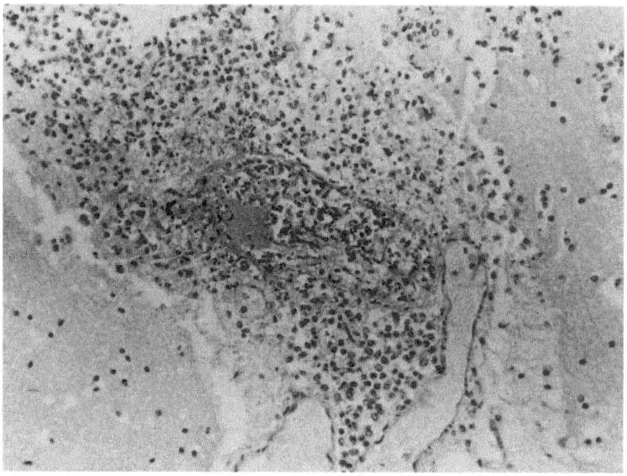

Fig. XIII.17. Fungal infection of the brain. Mycelia are seen in and around the blood vessels. H & E, ×250

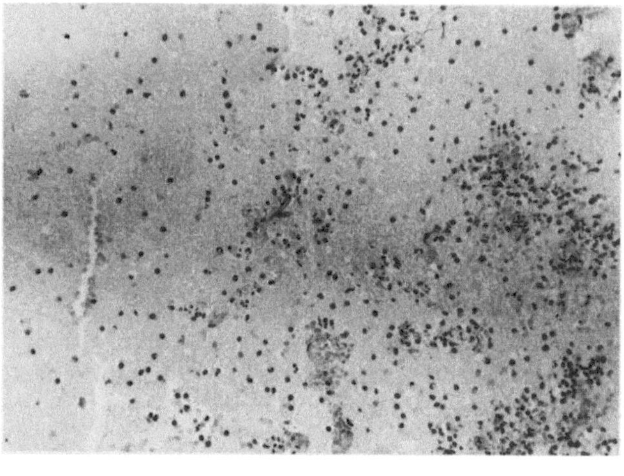

Fig. XIII.18. Fungal infection of the brain. Vascular congestion, inflammatory exudate, and mycelia are seen. H & E, ×250

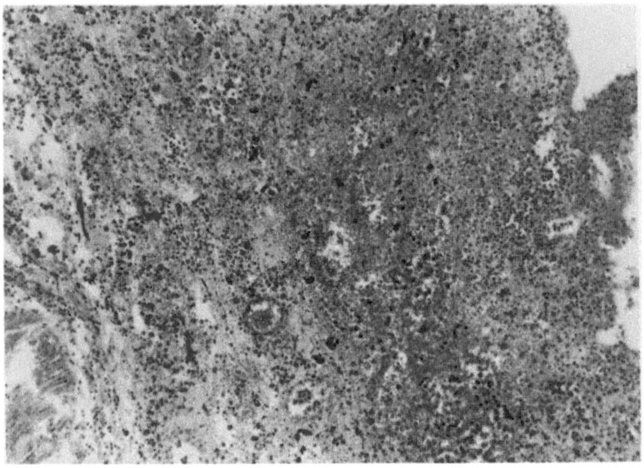

Fig. XIII.19. Necrosis, hemorrhage, and numerous inflammatory cells in the mucosa of the urinary bladder. H & E, ×125

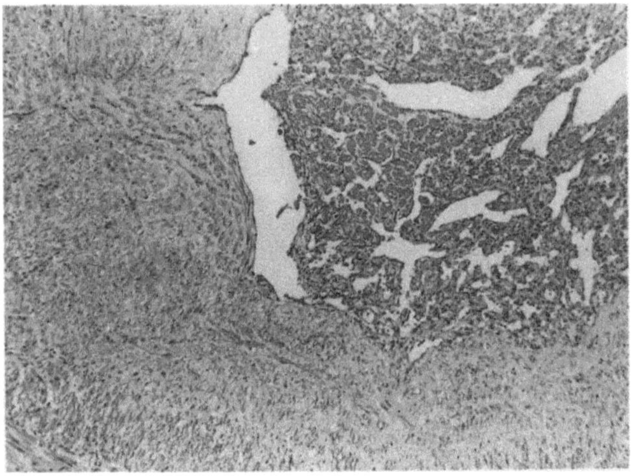

Fig. XIII.20. Organized, recanalized thrombus of the femoral vein. The smooth muscle of the vascular wall and part of the endothelium are intact. The thrombus is attached to the other part of the endothelium. H & E, ×125

13 cases of edema of the brain and 14 cases of congestion of the brain. When there was congestion of small cerebral vessels, red blood cells agglutinated and formed a mass of homogeneous, amorphous, hyaline material, indicating stasis of the blood flow or thrombus formation in the capillaries of the brain.

2.10 Bladder

Acute inflammation of the urinary bladder wall was present in all of our autopsy cases (Fig. XIII.19), and mucosal hemorrhage or ulceration of the mucosa was also frequently seen. In individual cases this was due to irritation by catheterization, but most of the inflammatory changes were related to septicemia or wound sepsis.

2.11 Serosa and Mucosa

Numerous petechial hemorrhages of conjunctiva, endocardium, epicardium, peritoneum, intestinal mucosa, and mucosa of the renal pelvis were frequently seen in patients with septicemia or wound sepsis.

2.12 Thrombosis of the Femoral Vein

Thrombosis of the femoral vein was occasionally seen upon autopsy. Most cases involved were mixed thrombi. Recanalization after organization of the thrombus may alleviate the local circulatory disturbance (Fig. XIII.20).

Chapter XIV Plastic Surgery in Burns

Yang Zeng-nia

Translated by Chang Ti-sheng and Nyi Pao-chun

Plastic surgery constitutes an integral part of the treatment of burns. It is primarily concerned with dysfunction and disfigurement caused by cicatricial contraction after burn trauma. By transplanting tissues, function can be restored and disfigurement corrected so that the patient is able to resume his work and social activities sooner.

1 General Considerations

When skin is damaged by burn the process of wound healing and the degree of functional interference vary with the severity of tissue damage. In second degree burns, only the epithelium and part of the dermis are involved, so that the wound heals more rapidly because of easy reepithelialization. In such a case, only mild pigmentation or depigmentation occurs on the part involved unless the patient has a tendency to scar formation. In deep second degree or third degree burns in which the dermis or the entire skin and subcutaneous tissues are destroyed, the wound usually takes longer to heal. It undergoes a process of sloughing, granulating, progressive fibrosis, and ultimately scar formation. If proper measures have been taken to repair the defects, such as skin grafting or flap transplantation, cicatricial contraction will be minimized.

Scar formation is the result of contraction of granulation tissue and continuous growth of fibrous tissue. Histologically, scars contain a large amount of collagen with a thin layer of epithelium covering its surface. They are devoid of sebaceous glands, sweat glands, hair follicles, and lymphatics, which are often seen in normal skin. Scars are covered by several layers of epithelial cells, with no distinguishable dermal papillary layer. Clinically scar appears as a layer of bright, thin, and transparent epithelium which breaks down easily even with slight trauma and is usually called "scar epithelium."

1.1 Classification of Scars

There are usually two types of scar following burns, namely, atrophic and hypertrophic scars.

1.1.1 Atrophic Scar

This scar presents as depressed, pink, smooth, and glistening. It is usually located on joint surfaces or on the parts with bony prominence, such as around the knee, ankle, elbow, and wrist. The scar always adheres to the underlying bone, and tends to ulcerate after trauma. Once ulceration occurs it does not heal readily and becomes a chronic ulcer.

1.1.2 Hypertrophic Scar

This scar manifests itself as a raised, dense, and hard mass which in its early stage has a red, engorged appearance with capillary proliferation. In its advanced stage it becomes brown, soft, and flat, although it is still raised from the surface of the surrounding skin.

Hypertrophic scar is often encountered in deep second degree burns or in chemical burns such as those caused by acid and alkali. The dermis of the skin is always involved. However, the development of hypertrophic scar is closely related to the following factors: infection of the wound, secondary trauma to the wound after it has healed, and interference with venous drainage when the limbs are in a "hanging down" position.

Hypertrophic scar and keloid may have similar clinical signs but they are different from each other in nature and prognosis. Keloid is often seen over the ear lobe, sternal region, and shoulder. It presents as a raised, hard, bright red mass, and its base often creeps into the normal skin around it in a way which resembles the legs of a crab; it is therefore called "crab-like tumor" in traditional Chinese medical terminology. Itching and pain are its two main symptoms. When excised it recurs readily. Differential diagnosis between these two entities depends on case history and pathologic section.

1.2 Scar Contraction

Cicatricial contraction over a joint will often distort the surrounding normal skin, resulting in the limitation of joint extending and flexing motion. When this condition exists for a prolonged period, the tendon, the ligament, and the capsule of the joint will become fibrotic. In severe cases, dislocation of the joint or bone deformity usually follows. If cicatricial contraction occurs in regions where there is little subcutaneous tissue between the body surface and the underlying bone, i.e., frontal or anterior tibial regions and the lateral aspect of ankle, it tends to break and cannot heal again because of poor blood supply. It then finally becomes a chronic ulcer. Adequate treatment includes wide excision of the scar and ulcer, and application of a free skin graft or a pedicle flap, depending on the blood supply of the recipient bed.

1.2.1 Timing of Surgery

The most suitable time for operation is 6 months post burn because at that time the scar is stable, with less engorgement and hypertrophic reaction, and becomes soft and brown. However, when the hand has been burned and there is severe cicatricial contraction which has already caused dislocation of the joints, fibrosis of the tendons, and other deformities, the operation should be carried out earlier in order to restore better function. Ectropion of the eyelids and microstomia arising from cicatricial contraction also deserve early operation.

1.2.2 Principles of Surgery

1.2.2.1 Formulating the Operative Plan

The severity of dysfunction caused by cicatricial contraction depends on the degree and location of burn, the compensation of adjacent skin, and the fibrosis of deep structures as well as the degree of damage to bones, nerves, tendons, and other tissues. Careful preoperative evaluation of the patient is important for the formation of an operative plan. For those patient whose bones, joints, nerves, or tendons are involved, radical scar excision followed by flap repair must precede the secondary reparative operation on deep structures. The operation should be carefully staged, especially in those patients with extensive burns as donor areas in these patients are scarce. One must make economical use of the scarce donor areas. Preoperative examination of patient's vital organs and general condition should be as thorough as possible, and the necessary preoperative preparation should then be made. Priority of operation is given to areas such as the perioral region and the neck as they are important to the maintenance of adequate air passage and feeding. This will also enable the patient to undergo multiple subsequent operations under favorable conditions.

1.2.2.2 Release of Contraction

Contraction occurs in all directions, and incision should begin at the part at which contraction is most tight. The incision is placed perpendicular to the line of contraction and, as it is deepened, all the fibrotic fascia must be excised in order to release the affected normal tissue.

When tendons, ligaments, and joint capsules are involved in the contraction it is advisable to release them first by dissection, but in severe cases it is sometimes necessary to divide part of those structures which are not of vital importance, e.g., the adductor muscle of the thumb and accessory ligaments of metacarpophalangeal and interphalangeal joints, before complete relief can be achieved.

Cicatricial contraction on the face has a close relationship with the direction of muscular activity. The face is usually divided in to several zones for the application of skin grafts, namely, the frontal palpebral, nasal, perioral, and buccal. The suture line of the graft should be so arranged that it is hidden in the nasolabial fold, in the periorbital and submandibular regions, and in the hairline. One should also avoid a suture line passing transversely across the face, the middle of the nose, or the frontal region. In this way recurrence of linear contraction can be prevented, and the patient can have a face with a normal appearance.

1.2.2.3 Wound Care

The wound resulting from excision of scar is covered with a split-thickness or full-thickness free skin graft. In deep burns where bones, nerves, and tendons are involved, the scar should be replaced with a flap prior to secondary repair. With regard to repair of the face, a graft with a good color match and less tendency toward pigmentation and contraction is preferred, while for defects at the tip of a finger or on the plantar surface of a foot, where weight bearing is to be expected, a full-thickness graft or pedicle flap is more satisfactory as they are more durable.

1.3 Cutting of Skin Graft

1.3.1 Partial-Thickness Grafts

With regard to cutting a graft with a Humby's knife or a Padgett-Hood dermatome, the reader is referred to Sect. 4 in Chap. IV.

1.3.2 Full-Thickness Grafts

Full-thickness graft of a small size can be obtained from the postauricular or supraclavicular region or from the inner aspect of the upper arm.

After excision of the scar and total release of contraction, a sterile paper pattern is made from the defect, corresponding to it exactly in size and shape. With this pattern placed on the donor site as a guide, a full-thickness graft

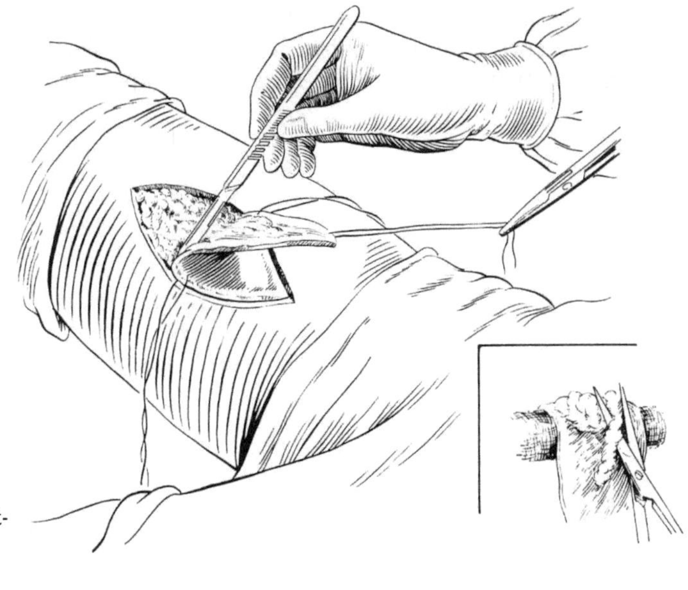

Fig. XIV.1. Method of cutting a full-thickness graft

is cut. To facilitate the procedure a traction suture is made at the tip of the graft and a roll of gauze is placed under it as a cushion. With his left hand pulling the traction suture tight, the surgeon cuts the graft with his right hand at a plane between the skin and the subcutaneous fat. The graft can also be dissected with some of the subcutaneous fat attached to it; it is then placed upside down on the surgeon's finger and the fat is nipped off with a pair of scissors. When a large sheet of full-thickness graft is needed, a dermatome is recommended. The donor site is then covered with an intermediate split-thickness graft (Fig. XIV.1).

1.4 Z-plasty

Z-plasty is one of the popular methods used in plastic surgery. It is indicated for linear and webbed cicatricial contractions. The principle of performing it is to excise the scar and then to make a Z-shaped incision on the surrounding skin. The two triangular flaps thus formed are transposed.

The skin around the linear scar should be pliable, without engorgement or ulcer. With the linear scar as the common axis, two triangular flaps of equal size are designed, each at an angle of 60° to the axis. A skin incision is made along the line of the design and the two triangular flaps are elevated, transposed, and sutured in place (Fig. XIV.2).

It should be noted, however, that too great an angle will render transposition of the two flaps impossible, while too small an angle will impair the blood supply and cause necrosis of the tip. When the linear scar is too long for a single Z-plasty, multiple Z-plasties are indicated.

Webbed scar often occurs around the joints, such as areas over the neck, axilla, elbow, and popliteal region. The development of a web depends on two factors, i.e., the pulling action of the joint movement and the stretching of the elastic fibers of the adjacent normal skin. It is always located on the flexion aspect of the joint and usually causes limitation of the joint movement. The contracting force of the web is greatest along its free border.

For the correction of webbed scars with a Z-plasty the principle of design is similar to that in the case of linear scars, apart from the fact that the two

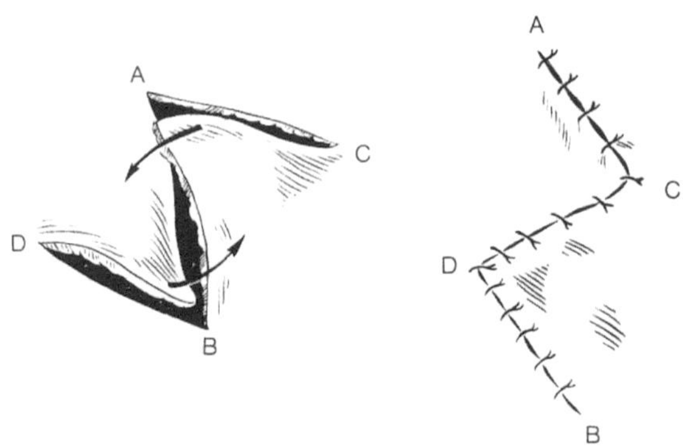

Fig. XIV.2. The design of a Z-plasty

triangles are not on the same plane. When the two triangular flaps are elevated and transposed the contraction is released. Sometimes there is a gap between the two flaps after they have been transposed. This gap can be covered with a free skingraft. When splitting the web one should divide it into two equal halves. As the subcutaneous fat is very thin, care should also be taken not to perforate it or to damage the subdermal plexus, for this will jeopardize the blood supply to the flap and necrosis is inevitable.

1.5 Skin Tubes

1.5.1 Indications

The indications for tube repair are (1) deep burns with involvement of subcutaneous fat and bone, (2) electric burns with involvement of tendons, nerves and joints, (3) loss of thumb or penis, (4) amputation of the nose or ear, and (5) other facial deformities which require reconstruction of contour.

On designing a tube one should place its axis parallel to the main vessels of the skin. The ratio of length to breadth is about 3:1. (This ratio can be increased if the tube includes a known artery.)

1.5.2 Complications of Design and Transfer

The chief complications are impairment of blood supply and infection. The impairment may be arterial or venous in nature. Incompetence of arterial supply is evidenced by pale color and low temperature at the middle portion of the tube. Most cases are caused by transient vascular spasm, and in such an event one must wait until the blood supply is established before it can be safely transferred. Interference with venous drainage is characterized by cyanosis of the middle porton of the tube.

The factors which may lead to vascular impairment are (1) improper design, especially in relation to the length–breadth ratio, (2) excessive adipose tissue within the tube, failure to leave room inside the tube for postoperative swelling, (3) undue tension on the tube when it is sutured to too large a wound, and (4) trauma from improper handling. With regard to hemodynamics, it can be seen that owing to the absence of nerve control, the blood vessels within the tube are in a state of dilatation and the blood flow slows down. This factor together with the factors mentioned above are responsible for the stagnation of the blood flow as well as the formation of thrombi which eventually lead to necrosis of the tube.

Therefore, design and timing of transfer of the tube must be strictly observed. Emphasis should be placed on prevention, but once interference with venous drainage happens one should immediately establish the cause. After all possible technical errors have been ruled out, low molecular dextran (molecular weight 20,000) together with a small dose of corticosteroid should be administered intravenously; alternatively the patient should be treated with hyperbaric oxygen therapy to improve the circulation.

1.6 Free Flaps

In recent years, with the advancements in microvascular surgery and replantation of amputated limbs, it has become possible to transplant successfully a free flap through microvascular anastomosis of known vessels (cf. Sect. 11 in this chapter).

2 Cicatricial Contraction of the Face

Deep burns of the face often cause hypertrophic cicatricial contraction, resulting in ectropion of eyelids, eversion of lips, microstomia, defects of the ears, disfigurement, etc., all of which make it difficult for the victim to lead a normal life.

2.1 Dysfunction Caused by Facial Cicatricial Contraction and Its Repair

Facial hypertrophic scar often covers an area extending from the tragus on one side, across the face to the tragus on the opposite side. Due to eversion of the lips, the patient has difficulty in opening his mouth and sometimes even drooling occurs.

2.1.1 Repair with a Large Sheet of Skin Graft

After excision of the scar subsequent to its stabilization, an extraordinarily large sheet of skin graft, about 0.40 mm–0.50 mm in thickness and 30 cm × 10 cm in area, removed with a specially designed dermatome from the back of the body, is applied to the face. It should be emphasized that the graft is applied as a whole piece and the suture lines are so arranged that they lie in a favorable way. Thick graft is preferred in order to reduce postoperative contraction and pigmentation (Fig. XIV.3).

As there is no distinguishable connective tissue between the scar tissue and the subcutaneous fat in the face, the dissection plane should be kept close to the underface of the scar if a level and plump surface of the recipient bed is to be expected. Neglect of this point will result in damage to the intactness of expression muscles and the fat and doubtlessly will have an ill-effect on the outcome of the operation.

Bleeding is often copious when operating on the face, but, to lessen foreign body reaction postoperatively only active bleeding points need to be ligated with silk, while other oozings are preferably stopped by pressure with hot saline compresses. Alternatively a dry operative field can be obtained by infiltration of 0.25% procaine solution mixed with 1 : 1,000 epinephrine into the subcutaneous tissue. One must be aware of the disadvantage of this method, i.e., a subsequent delayed vasodilatation may occasionally cause a hematoma under the graft.

Fig. XIV.3. **a** Cicatricial contraction of the face subsequent to flame burns. **b, c** Postoperative appearance. A sheet of skin 300 cm^2 large and 0.5 mm thick was taken from the back and transplanted to an area extending from one cheek to the other

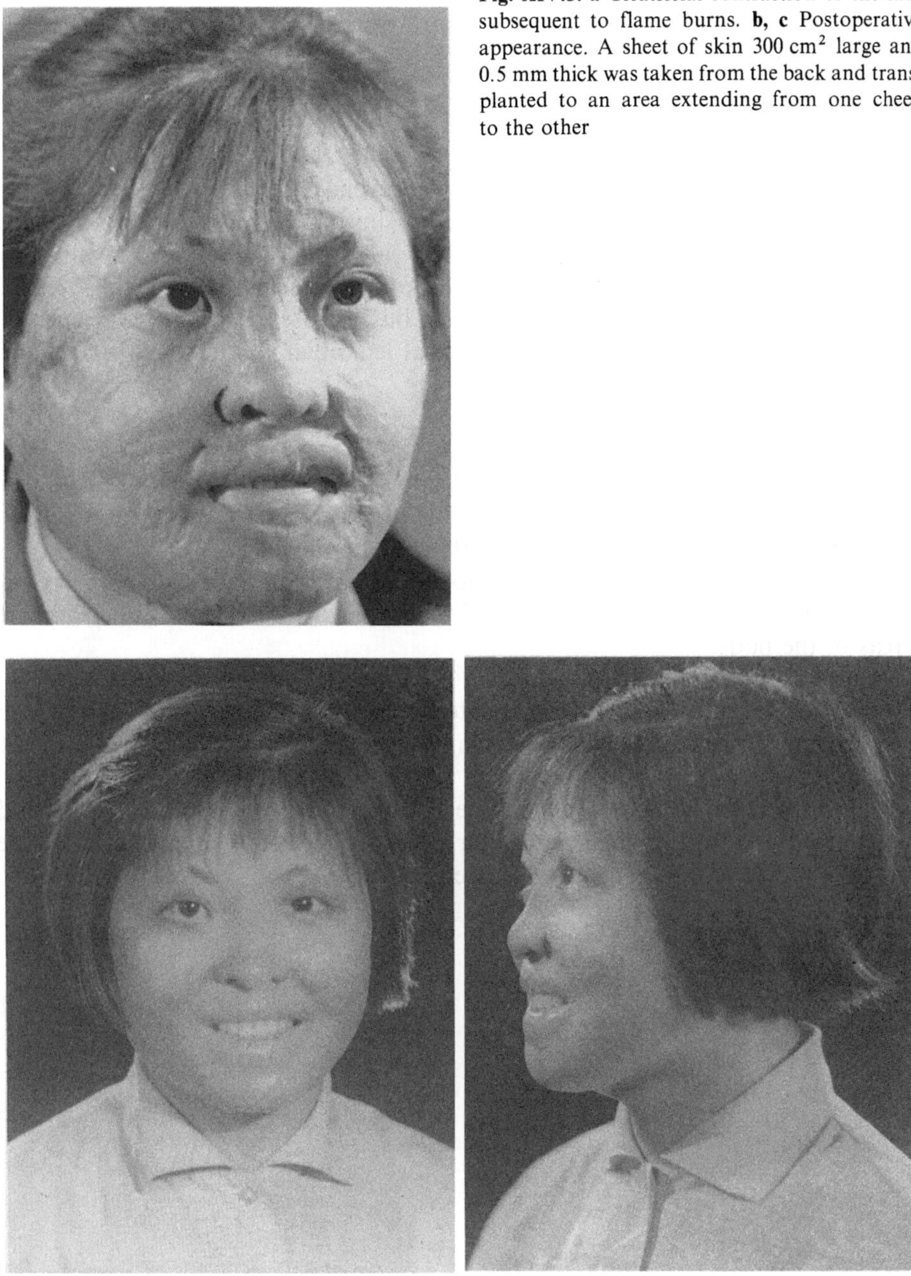

a b c

2.1.2 Repair with a Tube Flap

For the repair of deep facial burns involving muscle and bone it is usually necessary to use distant tubes such as thoracodeltoid or abdomino-thoracic tubes. The advantages of tube repair are better facial contour, less pigmentation, good color match, and softness of the part. Tubes taken from obese patients often have thick subcutaneous adipose tissue and may appear too bulky. These flaps usually need to be thinned out several times before an acceptable result can be achieved.

2.2 Ectropion of the Eyelids

Facial burn often involves the skin of the eyelids. Ectropion of the eyelids may also be indirectly caused by cicatricial contraction of frontal, nasolabial, and cheek regions. Ectropion of the lower lids is sometimes accompanied by epiphora due to failure of contact of the puncta lacrimalia with the eyeball, while ectropion of both upper and lower lids exposes the cornea, sooner or later leading to keratitis, ulceration, corneal leukoplakia, and even perforation as a result of dryness.

Operative Procedure

V-Y procedure and Z-plasty are only indicated for mild ectropions due to linear cicatricial contraction; they are not suitable for more extensive and severe ectropions. For the latter, full-thickness grafts are recommended.

Full-thickness grafts are usually removed from postauricular or supraclavicular regions, from the medial aspect of the upper arm, or from other suitable areas of the body.

The *key points* of the procedure are listed below:

1. The donor area is first infiltrated with procaine solution mixed with epinephrine to reduce bleeding. Bleeding should be stopped by pressure rather than by ligation.

2. An incision is made along a line 2 mm–3 mm from the lid margin and is extended beyond the inner and outer canthi. The scar is excised in a shuttle shape; all fibrotic tissue must be released.

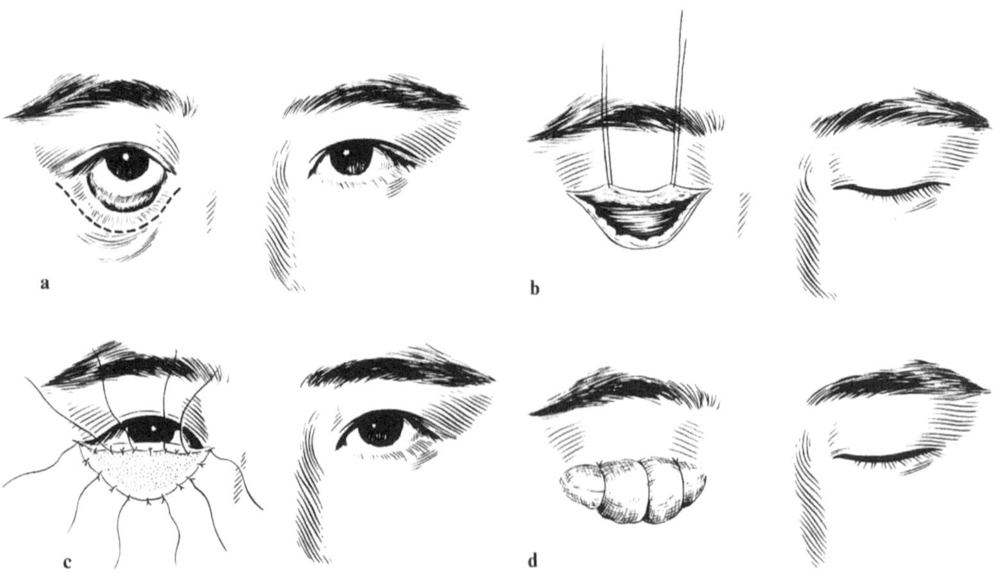

Fig. XIV.4a–d. Transplantation of full-thickness skin to correct ectropion of the eyelid

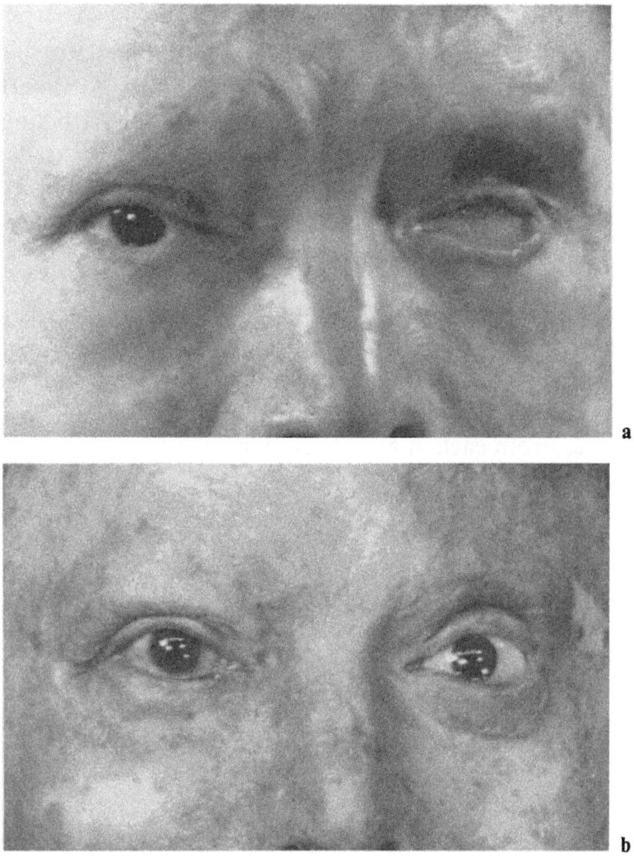

Fig. XIV.5. a Preoperative and **b** postoperative appearance after burns of the face. The left eyeball had been burned and extracted, and there was ectropion of the lower eyelid. After repair by means of a full-thickness graft an ocular prosthesis was inserted

3. Three traction sutures are inserted into the lid margin. Pulling tightly on these sutures, the operator cuts the fibrous tissue with a slight touch of the scapel tip. In this way the tarsal plate can easily be reduced to its original state once all fibrous tissue is divided. The lids can then be closed.

4. Excessive depth of dissection in the upper lid may injure the levator muscle, resulting in ptosis of the lid, while in the lower lid it will damage the orbicular muscle of the eye, forming an undesirable groove.

5. A paper pattern is made from the defect. Using it as a guide, a full-thickness graft similar in size and shape is removed from the donor site and applied to the wound. The graft is then secured with a tie-over dressing (Fig. XIV.4).

6. When there is ectropion of both upper and lower lids, an oval-shaped full-thickness graft is first obtained. After this, a strip of shuttle-shaped tissue, 0.3 cm wide, is removed from the center of the graft, to form a new normal fissure of palpebrae. The graft is then applied, sutured in place, and secured with a tie-over dressing.

7. Ordinarily no tarsorrhaphy is needed and recurrence is unlikely provided that the graft is big enough (Fig. XIV.5).

2.3 Microstomia

Perioral cicatricial contraction may occur unilaterally or bilaterally. Cicatricial contraction at the corners of the mouth may interfere with the opening of the mouth to such an extent that only the fifth finger (digitus minimus) can be inserted. The situation is worse if the patient has simultaneous atresia of the anterior nares and has to rely on this small opening for his breathing. Early operation should be performed in such cases.

Operative Procedure

1. With the patient's eyes looking forward, two parallel lines are drawn perpendicularly downward from his pupils. The future angles of the mouth are on these lines (Fig. XIV.6). (Normally, the angles of the mouth are within these two lines.)

2. From each angle a triangular piece of scar is removed, leaving the mucosa untouched (Fig. XIV.7a).

3. The mucosa is then cut in the form of a transverse Y, with its bifid end pointing outward, thus forming three mucosal flaps (Fig. XIV.7b).

4. The mucosal flap within the bifid limbs of the Y is turned laterally to be sutured to the wound edge, thus forming the plicae oris. The other two flaps are also sutured to the skin edge, superiorly and inferiorly respectively. The mouth is now enlarged (Fig. XIV.7c, d).

The following are the *key points* of the procedure:

1. Attention should be paid to the symmetry when designing the angles of the mouth.

2. If there is extensive scar around the mouth, the above-mentioned procedure may not be adequate. In such a case, it is sometimes necessary to excise all the scar and replace it with a skin graft before a functional mouth can be expected.

3. When a patient who has concomitant nostril atresia is operated on, great care must be taken to prevent the patient from being choked by blood during the operation, as he can only breathe through his mouth.

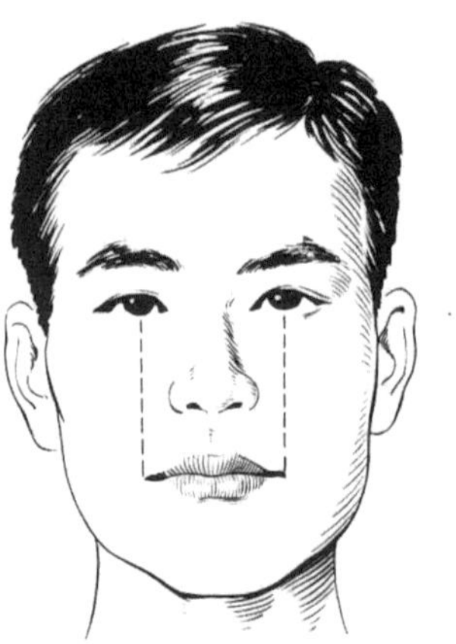

Fig. XIV.6. Locating the angles of the mouth

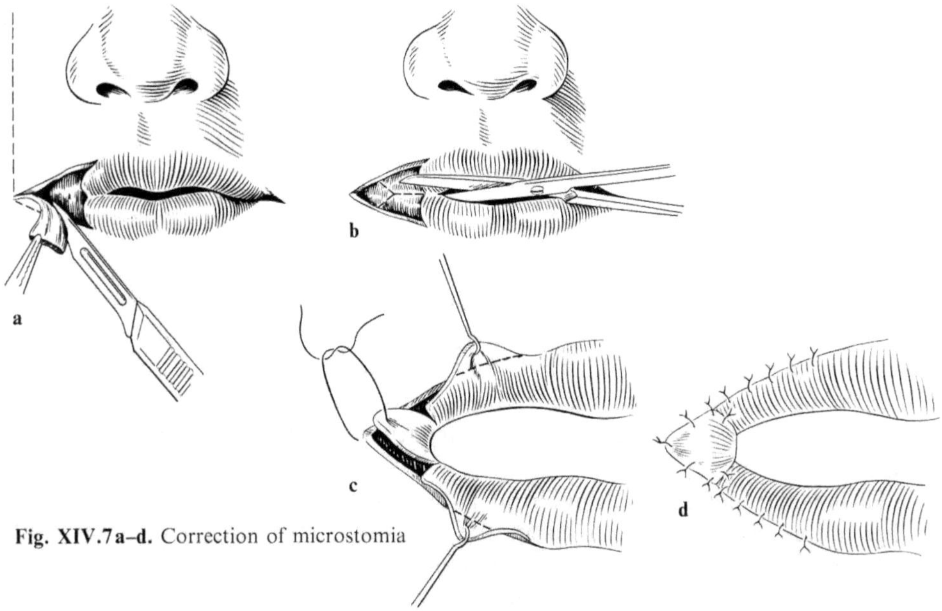

Fig. XIV.7a–d. Correction of microstomia

2.4 Nostril Atresia

Nostril atresia may be due to (a) cicatricial contraction of burns of the face and perioral region, complicated by infection, (b) burns of the respiratory tract by flame, or (c) chemical burn of the vestibule of the nose. Cicatricial contraction is often situated in the vestibule, and the nostril rim is reduced by the constricting action of the scar around it. For these two reasons the vestibule is often blocked. The columella is displaced, and the alae are deformed and collapsed.

Operative Procedure

1. Bilateral infraorbital nerves are blocked with anesthetic. Suction apparatus must be at hand because the patient may be choked by breathing in blood during the operation.

2. The scar is excised circumferentially along the nostril rim. Great care should be taken to avoid injury to the alar cartilage. The scar is often found situated 1 cm–2 cm deep in the vestibule (Fig. XIV.8a).

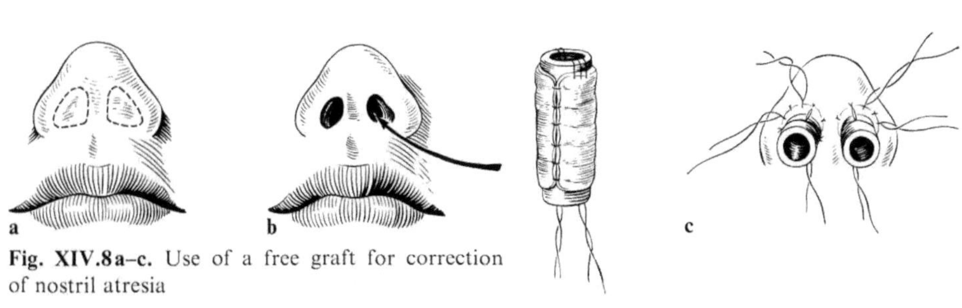

Fig. XIV.8a–c. Use of a free graft for correction of nostril atresia

3. A piece of skin graft is wrapped inside out on a plastic tube which is inserted into the nostril. One must ensure that the graft contacts snugly with the raw surface within the nostril. The plastic tube is removed 7–9 days postoperatively, and a normal nostril is thus formed (Fig. XIV.8b).

4. Another solid plastic tube is worn in the nostril to prevent contraction of the graft for some time after operation (Fig. XIV.8c).

2.5 Partial or Total Loss of the Nose

Alar defects and partial loss of the nose are more common than total loss of the nose in facial burns, and penetrating wounds are seen only in electric burns. In these patients, cold wind, dust, or other foreign bodies may directly enter the upper respiratory tract, giving rise to infection in this region. Reconstruction of the nose is therefore necessary for physiologic as well as cosmetic reasons.

Partial alar defect resulting from a burn may generally be repaired with either a free skin graft or a composite graft from the ear. Sometimes both ears are destroyed by burns and no composite graft is available, in which case a pedicled flap from other regions may be used.

2.5.1 Alar Defects

Operative Procedure

1. A sickle-shape flap is designed at the recess of the hairline on the same side as the defect, lying along the course of the posterior branch of the temporal artery. The flap consists of hair-bearing scalp, except for the distal portion, which is actually the hairless frontal skin flap. It is this portion that is used for the repair of the alar defect. As the flap contains a known artery and its accompanying vein, the length–breadth ratio may exceed that of a conventional flap (Fig. XIV.9a).

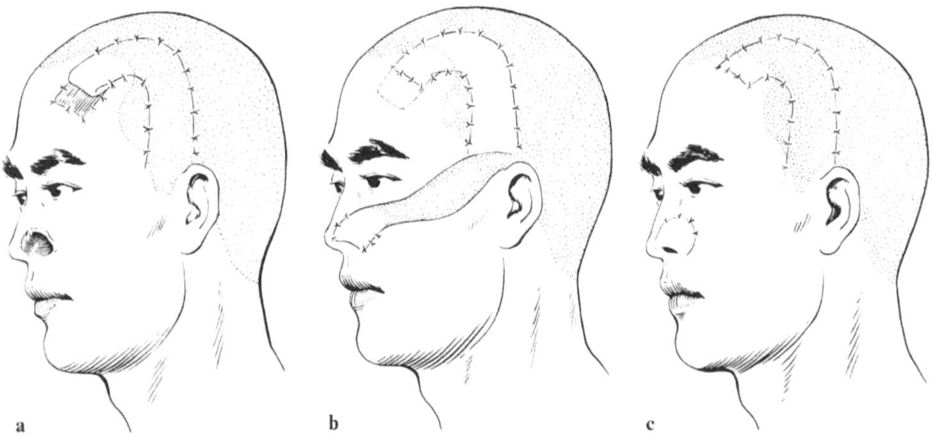

a b c

Fig. XIV.9a–c. Repair of an alar defect by means of a pedicle flap

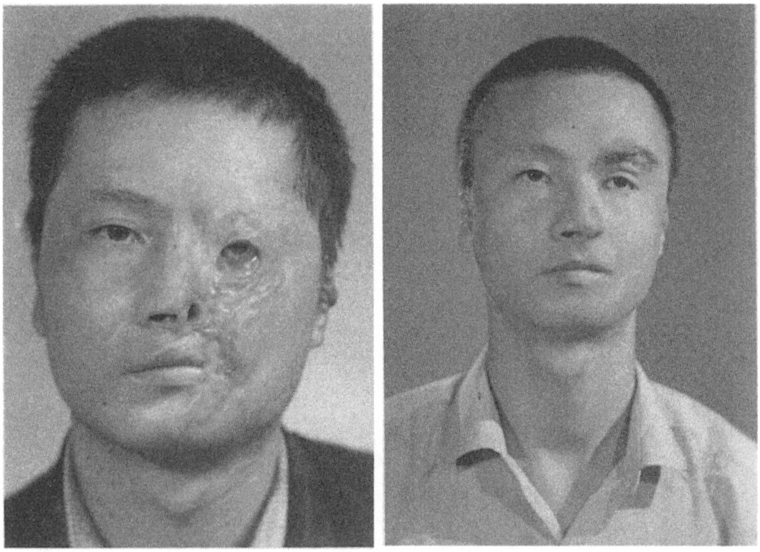

Fig. XIV.10. a Postburn facial deformity involving loss of the left eyebrow and a partial alar defect. b Appearance after repair of (a) the facial deformity by means of a full-thickness graft, (b) the eyebrow by means of a temporal island flap, and (c) the alar defect by means of a pedicle flap

2. The distal part of the flap is either folded on itself to make the lining or lined with a skingraft in a previous operation. The length of the flap should be sufficient to reach the alar defect without tension (Fig. XIV.9b).

3. The donor area on the scalp is temporarily skin grafted. When the distal portion of the flap takes well on the alar defect, the flap is divided and the remaining part is returned to the donor site. Apart from some skin-grafted area at the recess of the hairline, there is no other visible scar on the scalp, as the scar is hidden in the hair (Figs. XIV.9c, XIV.10).

2.5.2 Subtotal and Total Loss

In patients with severe burns involving the face, upper extremity, trunk, and other regions, there is usually no healthy tissue available from the frontal and supraclavicular regions or upper arm. The tube for reconstruction has to be taken from the abdomen or the chest, but skin from these areas has a poor color match and contains too much subcutaneous fat, which may make the nose appear too bulky. Removal of some of the fat from the tube becomes necessary in a second operation to produce a nose of normal size. However, skin from the thoracoclavicular regions has a better color match and may be used. It should be noted that when a tube is used to reconstruct the nose, it will shrink considerably after the operation, so it is preferable to construct the nose slightly larger than normal. Six months after the operation some revisions may be needed to improve the appearance.

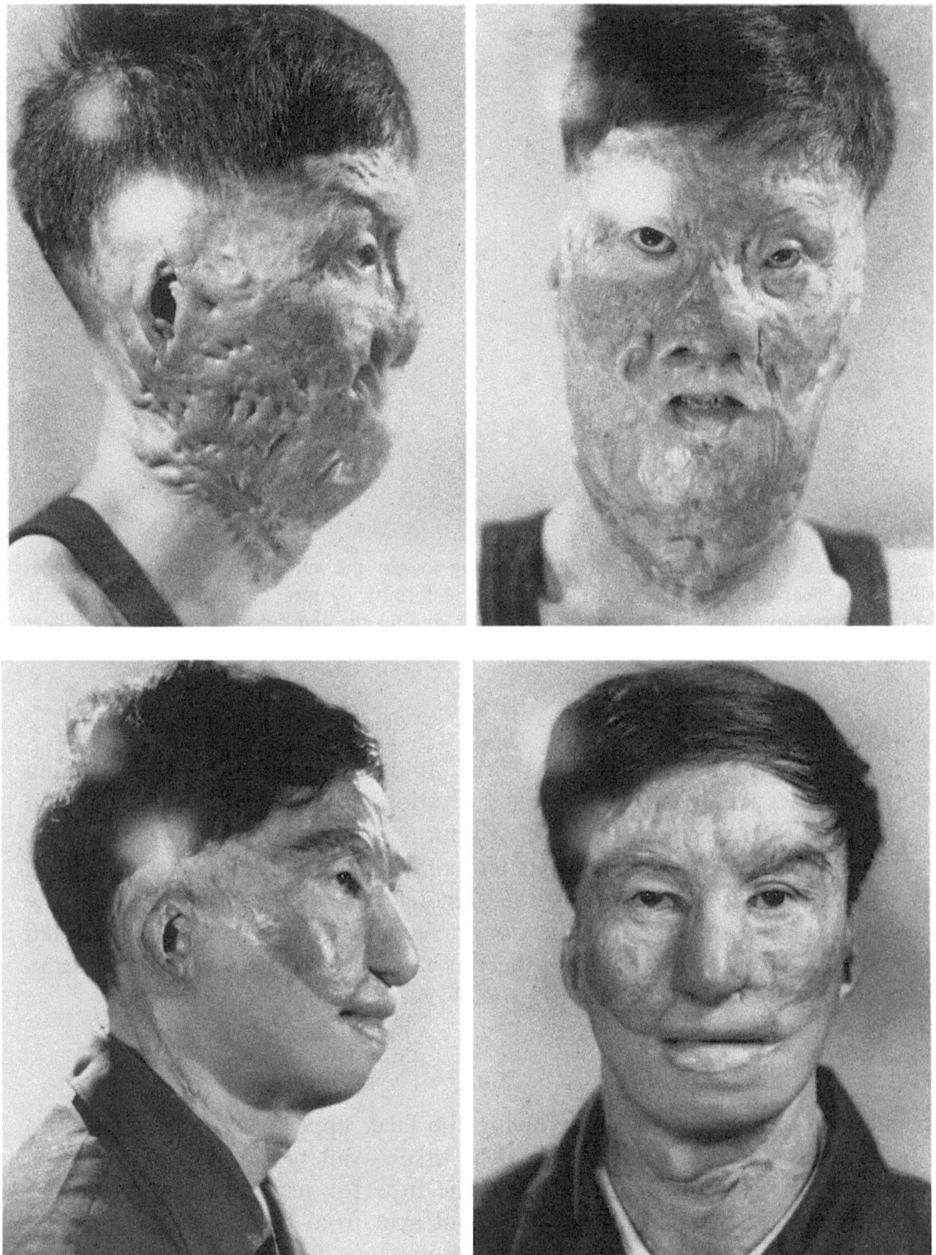

a b c d

Fig. XIV.11. **a, b** Chemical burn of the face. **c, d** Appearance after repair of the face with a pedicle tube and total reconstruction of the nose

Operative Procedure

1. A tube 16 cm long and 8 cm–9 cm wide is constructed at the flank of the abdominal wall because there is less adipose tissue there. The upper portion of the tube is purposely made slightly narrower than the lower portion. In doing so, care should be taken not to jeopardize its blood supply.

2. Three weeks later the lower end of the tube is divided and transplanted to the wrist, which serves as a carrier. After another 3 weeks the other end is divided and transplanted to the base of the nose, that is, a site just below the glabella.

3. The tube must remain there for more than 4 weeks before adequate blood supply can be established. Only when necrosis of the distal portion is unlikely can the tube be used to construct the new nose.

4. The lining of the new nose may be taken from the nasal base if there is enough tissue in that area; in such a case, the tube may be designed a little shorter. Alternatively the lining is procured by folding up the distal portion of the tube.

5. After 4–5 weeks have elapsed, the tube is opened longitudinally along its suture line. Any redundant fat or residual scar tissue is meticulously removed, and care is taken not to damage the subdermal vascular plexus.

6. The columella is formed from the folded part of the flap by making two parallel incisions 6 mm–8 mm apart. The tip of the new columella is sutured to the wound at the piriform aperture, which is the site of the original columella. The two alae are then sutured in place, proceeding from the inside to the outside.

7. After all the sutures have been completed, a mattress suture with a cushion under it is placed at the dorsum of the new nose in order to maintain the shape of a normal nose. Two plastic tubes are inserted into the nostrils for support and breathing (Fig. XIV.11).

2.6 Defects of the Ear

Both ears are usually involved in burns of the face. Defects of the ear frame occur as a result of chondritis, which usually leads to necrosis of the cartilage. The cartilage has to be removed once it becomes necrotic.

The common defect in a burned ear is loss of the helix, while the concha and the scapha are spared. Sometimes the ear adheres to the mastoid region, with disappearance of the angle between the ear and the skull, and the patient finds it difficult to wear glasses or a mask. In severe cases the upper third or even the whole ear is absent.

2.6.1 Repair of Ear Defects

When the undamaged cartilage is covered with only a thin layer of scar tissue it tends to break and become infected. Repair is therefore necessary.

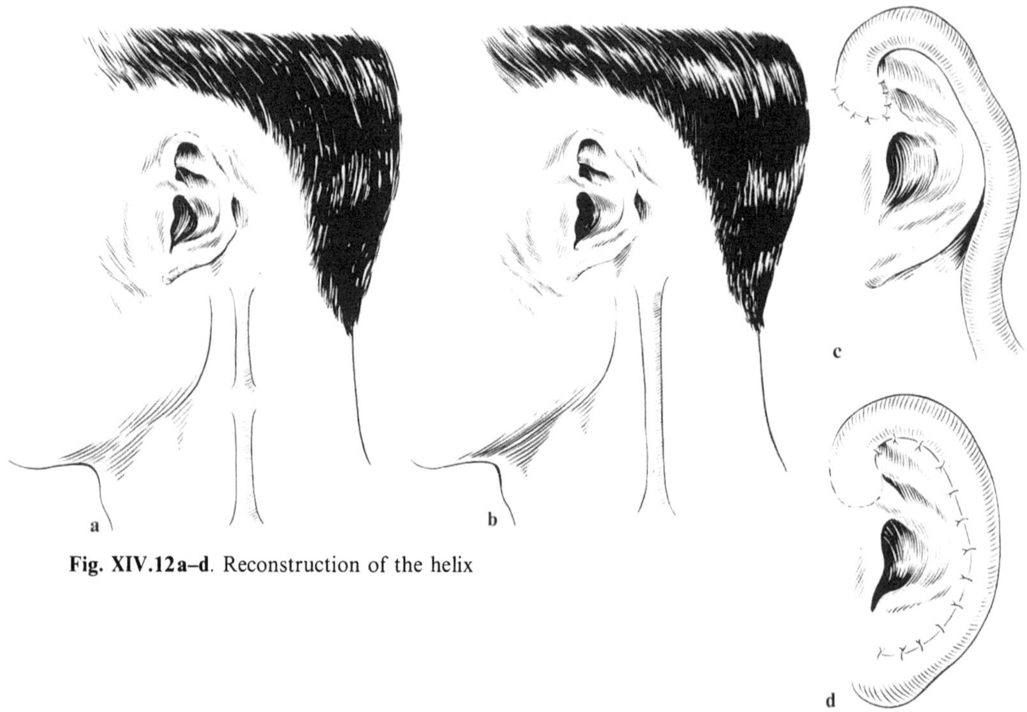

Fig. XIV.12a–d. Reconstruction of the helix

Operative Procedure

1. A tube 13 cm–14 cm long and 2 cm–3 cm in circumference is first constructed in the postauricular area obliquely downward to the neck. As the tube is usually long and narrow it is wise to leave a skin bridge at its middle portion to avoid necrosis. The skin bridge is raised and tubed 3 weeks later (Fig. XIV.12a, b).

2. Another 3 weeks later, the lower end of the tube is transplanted to a spot just above the tragus, which is actually the starting point of the helix (Fig. XIV.12c).

3. After circulation has been established, the tube is opened longitudinally and sutured to the rim of the ear (Fig. XIV.12d).

2.6.2 Scar Adhesion Between the Ear and the Mastoid Region

Infection and cicatricial contraction are common causes of adhesion between the ear and the mastoid region. The ear loses its normal contour, and the angle between it and the skull disappears.

Operative Procedure

If the absent part of the ear cartilage is not large and the concha and antihelix are still present, it is only necessary to excise the scar and cover the resulting wound with an intermediate thickness skin graft which is secured by a tie-over dressing. After the graft has taken well, the patient is advised to wear a splint over the area to prevent secondary contraction of the graft (Fig. XIV.13).

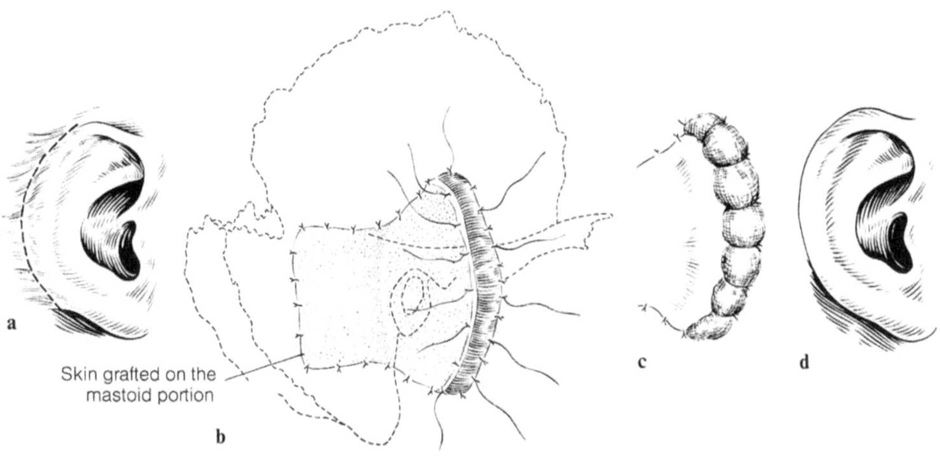

Fig. XIV.13a–d. Repair of adhesion between the ear and the mastoid region

3 Cicatricial Contraction of the Neck

Patients with cicatricial contraction of the neck not only find it difficult to extend and rotate their neck but may also have eversion of the lower lip, ectropion of the lower eyelid, and deformity of the mandible.

3.1 Classification

Cicatricial contraction of the neck may be divided into three types according to the degree of severity:

Type 1: Superficial cicatricial contraction of the neck. In second degree burns when only the superficial layer of the dermis is affected, the resulting scar is often flat. Cicatricial contraction, if any, is also slight, and mentocervical deformity is not severe. Though the motion of the neck is somewhat limited, there is no eversion of the lower lip and the patient experiences no difficulty in extending his neck. Most of the scars gradually soften and become linear or a web as a result of persistent stretching action and compensation of the adjacent normal skin.

Typ 2: Mild cicatricial contraction of the neck. Deep second degree burns of the neck complicated by infection may produce a flat or masslike hypertrophic scar which is dense and hard. The patient usually complains of itching and pricking. This scar often undergoes a vicious process of breaking and healing, but becomes progressively thicker. There is limitation of neck motion and eversion of the lower lip, and other deformities are also present.

Type 3: Severe cicatricial contraction of the neck. In this type the burned area often covers the face, the neck, the chin, and other parts. Deep structures of the neck are also affected. In the late stage there is always severe cicatricial contraction between the chin and the neck so that the chin is actually bound down to the chest; this is the so-called thoracomental adhesion deformity.

The angle between the chin and the neck often disappears in profile view. The patient has difficulty in turning his neck. Sometimes even drooling occurs owing to severe eversion of lower lip. Closing of the eyes is also interfered with, because of secondary ectropion of the lower lid, which is pulled down by cicatricial contraction over the neck. If the patient sustains the burn before adolescence he will have *micrognathia*.

3.2 Surgical Treatment

General anesthesia becomes difficult because the patient cannot extend his neck and open his mouth. Therefore, maintenance of an adequate airway is difficult and accidents are likely (see Chap. XV).

3.2.1 Z-plasty

With the neck passively extended so that the scar web can easily be seen, a z-plasty is designed. Skin incision is performed as designed (Fig. XIV.14a), and when the two triangular flaps are transposed the cicatricial contraction is released (Fig. XIV.14b). Investigation of the blood supply of the surrounding skin and evaluation of its pliability prior to operation will help to predict the operative outcome.

3.2.2 Free Skin Graft

Most cases of cicatricial contraction of the neck are treated with free skin graft. Special attention should be paid to the anatomic features of the neck. As skin graft over the neck has a great tendency to contract postoperatively, a specially designed splint must be worn for a long period after operation if a good result is to be obtained. If an intermediate thickness skin graft is chosen (not thinner than 0.4 mm) for neck surgery, the following technical points deserve emphasis:

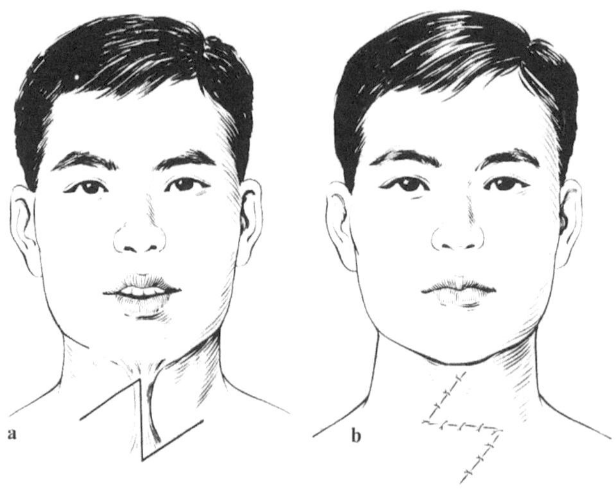

Fig. XIV.14a, b. Repair of linear or web cicatricial contraction of the neck by means of a Z-plasty

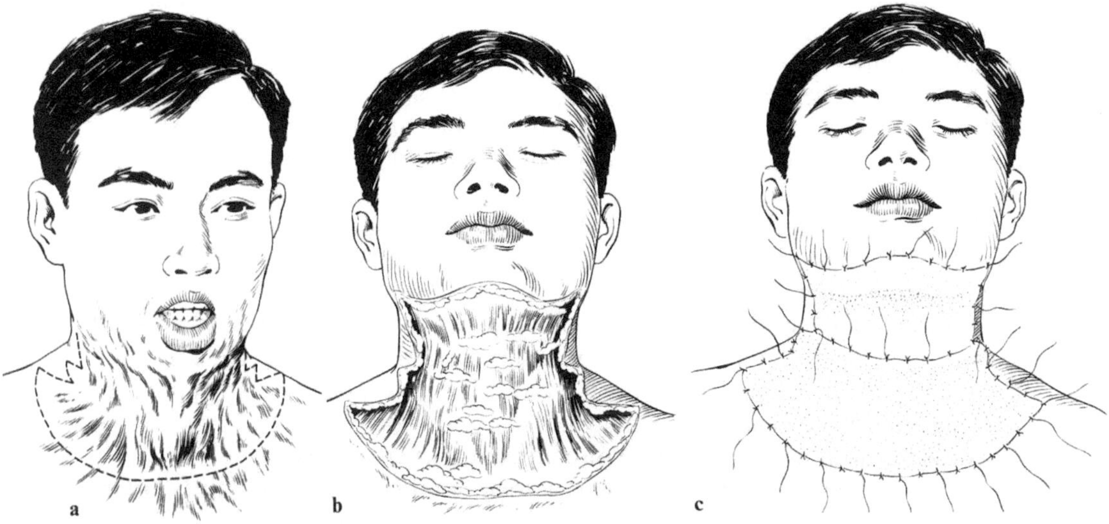

Fig. XIV.15a–c. Use of a free graft for repair of cicatricial contraction of the neck

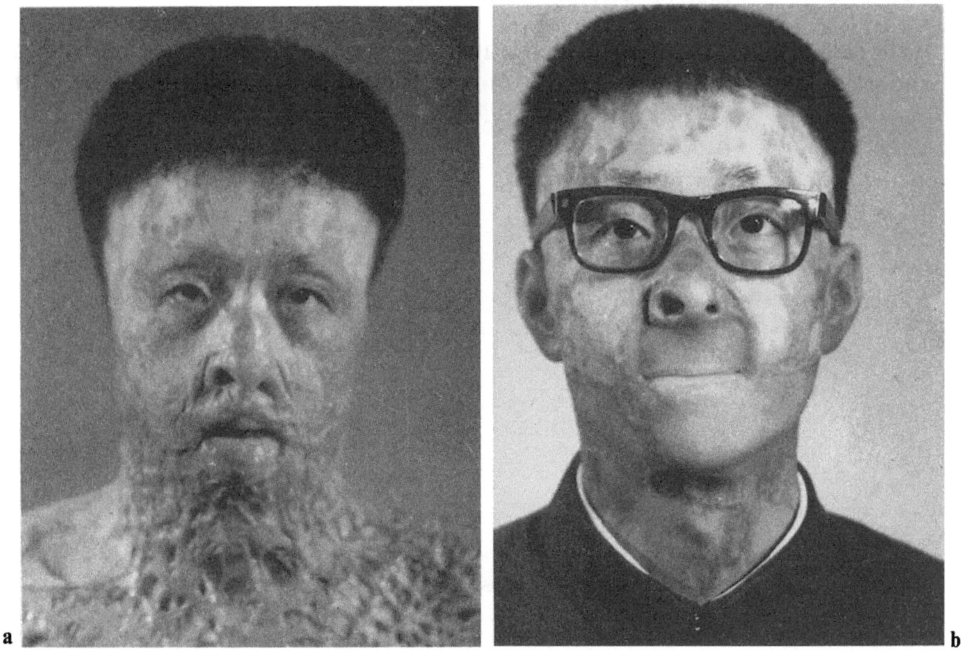

Fig. XIV.16. a Severe scar contraction of the neck causing chin–chest fusion. **b** Appearance after excision of the scar tissue and grafting of a large sheet of full-thickness (0.5 mm) graft

1. The platysma always undergoes fibrosis because of long-standing limitation of neck movement; consequently it must be excised to gain full release of the contracture.

2. Scar excision must be radical and hemostasis complete. The recipient bed is made as even as possible and care should be taken to make zig-zag incisions along the margin of the wound to avoid postoperative linear contraction.

3. The tension on the skin graft should be such that the skin lies in close contact with the recipient bed. A tie-over dressing is applied to avoid postoperative hematoma (Fig. XIV.15).

4. Postoperatively the neck is immobilized in a combined cervico-thoraco-axillary dressing without causing unnecessary discomfort to the patient. The patient is put on a liquid diet for 3–5 days after the operation to minimize chewing and swallowing movements.

Measures to prevent recurrence of contraction after surgery:

1. The patient is advised to wear a foam rubber splint constantly after the operation. The neck is extended when the patient lies on his bed. When he is ambulant he should perform neck exercises as a complement to physiotherapy.

2. A collar made of foam rubber or metal is worn for a period of 6–12 months.

If these preventive measures are taken, the outcome of the operation will be quite rewarding (Fig. XIV.16).

3.2.3 Tubes or Flaps for Repair of the Neck

If the skin around the hypertrophic scar is pliable and has good vascularization and color match, it can be used as a flap for the repair. The advantages of

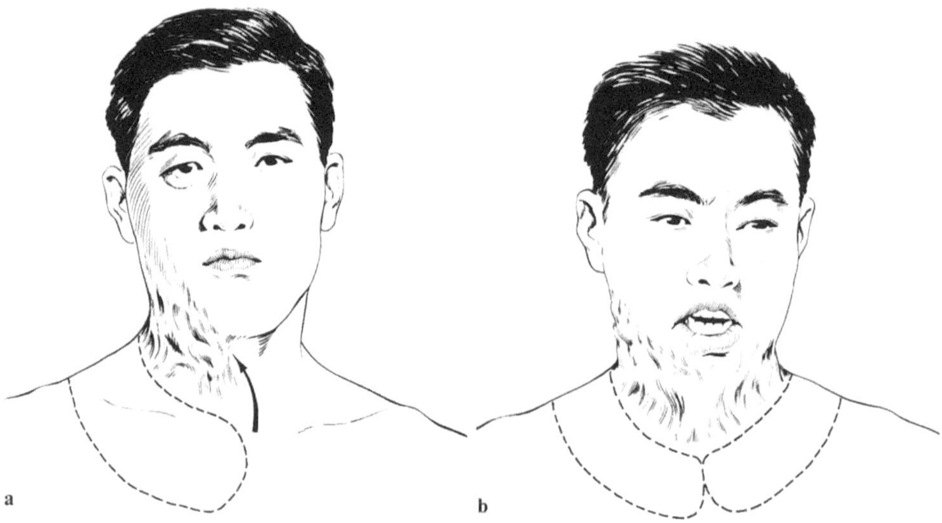

Fig. XIV.17a, b. Supraclavicular flap

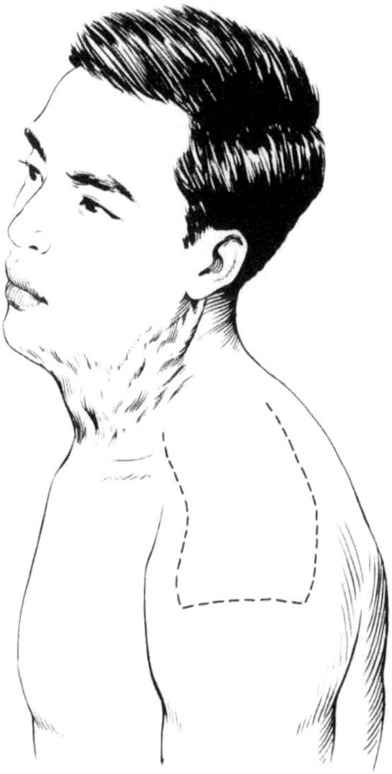

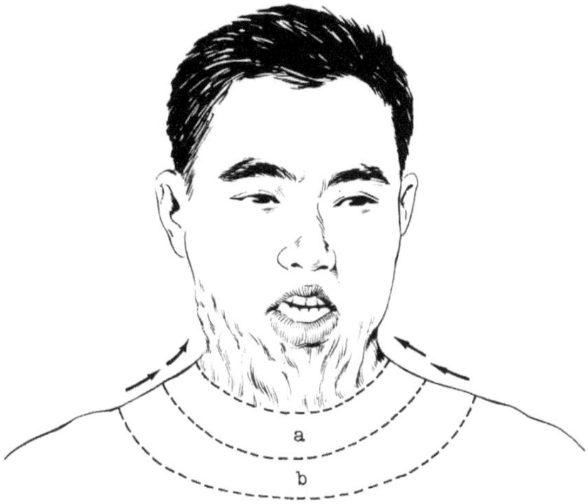

Fig. XIV.19. Bipedicle flap

◁**Fig. XIV.18.** Acromial flap

tube or flap repair are their good color match and soft texture, their fullness in appearance, and their lack of tendency to pigmentation and recurrence of contraction. They are frequently used in the treatment of cicatricial contraction of the neck. On the other hand, they need multiple operations and the course of treatment is prolonged.

The following flaps are commonly used:

1. A *supraclavicular flap:* After excision of the scar, a flap of the same size as the defect is designed over the supraclavicular region, having a length-breadth ratio of 2:1. It is raised and swung toward the mentocervical region to cover the defect (Fig. XIV.17a). The secondary defect is covered with a free graft. If a single flap is not big enough, double flaps from both sides are recommended (Fig. XIV.17b).

2. *An acromial flap:* If the flap is not available from supraclavicular region or the chest, it can be taken from the acromial area (Fig. XIV.18). However, the flap in this area has the shortcoming of too great a rotationary angle, which will cause kinking of the pedicle and jeopardize the blood supply. This shortcoming deserves careful consideration if use of an acromial flap is planned. The secondary defect is covered with a free graft.

3. *A bipedicled flap:* If the scar of the neck is extensive but the skin over the subclavicular area is normal, a bipedicled flap can be designed on this area, the length-breadth ratio being 3:1. This flap is elevated at a plane superficial to the fascia and is lifted to the neck to cover the defect (Fig. XIV.19). The donor area is covered with a free graft or another bipedicle flap.

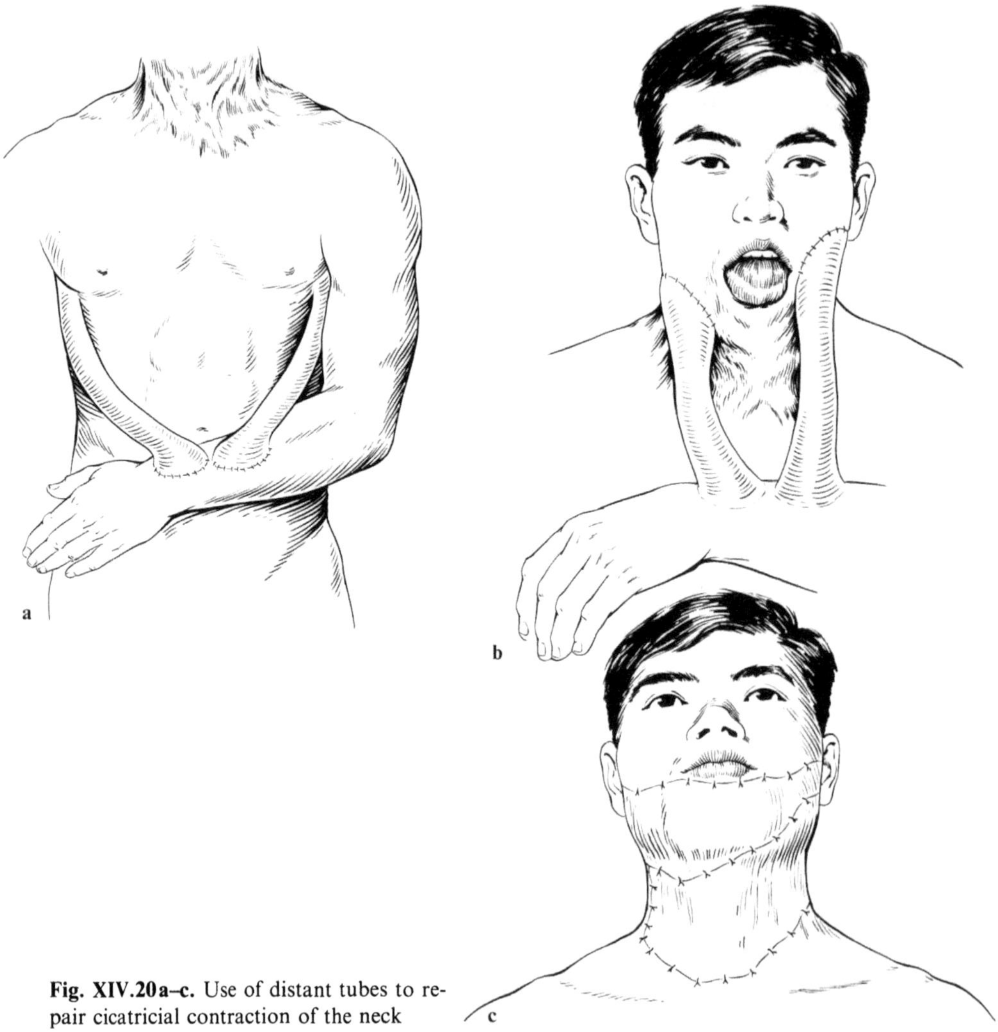

Fig. XIV.20a–c. Use of distant tubes to repair cicatricial contraction of the neck

Shortcomings of this bipedicle flap are (a) there is usually a dog-ear at the pedicle which needs to be dealt with later, (b) when it is slid to cover the protruding chin it will not only obliterate the mentocervical angle, resulting in an unsatisfactory appearance, but will also interfere with extension of the neck, (c) in female patients the upper part of the breast may be involved in the flap, and (d) the operation involves a greater risk because of its extensiveness.

4. *A tube:* In severe cases distant tubes may be required. These tubes are taken from both sides of the chest and the abdomen and are about 30 cm in length (Fig. XIV.20a). When blood supply has been established the tubes are transplanted to the neck via the forearm as the carrier (Fig. XIV.20b). They are not placed at the same level; rather one is placed higher than the other. When they are opened up they may cross each other to cover the wound (Fig. XIV.20c). The result is quite satisfactory because of good contour and color match.

4 Cicatricial Contraction of the Axilla

4.1 Classification

Clinically burn scar contraction of the axilla is divided into three types:

Type 1: Scar web of the axilla: Subcutaneous fat in the anterior wall (clavicothoracic wall) and posterior wall (scapular wall) of the axilla is usually scanty. In burns of this area there is often a small piece of normal skin spared at the top of the axillary dome. As the scar in this area is subject to the stretching action of the upper limb, the adjacent normal skin usually compensates to form a web over the anterior wall or the posterior wall. This condition occurs more often in children than in adults. As the child grows, his bones become longer. At the same time compensation by the adjacent skin takes place as the scar becomes soft. This process continues for years and a web is gradually formed at the axilla. This scar web is soft and pliable, has a good blood supply and color match, and contains thin subcutaneous fat. Hence it may serve for a Z-plasty.

Type 2: Scar adhesion between upper arm and the chest wall. This type usually occurs when the medial aspect of the upper arm as well as the adjacent chest wall is burned. Constant rubbing between the chest wall and the upper arm causes ulceration over the scars. The scars gradually become hypertrophic as a vicious process of healing and ulceration takes place. Finally the anterior and the posterior walls adhere to each other, thus obliterating the axillary fossa.

The scar covers an area from the anterior wall of the axilla to the twelfth rib and medial side of the elbow. The breast is displaced laterally, with complete loss of arm activity.

Type 3: In this type the upper arm, the lateral side of the chest, and the elbow (often in flexing position) are embodied in a mass of scar. This is the most severe type, usually seen in extensive burns which include the upper arm, the chest wall, and the elbow. The patient can neither abduct and raise his arm nor move his arm forward and backward. He is also unable to extend his elbow joint.

4.2 Infection

In patients with cicatricial contraction involving the upper arm and the chest wall, the anterior and posterior walls of the axilla often become fused so that a dead space is formed in the axillary fossa with a piece of normal skin enclosed in it. Secretion from the sweat glands and hair follicles of this piece of skin cannot find its way out, thus inevitably inducing infection, usually with the piece of skin as a nucleus. Pus tends to collect in this dead space, and the patient has a high fever, chills, and polynucleosis. The skin around the armpit becomes red and edematous, and there is always pain over this area. The amount of pus increases rapidly. Finally the pus breaks through a weak point and an infective sinus is formed. This sinus does not heal for a long time. Incision and evacuation of the pus together with the administration of antibiotics

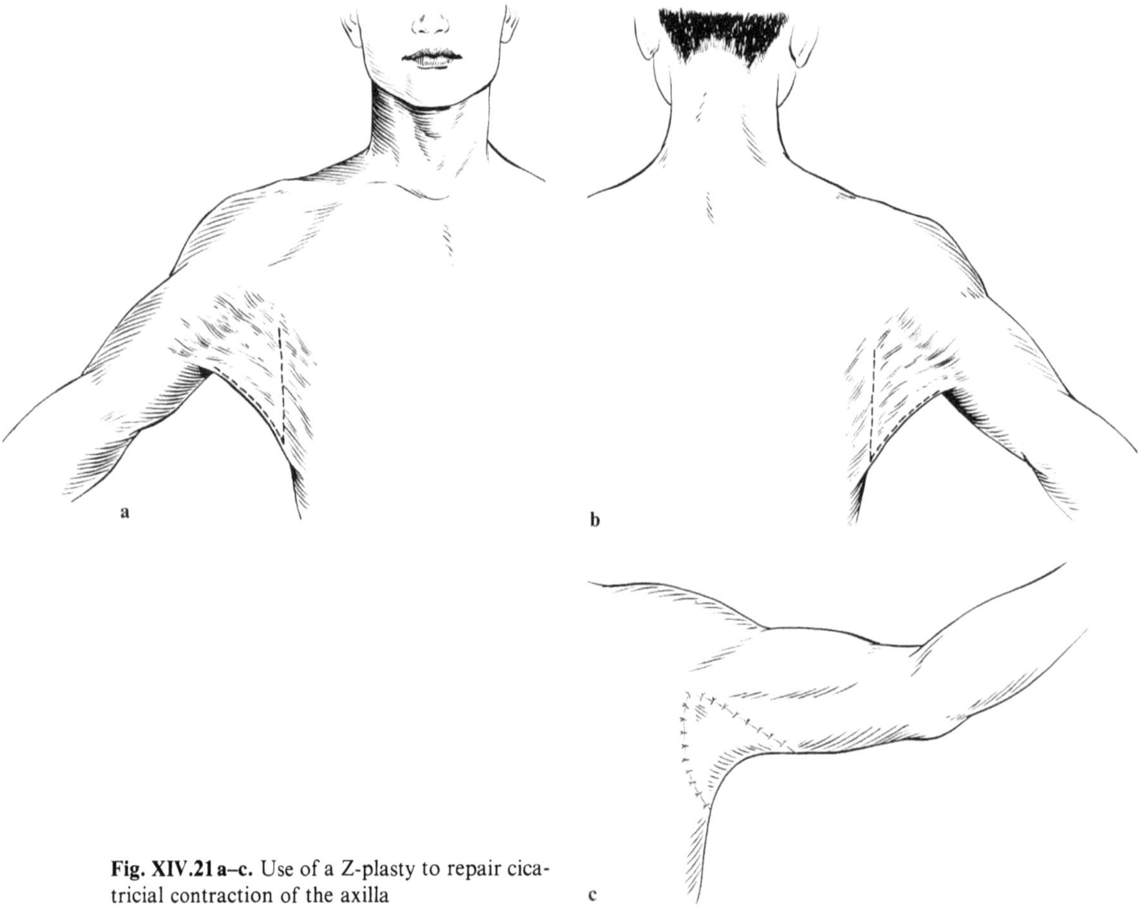

Fig. XIV.21 a–c. Use of a Z-plasty to repair cicatricial contraction of the axilla

only stop the infection temporarily – they can never prevent its recurrence. The only way to eradicate it is to open up the dead space, excise the piece of skin and the scar, cleanse the wound, and apply a large sheet of skin graft to the wound with the upper arm fully abducted.

4.3 Surgical Treatment

4.3.1 Z-plasty

With the upper arm as fully abducted as possible and the web stretched, a Z-plasty is performed with its axis lying along the free border of the web. Dissection of the flaps should be confined to a plane just superficial to the fascia. Once all fibrous tissue is excised, the upper arm is able to abduct. The two triangular flaps are then transposed and sutured in place to complete the procedure (Fig. XIV.21).

4.3.2 Transplantation of Free Skin Graft

1. The procedure begins with radical excision of all scars. The incision should go beyond the anterior and posterior lines of the axilla, downward to the twelfth rib, and laterally to the middle third of the medial aspect of the upper arm

2. At the top, the incision crosses both the anterior and posterior walls of the axilla and then turns upward to reach the shoulder. Only in doing so can the upper arm be fully abducted without difficulty.

3. The incision must be zig-zag while crossing the anterior and posterior walls in order to prevent postoperative linear scar contraction.

4. The upper arm must be held in a fully abducted position, preferably at a right angle to the body, before proceeding with the operation. Incision should begin from the part which has the greatest tension. It should be noted that undue traction on the upper limb while the patient is under anesthesia is likely to cause injury to the brachial plexus.

5. Structures that constitute the base of the armpit are skin, subcutaneous fat, and axillary fascia. The fascia is dense but without distinguishable cleavage. If cicatricial contraction is not severe the fascia is preferably left untouched, so that a level recipient bed can be created. To go too deep into the axillary triangle has no effect on further releasing the scar; on the contrary, it involves the risk of injuring the brachial plexus. Moreover, the recipient bed will have an irregular surface which is unfavorable for a pressure dressing. Hence, radical excision of all pathologic tissue is not indicated for this area.

6. A tie-over dressing is preferred for the area. The upper arm is immobilized in abduction at a right angle to the body by a splint. In order to prevent postoperative contraction of the graft the patient is advised to assume a position with his arm fully abducted when he is in bed. When he is ambulant he must exercise his arm diligently. Physiotherapy may be supplemented.

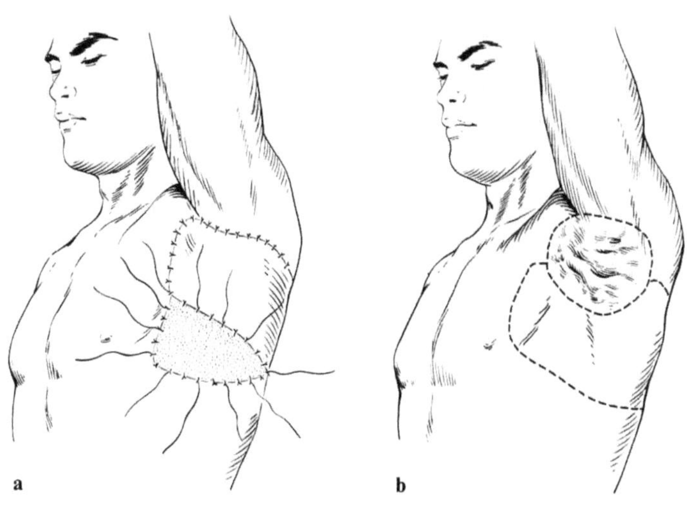

Fig. XIV.22a, b. Repair of cicatricial contraction of the axilla by means of an adjacent pedicle flap

4.3.3 Repair with a Pedicle Flap

For deep burns in this area, such as those caused by electricity and radiation, repair with a pedicle flap from the adjacent area should be considered since a free skin graft may not meet the requirements. The donor area is covered with a skin graft (Fig. XIV.22).

5 Cicatricial Contraction of the Elbow

Cicatricial contraction can be situated anterior or posterior to the elbow joint. Sometimes it may present as a circumferential hypertrophic scar over the elbow. The skin over the cubital fossa is thin and the subcutaneous fat scanty. Main vessels and nerves of the upper limb course medially to the biceps brachii into the cubital fossa. The skin and subcutaneous fat at the back of the elbow joint is, however, thicker. The ulnar nerve passes medial to the olecranon. Clinically, burn cicatricial contraction is often located in front of the elbow joint, probably due to its anatomic features. Cicatricial contraction at the back of the elbow joint is rare, except in electric burns.

A long-standing superficial second degree burn scar in front of the elbow joint tends to become a soft web, owing to the stretching action of the joint and compensation of the normal skin around it. In children the scar web is usually long and pliable (Fig. XIV.23).

This scar web can be satisfactorily treated with a Z-plasty. If there is a gap between the two triangular flaps after they have been transposed, the gap may be covered with a skin graft (Fig. XIV.24).

Extensive hypertrophic scars caused by deep second degree or third degree burns are usually thick and dense. Wide excision of the scar is necessary prior to skin grafting. Sometimes deep structures which have undergone fibrotic changes may jut out and pass longitudinally across the cubital fossa. Such structures will interfere with extension of the elbow joint, even though the overlying scar has been excised. In such cases all the fibrotic tissue, including some unimportant tendons, should be excised. If, after all these efforts, the elbow joint still can not be extended, as often occurs in severe cases, it is preferable to place the joint in about 120°–140° flexion and then cover the wound with a graft. The patient is advised to exercise his joint diligently and usually full extension can be gained.

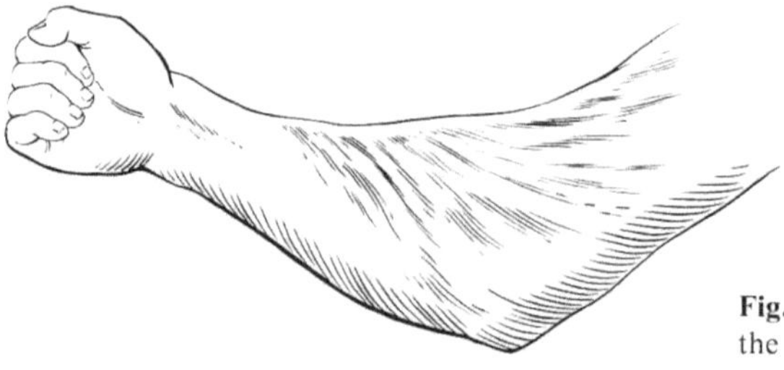

Fig. XIV.23. Web cicatricial contraction of the elbow

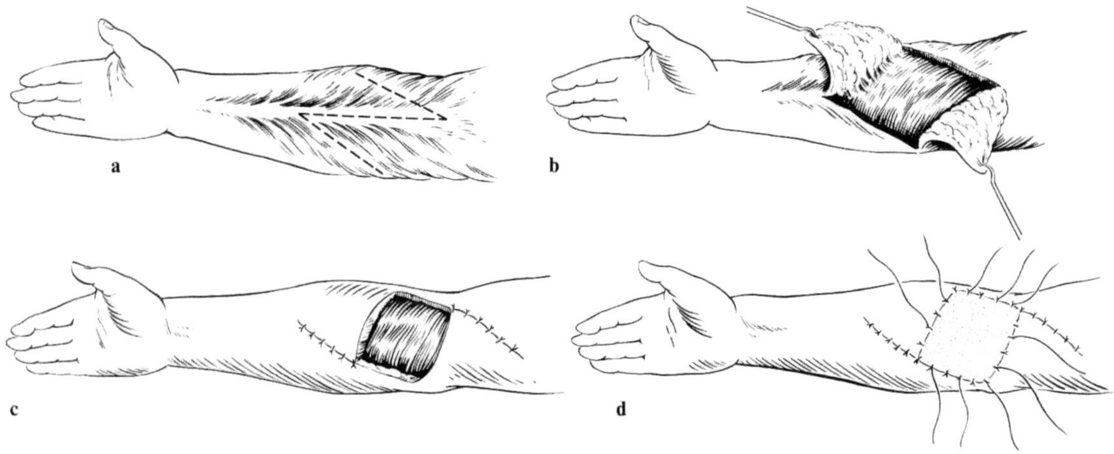

Fig. XIV.24a–d. Use of a Z-plasty for repair of scar web of the elbow

An attempt to extend the joint by undue force may cause spasm of vessels and sometimes even injury to nerves and other structures. A second operation may make possible full extension of most of the joints that cannot be fully extended after the first operation.

Burns at the back of the elbow joint occasionally expose the olecranon, which usually requires a flap from the adjacent region for its coverage. If the flap is designed on the chest wall, the elbow should be brought to it and secured in place for about 3 weeks before the pedicle of the flap is divided.

6 Cicatricial Contraction of the Hand

The incidence of burn cicatricial contraction of the hand is higher than that of the other parts of the body. Functions of the hand such as opposing, grasping, and holding are often lost. The patient can neither work nor live a normal life.

The skin on the dorsum of the hand is looser than that on the volar surface. As there is only a thin layer of subcutaneous fat in the dorsum of the hand, extensor tendons and joint capsules lie very close to the overlying skin. Hence, burns on the dorsum of the hand are likely to involve and destroy these two deep structures. If the eschar of a third degree burn is allowed to separate by itself and no skin graft is applied to the wound, repeated infection will cause progressive fibrosis, which will end in severe cicatricial contraction. Clinically, a clawhand is the typical example of this condition – DIP and MP joints are in hyperextension deformity while PIP joints are in flexion deformity and the first web is considerably narrowed.

The skin and subcutaneous fat of the volar surface of the hand are thicker, so that burns in this area seldom involve tendons or joints, an exception being electric burns. However, if cicatricial contraction is left untreated, secondary

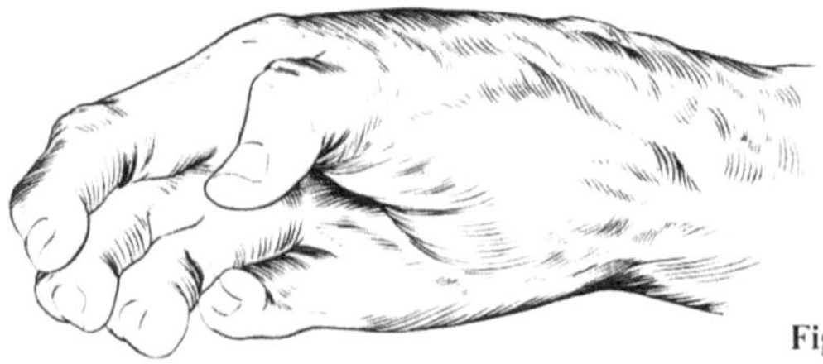

Fig. XIV.25. Cicatricial contraction of the palm

deformities such as fibrosis of the aponeurosis palmaris and shortening of tendons, nerves, and vessels will result. This renders late repair difficult (Fig. XIV.25).

6.1 Classification of Burn Cicatricial Contraction on the Dorsum of the Hand

Cicatricial contraction on the dorsum of the hand may be classified as mild, moderate, and severe, according to the degree of contraction and pathologic changes of the tissue.

6.1.1 Mild Form

Scar is confined to the superfical layer, with mild fibrosis of deep structures. The joints are deformed but they still retain a certain range of motion. The deformity is easily corrected once the scar has been excised. The resulting wound is covered with a skin graft.

6.1.2 Moderate Form

The whole thickness of the skin is destroyed and deep structures such as tendons and joint capsules are also affected. The clinical appearance of the deformed hand leads to it being termed "clawhand" (Fig. XIV.26).

1. The metacarpophalangeal joint is in extreme dorsiflexion, with complete or incomplete dislocation of the joint and palmar displacement of the metacarpal head, often accompanied by disappearance of the palmar arch.

2. The transverse distance of the dorsal surface is decreased, with the first and fifth metacarpal bones crowding centripetally toward the third one.

3. The thumb is adducted and comes into line with the other four fingers.

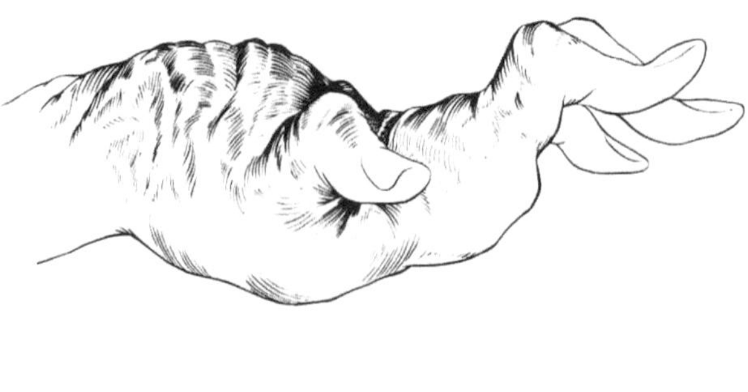

Fig. XIV.26. Clawhand deformity

The first web is narrowed, with subluxation of the MP joint of the thumb.

4. Proximal interphalangeal joints are in flexion or ankylosed while DIP joints are in full extension.

Clawhand is the result of the continuous pulling action of scar over the joints. Apart from joint deformities, thickening of joint capsules, intraarticular adhesions, and shortening of collateral ligaments and tendons also occur. In a long-standing case there will also be accompanying bone deformities due to persistent compression by the scar.

The pathologic changes of joints and tendons are most marked in this form. The aim of repair is to restore joint functions such as opposing, grasping, and holding. Descriptions of the pathologic changes of joints, capsules, and collateral ligaments are as follows:

1. *Ankylosis of IP joints:* When the skin on the dorsal surface of the hand and the capsules of IP joints are destroyed simultaneously by burns, intraarticular infection is always a complication. This may lead to destruction of cartilage and rupture of the central slip of the tendon of the extensor muscle. These factors, combined with shortening of flexor tendons and palmar displacement of the collateral ligaments, contribute to ankylosis of PIP joints in a flexion position.

2. *Contracture of joint capsules:* Normally, when a PIP joint extends, the palmar part of its capsule is under tension and becomes slack when the PIP joint is flexed. Hence, if the PIP joint is fixed in flexion for a prolonged period, this part of the capsule gradually becomes shortened and the joint can no longer be extended.

3. *Contracture of the collateral ligament:* Normally, the collateral ligament of the MP joint is loose when the joint extends and becomes tense when it flexes. Hence, if the MP joint is immobilized in extension for a prolonged period by cicatricial contraction on the dorsal surface of the hand, the collateral ligament will undergo fibrosis and become shortened. This interferes considerably with the opposing and grasping function of the hand.

In the moderate form of cicatricial contraction mere excision of the scar is apparently inadequate. All the pathologic changes of deep structures should be dealt with at the same time if a good operative result is to be achieved.

6.1.3 Severe Form

If a hand is injured by a hot roller or is immobilized in a nonfunctional position for too long, all of the intrinsic muscles will be likely to undergo atrophy. In such a case the hand will still lose all of its functions even if cicatricial contraction is not severe, and the outcome of surgery will often be poor.

6.2 Treatment

In mild cases, after excision of the scar and correction of the deformity by manipulation with the patient under anesthesia, the wound should be covered with a large sheet of intermediate thickness skin graft. In moderate or severe

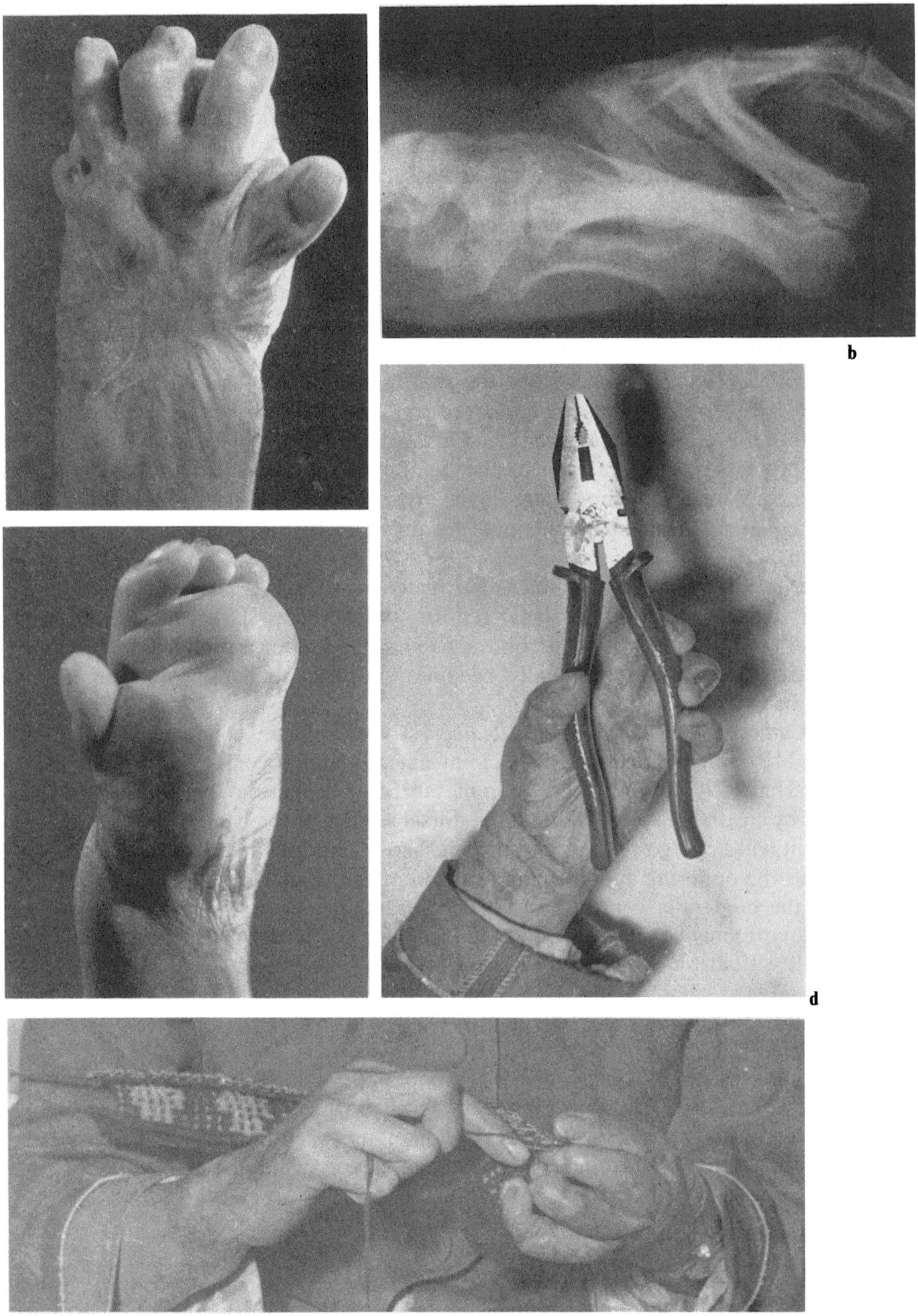

a b c d e

cases, the operation may include arthroplasty, transposition of tendons, excision of collateral ligaments, etc. Sometimes a distant tube is required and should be prepared in advance. The operative steps for repair of deep structures are as follows:

6.2.1 Reduction of the MP Joint

Hyperextension deformity of the MP joint is usually prominent in cicatricial contraction of a burned hand.

6.2.1.1 Reduction by Manipulation

After excision of the scar and with the patient under anesthesia, the deformed MP joint is reduced by manipulation to a position of opposition. With the use of a "pull-push" method to release tissue contraction, the operator can successfully reduce the subluxated joint. Undue force should be avoided, otherwise the joint capsule and ligament may be torn or even a buttonhole rupture of the capsule of the MP joint will result. In severe cases, it is often impossible to restore the opposing function of the hand with one operation, and staged operations are needed. In the first operation the joint is reduced to a certain degree of flexion and maintained in this position with a Kirschner wire, and a skin graft is applied on the wound. As soon as the graft has taken well the patient is advised to exercise the joint to overcome stiffness of the joint and ligament. Six months after the first operation, a similar procedure is carried out on the hand to obtain complete reduction of the joint.

The advantages of staged procedures are:

1. It is possible to use a free skin graft instead of a more complicated tube.

2. Excision of the joint capsule and collateral ligament is avoided so that stability of the joint is maintained. The use of a tube can be avoided in most cases of clawhand if staged operations are adopted (Fig. XIV.27).

6.2.1.2 Excision of the Collateral Ligament

The collateral ligament arises from the dorsal aspect of the metacarpal bone and inserts into the first phalanx at its proximal palmar aspect. When the MP joint extends, the collateral ligament relaxes, and when the MP joint flexes, it tightens. If the MP joint is immobilized in extension for a long time, the collateral ligament will become fibrotic and shortened so that flexion of it is impossible. Generally, excision of the collateral ligament becomes necessary only when an attempt to reduce the MP joint by manipulation has failed.

◁ **Fig. XIV.27. a–c** Severe clawhand deformity (present for 20 years) in a 23-year-old female. **d, e** Reconstructive surgery included excision of the scar tissue, plastic repair of the finger webs, reduction of MP joints, and fushion of the IP joints of the 2nd, 3rd, and 4th fingers. Six months postoperatively the patient is seen to have recovered most of the function of her left hand

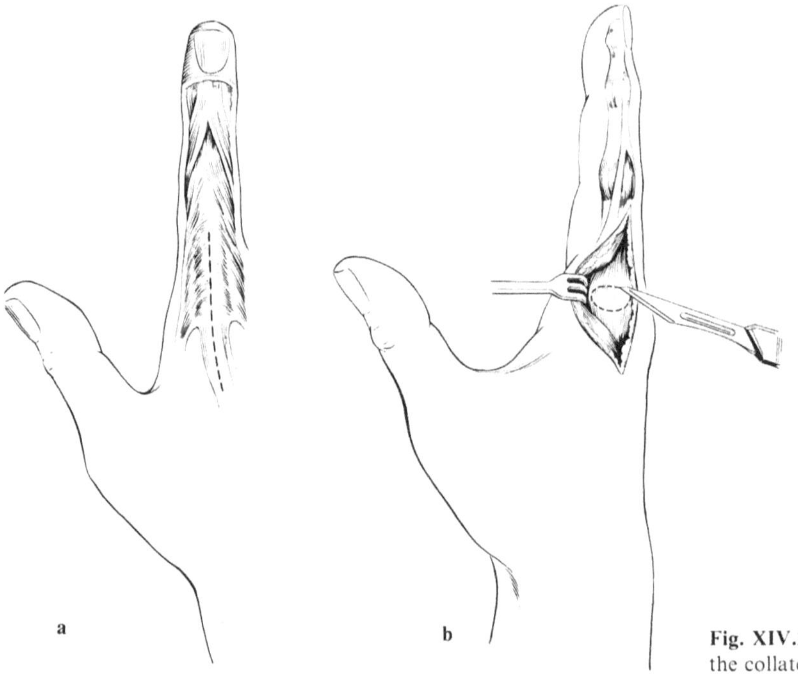

Fig. XIV.28a, b. Excision of the collateral ligament

Excision will have an adverse effect on stability of the MP joint, so it should not be performed routinely (Fig. XIV.28).

6.2.1.3 Handling of Extensors

Shortening of the extensors often hinders successful reduction of the MP joint. Lengthening of the extensors is generally reserved for severe shortening of the extensors of the thumb. As for the other fingers, a releasing procedure sometimes suffices. When lengthening is necessary, the exposed tendons should be covered with surrounding soft tissue before a skin graft is applied, for the skin graft will not take on a bare tendon.

6.2.1.4 Arthroplasty

In long-standing cases involving hyperextension of the MP joint, a depression is often present around the dorsal aspect of the metacarpal head owing to persistent compression from the base of the proximal phalanx. Sometimes complete dislocation of MP joint is also encountered. In such an instance, the deformity is usually difficult to correct and resection of the metacarpal head or arthroplasty may be required (Fig. XIV.29).

6.2.2 Arthrodesis of IP Joints

In deep burns on the dorsal surface of the fingers, extensors together with IP joint capsules are often destroyed. Balance of the finger flexor-extensor

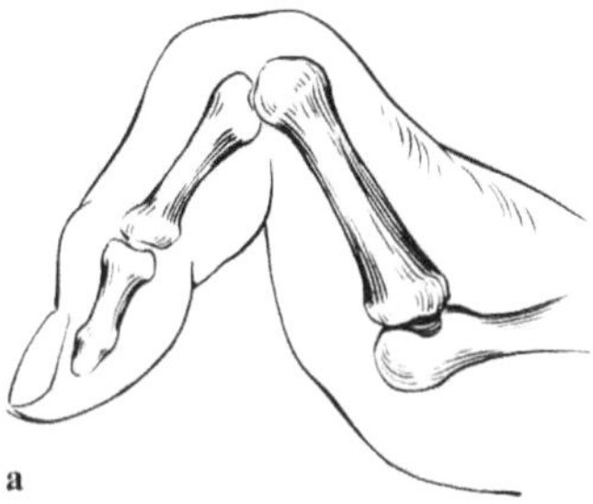

a

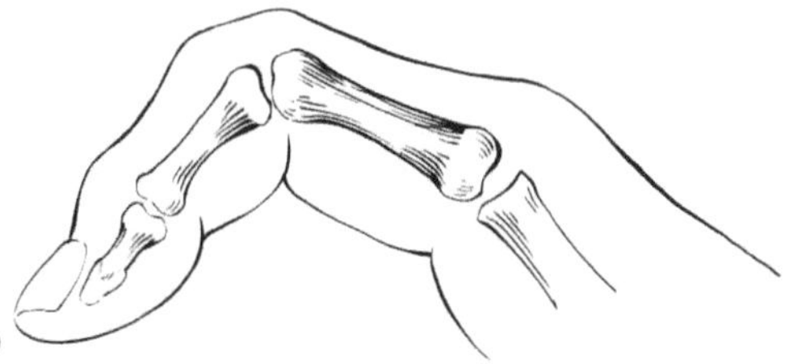

b

Fig. XIV.29. Arthroplasty of the MP joint

mechanism is lost, so that IP joints are in flexion deformity owing to the stronger action of the flexor. Occasionally even the joint cartilage is destroyed, and the joint becomes ankylosed. Distal interphalangeal joints are often hyperextended owing to rupture of the central slip and the strong action of the contracted lateral slips.

For this deformity it is always necessary to resect a wedge from the bone and perform a functional arthrodesis. The joint is then held with a Kirschner wire for about 6 weeks (Fig. XIV.30)

By contrast, hyperextension deformity of a DIP joint by scar contraction only requires excision of the scar and application of a free skin graft and transfixation of the joint with a Kirschner wire to keep it in a functional position. Bone resection is rarely necessary.

The angle of functional arthrodesis of an IP joint is about 120° in flexion. Care should be taken not to resect too much bone, otherwise the finger will be too short. The amount of bone resected should be limited to just enough to facilitate approximation of the two cut ends.

6.2.3 Adduction Deformity of the Thumb

Cicatricial contraction of the area between the thumb and the index finger usually results in adduction deformity, and the opponent action of the thumb is lost. The reconstructive surgery includes excision of all the scar and the contracted fascia and covering of the wound by means of partial-thickness graft or a distant tube. Web of the thumb should be cut open down to the palm in order to eliminate completely the adduction deformity of the thumb. If there is contraction of the adductor pollicis and the first interosseous muscles, the transverse head of the adductor pollicis and the point of insertion of the

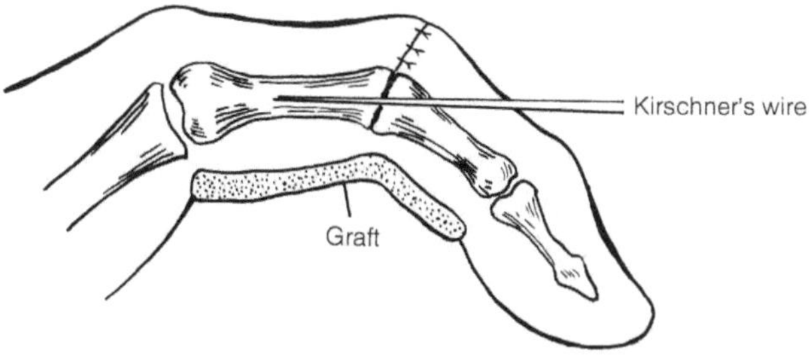

Fig. XIV.30. Arthrodesis of the IP joint

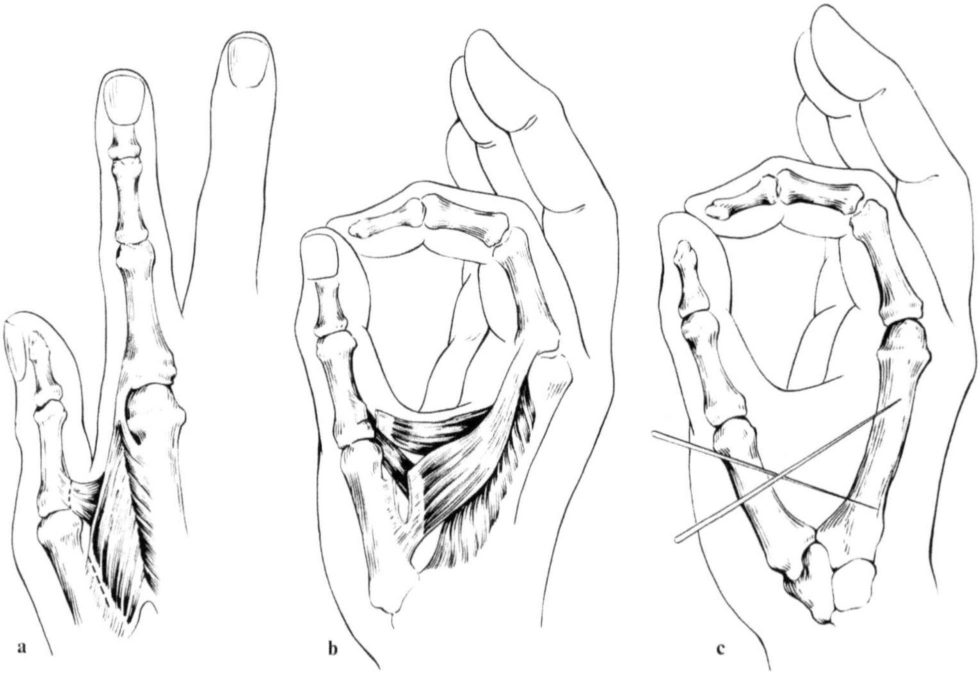

Fig. XIV.31. a Adduction deformity of the thumb. **b** Severance of the transverse head of the adductor muscle of the thumb and of the point of insertion of the first interosseous muscle. **c** Transfixing the first and second metacarpal bones to secure the abducent and opponent position of the thumb

first interosseous muscles must be cut. Never sever the oblique head of the adductor muscle, otherwise the adduction function of the thumb will be lost (Fig. XIV.31 a, b).

In very severe cases, in order to prevent the recurrence of the deformity, stainless steel wires should be transfixed through the first and the second metacarpal bones to fix the thumb in the extreme abducent and opponent position (Fig. XIV.31 c).

7 Cicatricial Contraction over the Perineum

7.1 Deformities

Postburn cicatricial contraction over the perineum is commonly seen in children. The simple form manifests as pliable web scars crossing between the thighs. These web scars are usually located transversely at the front and back of the anus, causing limitation of separation, abduction, and other movements of the lower extremities. The anal region cannot be cleaned easily after defecation. The scar web tends to become ulcerated owing to irritation during walking. After repeated ulcerations, the scars may become thick and hypertrophic. Circular contractions may sometimes be formed around the external genital area, and the penis or vagina and the anal region may be concealed in a scarred "diverticulum" from which urine, feces, and even menses pass out. The severe form of contraction of the perineum may result in anal stenosis or even obstruction. If the patient has burns over the lower extremities at the same time, the scar may extend from the perineum down to the inner aspects of the thighs, resulting in flexion contraction of the popliteal fossa. In such a case, the patient is unable to walk and will be bedridden. Burns over the perineum may also involve the penis, scrotum, labia majora, etc. If the penis is involved, it may adhere to the lower abdominal wall, resulting in malposition of the urethral opening. In this condition, normal urination and sexual function is greatly disturbed. However, the corpus cavernosum is seldom involved, except in the case of electric burn.

7.2 Principles of Treatment

For the simple form of perineal cicatricial contraction, various methods of surgical treatment may be selected according to the different conditions and degrees of cicatricial contraction. If the flap of the web which runs across transversely in front of or at the back of the anus is soft and pliable, Z-plasty or rotation flap operation may be used for the repair. The kind of operation is quite simple and a good result can be expected. However, Z-plasty is not indicated in a hard and hypertrophic web scar. The scar should be cut open or excised partially so as to separate the thighs in full abduction. The wound thus created is then grafted with a split-thickness free skin graft.

The cutting or excision of extensive scars over the perineum often results in an extensive open wound which should be covered immediately by skin grafting. In adults, 400 cm^2–600 cm^2 of skin graft (in some cases, even more) is usually needed.

Cicatricial contraction of the external genital organs usually involves the problem of skin loss of the scrotum. The principle of treatment is to reconstruct the scrotum. Free skin grafting over the testicles after they have been reduced to their normal position is the method of choice. Scrotum reconstruction by the skin tube method often results in a big sac which will interfere with the motion of the thighs.

After complete excision of the scar over the penis, the corpus cavernosum may be completely freed. A free circular skin graft may then be applied over the shaft of the penis. The grafted penis is dressed with encircling gauze sponges of sufficient bulk to support the organ. Stilbestrol is given routinely to prevent erection.

7.3 Operative Procedure and Pre- and Postoperative Care

The wound over the perineal region is easily contaminated by urine or feces. Therefore, preoperative care is of utmost importance: It is the key to the success of this reparative operation.

Constipation is common in patients with cicatricial contraction over the perineal region. It is advisable to start a soft diet a few days before the operation.

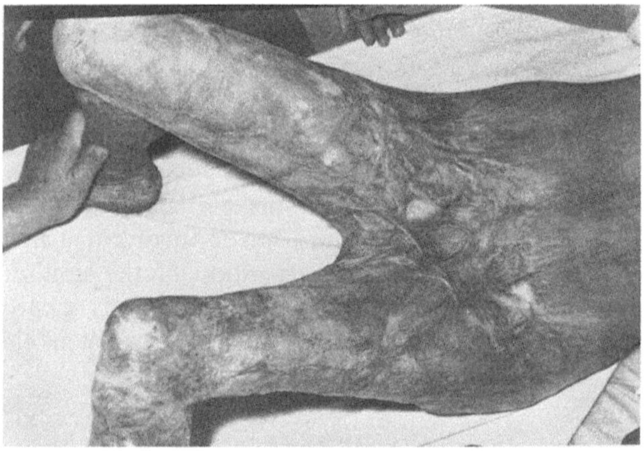

a

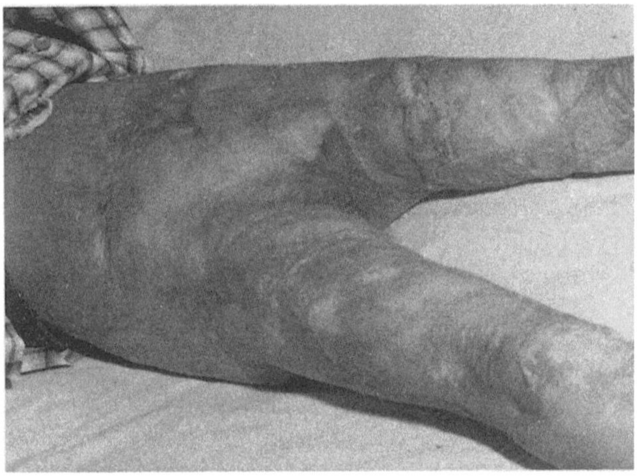

b

Fig. XIV.32. a Female, aged 19 years, with cicatricial contraction of the perineum present for 14 years following flame burns. **b** Appearance after exision of eschar and application of partial-thickness graft

Repeated saline enema should be carried out two to three times the night before operation.

Local irrigation should be performed through the small opening to clean away all the dirt and purulent discharge in the diverticulum. If the opening is extremely small, cleansing work may be carried out during the operation after the diverticulum has been cut open. Preoperatively, besides the routine skin cleansing procedures, every crease or depression of the scar should be carefully cleaned with soap and water.

Generally speaking, incisions are first made obliquely along the inguinal ligaments, where the cicatricial contraction is tightest, up to the anterior superior iliac spines. A transverse incision is then made to connect the upper ends of the two incisions. A part of the scar over pubis is excised so as to reduce the malposed umbilicus back to its original position. There is always a large piece of fibrotic fascia underneath the scar. This should be incised in order to release the lower extremities into full extension (Fig. XIV.32). The outline of the wound thus formed looks like a butterfly. In the paraperineal type of cicatricial contraction, after opening the diverticulum, one often discovers that the area around the penis or over the labia majora is covered with normal skin. This skin area should be well preserved in order to obtain better functional recovery.

After the operation, an indwelling catheter should be employed for 3–4 days in order to prevent any contamination of the wound. Liquid or soft diet is given for 1 week. Tincture camphor composita is given orally.

Temporary cystostomy or colostomy is not necessary except in the case of the central type of perineal contraction, which needs reconstruction of the penis. The skin graft is fixed by the common bolus dressing. The hip and knee joints should be immobilized by plaster of Paris cast with the thighs kept in abduction and at an angle of 60° to each other.

As there is always good blood circulation in the perineal area, the skin graft usually takes well, except when there is hematoma or infection. No change of dressing after operation in necessary. The stitches are removed on the 10th day after the operation.

Secondary contraction usually occurs after perineal skin grafting. Therefore, physical exercises should be started 2 weeks postoperatively. A plaster cast which maintains the legs in full abduction should be applied at night. Sleeping in a supine position is advised. All the above-mentioned measures are very important to the success of the operation; if they are neglected, the skin graft over the inguinal region tends to contract again within a short period.

8 Cicatricial Contraction of the Popliteal Fossa and Chronic Ulcer of the Leg

During early ambulation in patients with burns of the lower extremities, hindrance of venous return at the cicatricized site is often produced. Afterward the scar appears dark purple, and blisters, which may break and form small wounds, are formed in severe cases. When the leg is in a "hanging down" position, hindrance of venous return may increase the cicatricial hypertrophy. To prevent this the patient is advised to wear elastic bandages during early ambulation to reduce venous stasis. In a lying or retiring position the affected leg should be elevated to promote subsidence of edema and to reduce the cicatricial hypertrophy.

8.1 Cicatricial Contraction of the Popliteal Fossa

The skin at the popliteal fossa is relatively thin with little subcutaneous fat. Abrasion of the epithelium of a newly healed wound there may easily occur during movement. Repeated gaping of the scar causes progressive hypertrophy and gradually results in flexion deformity of the knee joint. In severe cases it is associated with contracture of the tendon, ligament, and joint capsule.

8.1.1 Treatment

If the scar is of the web or band type, Z-plasty or intermediate thickness free skin graft can usually be used to achieve repair. Z-plasty is indicated in longitudinal web-shaped scar of the popliteal fossa region with soft and well vascularized tissue flaps of both sides. If there is still some wound surface exposed after the repair, free skin graft may be used for coverage.

For severe cases with a large area of hypertrophic or contracted scars and flexion deformity of the knee joint, the contracted scars should be thoroughly excised to restore the joint in an extension position. After excision of the scars, no nerves and vessels exposed should be under tension, and all should be covered, if possible, by adjacent healthy tissues for protection. Forcible complete extension at one operation is to be avoided. At first the extension may be carried out to 120°–130°. After survival of the skin graft, complete extension may be gradually obtained through traction or walking exercises.

8.2 Chronic Ulcer of the Leg

After burns of a lower limb, chronic ulcers frequently occur at the anterior tibial regions, the ankle, the kneecap, etc. The ulcers have dense scar tissue at their periphery and base. The blood supply to the ulcer is very poor, and a thick layer of marginal cornification often develops and forms a barrier against the creeping of epithelial cells from the surrounding skin. Sometimes transient healing may be attained by means of bed rest, elevation of the affected limb, and local application of medication. Recurrence, however, is apt to occur.

8.2.1 Treatment

Chronic ulcer of the leg is usually surrounded by scar tissue with pigment deposits. Its blood supply is poor so that the transplanted skin does not easily survive. Before skin grafting, the patient should rest in bed and the affected extremity should be elevated to facilitate the subsidence of edema. The ulcer surface is compressed with 1:6,000 furacilin or antibiotic solution. Eczema of the surrounding skin, if any, should be treated beforehand. The ulcer and its surrounding scar, with pigment deposits, should be thoroughly excised, and the wound grafted with intermediate thickness free skin graft.

Chronic ulcer on a bony surface should be treated using a cross-leg skin flap or by transplanting a skin tube from a distant part of the body.

9 Cicatricial Contraction of the Foot

9.1 Signs

Cicatricial contraction at the dorsum of foot may cause dorsal flexion, dislocation or subluxation of the metatarsophalangeal joints, and plantar protrusion of the head of metatarsus to form clawfoot. Cicatricial contraction at the medial side of the ankle joint may lead to varus deformity of the joint in children, producing markedly changed bony contour. After the healing of deep burns of the toes, smooth atrophic scars are formed on the phalanges. These scars are tender to touch and ulcerate easily by friction with the shoe during walking. These ulcers often refuse to heal. Cicatricial contraction in the Achilles tendon region may produce shortening of the tendon, resulting in talipes equinus. After the cicatricial healing of deep burns under the foot, the scar in the heel region easily ulcerates upon weight bearing. The plantar fascia becomes shortened. Transverse arch of the foot is lost, resulting in pes cavus.

9.2 Principles of Treatment

1. Most of the cordlike scars on the dorsum of the foot and at the medial side of the ankle may be repaired by Z-plasty; orthopedic correction of bones is not necessary.

2. If there is a large area of hypertrophic scar on the dorsum of the foot and around the ankle joint, the scar should be excised. The subluxated metatarso-phalangeal joints must be reduced and fixed with stainless steel pins for 3 weeks. Free transplantation of a large piece of skin is used to cover the wound surface. Contracted and shortened tendons are separated by undermining dissection. Elongation of the tendons is required if reduction of the joints cannot be attained after the separation.

3. Clublike toes are formed by cicatricial contraction at the volar aspect of toes. The contracted scar is excised to facilitate reduction of the joints. The wound is covered by free skin graft. If it is difficult to reduce the dislocated interphalangeal joints, the principle of treatment is the same as that for clubtoes: the heads of proximal phalanges are excised. After proper reduction, the joints are fixed with stainless steel pins for 3 weeks.

4. After the loss of a toe, the defective stump of the metatarsal head is embedded in a layer of scar tissue. Once an ulcer is formed by abrasion, it will not heal readily. If there is any existing bony tip protrusion under the scar, pain is elicited upon touching any hard object or wearing a hard shoe. Such a scar must be repaired by cross-leg skin flap after its excision. The sharp bony protuberance should be suitably treated during the operation.

5. Prolonged contraction of the Achilles tendon is apt to cause distortion of the talocalcaneal and talonavicular joints, and even arthrodesis. Before the operation the movement of the joints must be examined. Most frequently the movements are good, and the treatment is to perform lengthening of the Achilles tendon after excising the contracted scar tissue. If excision of a large amount of scar and a lengthening operation are necessary, prior consideration should be given to the utilization of the adjacent skin pedicle for the coverage of the exposed Achilles tendon; free skin grafts can rarely survive. After the tendon lengthening operation, a plaster cast is made for fixation.

6. In cicatricial contracture under the foot, the adjacent skin is usually not used as a flap for repairing the defect after resection of an ulcerated scar. This is because of the thick corneous skin and the dense tissue there, which are unsuitable for undermining and render rotation of a flap difficult. Forcibly

suturing the wound together causes necrosis and thus enlarges the wound. Small localized ulcer may be treated by free full-thickness skin graft or repaired by cross-leg flap if possible. Cicatricial contraction of the whole plantar surface of the foot may be repaired using a skin tube transplanted from a distal site of the body. The operation is divided into three stages. In the first stage a skin tube is formed. In the second stage the tube is carried by hand to the sole of foot. In the third stage the tube is flattened. If the condition of the contralateral leg is adequate, a cross-leg skin pedicle flap may be employed for repairing the defect after excision of the entire plantar scar.

7. In cases of severe burn of the foot and ankle associated with talipes equinovarus, reduction of the part cannot usually be attained by simply excising the scar. It is necessary to transplant a skin tube from a distant region to the foot and ankle. The surrounding area is protected by the skin flap. Six months later triple arthrodesis (talocalcaneal, talonavicular, and talocuboidal joints) is performed to correct the talipes equinovarus deformity. For those patients with very extensive third degree burns a huge skin tube cannot be obtained: Once the scar tissue becomes soft and the local blood supply is good, triple arthrodesis can be performed straightforwardly. The therapeutic effect is fairly satisfactory.

10 Cicatricial Contraction After Very Extensive Third Degree Burns

After patients with burns exceeding 80% of the BSA, including third degree burns to more than 50%, have been cured, cicatricial contraction at the neck, axillae, elbows, dorsa of the hands, popliteal fossae, and other regions of the body often occur. After the wounds have healed, very little normal skin is left. Therefore after the scars have been excised, there is hardly any source of normal skin for autografting. Such cases have been considered as "incurables" in the past.

We have used large pieces of allografts with inlays of small pieces of autologous skins as a reparative procedure, and we have also taken soft flat scar as a donor area. In addition, "cicatricial skin tubes" have been transplanted from distant sites. All these measures are of aid in solving the problem of insufficient skin sources in reparative surgery of third degree burns.

10.1 Use of a Large Piece of Allograft with "Punched Windows" for Autologous Skin Inlays

After the excision of a large area of scar, when the resulting wound cannot be covered by a small amount of autograft, a large piece of allograft with punched windows for autologous skin inlays may be used for the coverage. This method offers a new way of solving the difficulty arising from insufficient source of autologous skin. When combined with the usage of "supplemental" autologous skin graft, the above-mentioned method not only gives functional restoration but also saves a large quantity of autologous skin. If too little autologous skin is inlaid, cicatricial contraction is apt to recur after the operation or the wound will refuse to heal on account of ulceration during movement. Under such circumstances, supplemental grafting with autologous skin is necessary. This method is useful for such sites as the neck, axillae, and elbows, but is not suitable for facial regions and the dorsa of the hands.

Plastic surgery for scars of large-area third degree burns should be postponed, usually until about 2 years after wound healing. This is due to the fact that it takes a long time for the remnant wound to heal, for the body to recover satisfactorily, and for cicatricial contraction to form. On considering reparative surgery, sufficient evaluation and thoughtful planning must be made with regard to the patient's general condition, preoperative preparation, postoperative care, etc. A detailed operative scheme should be mapped out, and an accurate calculation should be made concerning the quantity of skin needed for repair. A proper selection of the donor skin area should be made.

10.1.1 Preoperative Preparation

Fresh cadaver skin is prepared and preserved in an icebox at a temperature of 4 °C. (With regard to the selection and preparation of cadaver skin, see Appendix 2. For details of preparation of allograft with autologous skin inlays, see Chap. III.)

Before the operation the patient should have a general physical examination and all necessary laboratory data. The nourishment of patients with malnutrition and slow recuperation should be adjusted and supplemented to increase their strength. Any existing anemia should be corrected by blood transfusions 1–2 days before the operation. Routine preparation of the skin of the operative field is carried out. Usually the operation is not performed until the remnant wounds have healed. Wet compresses are applied preoperatively to old, hardhealing cicatricial ulcers, which are excised together with the scar tissue.

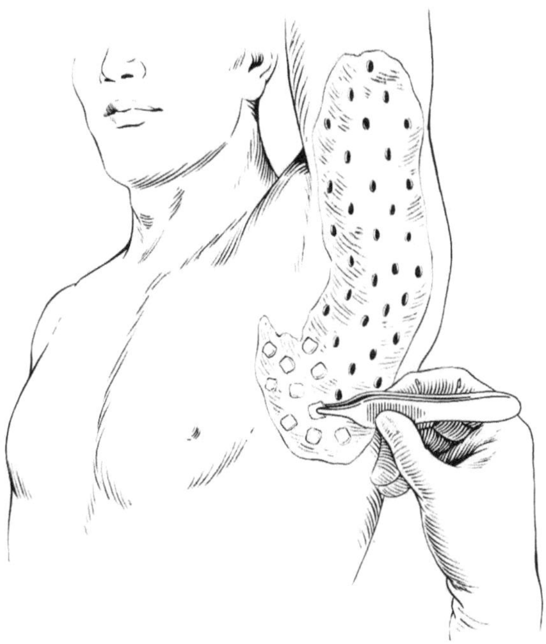

Fig. XIV.33. Intermingled transplantation

10.1.2 Operative Procedure

For scars of large-area burns the principle of resection aims at sufficient release of the contraction. Extensive excision of scar tissue is not to be recommended; the surrounding flat soft scar without functional interference should be preserved. The wound edge after excision should preferably be regular to facilitate suturing to the transplanted allograft.

After thoroughly checking the bleeding, the prepared piece of allograft is sutured to the wound surface. Pressure dressing is applied for fixation (Fig. XIV.33).

Four to five days after the operation, when the piece of allograft shows signs of survival, small pieces of autologous skin may be inserted and imbedded in the windows. The skin pieces should be as large as possible and the distances between them as close as possible. This will prevent secondary contraction after sloughing of the allograft.

The donor areas frequently used are superficially burned skin or the scalp after healing.

10.1.3 Postoperative Management

Stitches are removed 10 days later. When reparative operation is performed on the neck, the neck should be maintained in functional position by support or a collar. Small pieces of autologous skin are transplanted as soon as small wound surfaces appear following resolution of the allograft. Between 1 and 2 months after the survival of the grafted skin, continuous exfoliation appears clinically owing to gradual replacement of allograft by the proliferation of the autologous skin. Secondary contraction is dealt with by practising early movements. Splint support is given during the rest periods to prevent contraction. After secondary contraction becomes stabilized, autologous supplemental skin grafting is performed to release the contraction. This is done according to the functional interference of the principal site affected. Usually supplemental skin grafting is performed 6 months afterwards. Cure is expected after such a course of treatment.

Case Illustration. Male, aged 20. The patient had burns to 99% of the BSA, including third degree burns to 94%. Cicatricial contraction gradually occurred in the neck, axillae, and elbow regions. The lower lip became everted. Extension and rotation of the neck were impossible. Saliva dripped outward. Taking food by mouth was difficult. After excising the scar at the lower lip region, large pieces of punched allograft were placed on the neck. The donor site for autografts was the scalp, from which repeated donations of skin had been taken. The lower lip region was repaired by soft and flat full-thickness cicatricial pieces of skin from patient's back. Stitches were removed on the 7th postoperative day. Skin grafts survived well. The postoperative result 2 years later was satisfactory (Fig. XIV.34).

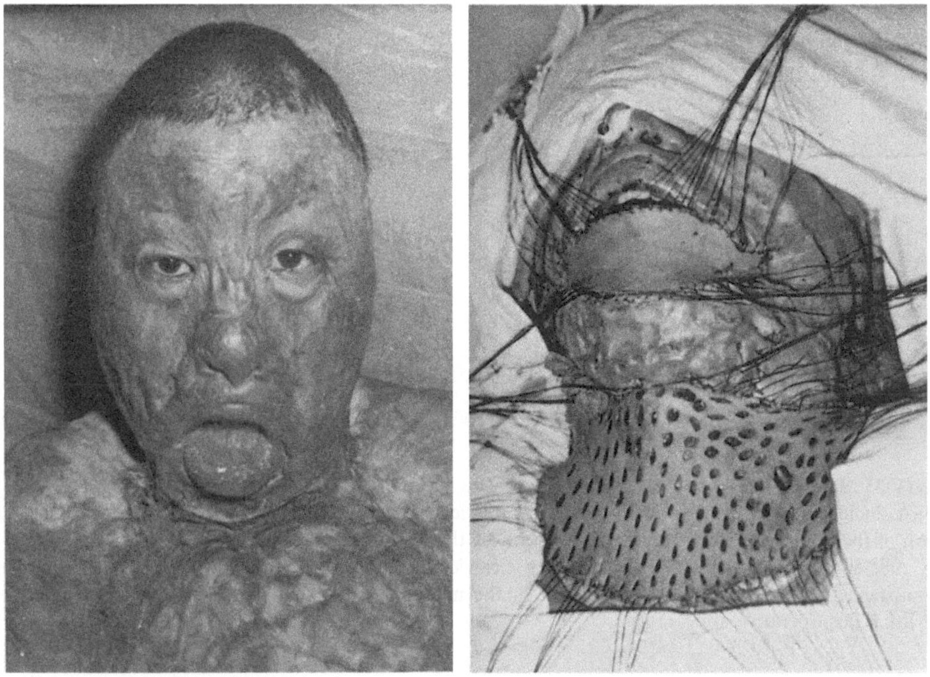

a b

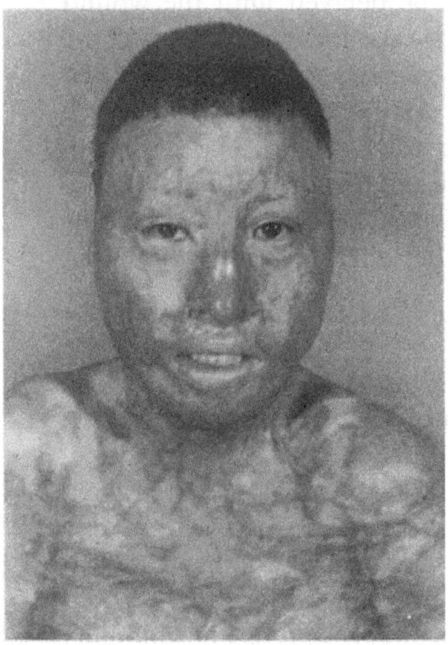

c

Fig. XIV.34. a Twenty-year-old male with burns to 99% of the BSA, including third degree burns to 94%. Cicatricial contraction of the neck occurred, resulting in chin–chest fusion and severe eversion of the lower lip. **b** The scar tissue was excised and intermingled transplantation of allografts and autologous grafts from the scalp performed. The lower lip was repaired using cicatricial grafts taken from patient's back. **c** Postoperative appearance

10.2 Distant Transplantation of Cicatricial Skin Tube

Cicatricial skin tube is prepared from the scar area healed by grafted granulation wound after a third degree burn. The tube is transplanted to the site with functional interference, or it may be used to repair tissue defect of the face.

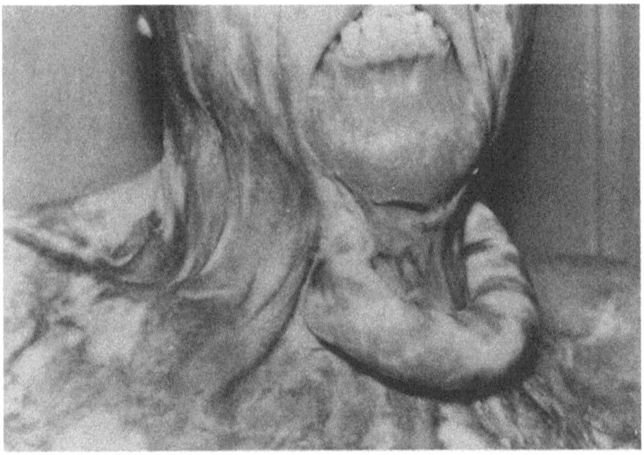
a

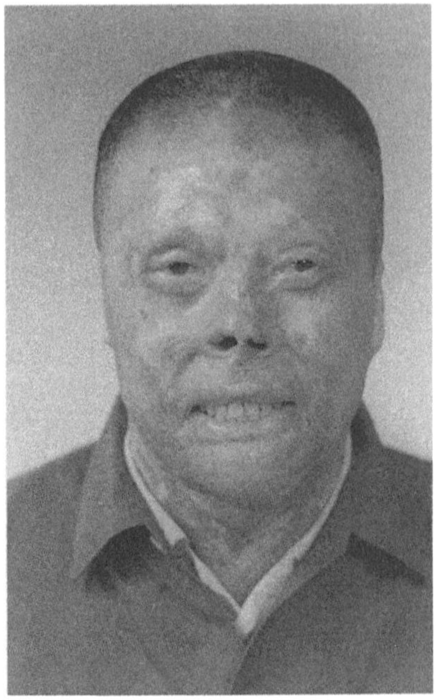
b

Fig. XIV.35. a Forty-one-year-old male with burns to 98% of the BSA, including third degree burns to 90%. Cicatricial contraction of the neck occurred, resulting in eversion of the lower lip. A tube was constructed on his back using cicatricial skin and transferred to the neck for reconstruction of the neck and lower lip. **b** Postoperative appearance

The preparation of the cicatricial skin tube must be delayed until the wound has been healed for more than 1 year. At that time, the local scar has become flat and soft with a good blood supply. After "loosening training" it is estimated that the skin pedicle can be rolled up to form a tube without interference of the circulation. The length-width ratio of the tube is the same as usual. After the tube is raised, the donor area is sutured together if possible, or it may be grafted with free skin grafts (stamp size). The cicatricial skin tube is usually used for a large deep tissue defect in the chin or neck region that cannot be cured by free graft of skin.

Case Illustration. Male, aged 41. The patient had burns to 98% of the BSA, including third degree burns to 90%. After wound healing, severe cicatricial contraction of the chin and neck regions appeared. The lower lip was everted, and the gum exposed. Saliva dripped outward. A skin tube was prepared from the scar healed at the back region after spontaneous eschar separation and skin grafting. The tube was rotated to the chin and neck regions to repair the contraction there. After the operation the lower lip was restored to its original position. The patient can now move his lips freely and has no difficulty in taking food by mouth (Fig. XIV.35).

10.3 Harvesting Free Cicatricial Skin Grafts

The reparative operation of a large area of third degree burn may be undertaken by harvesting free skin grafts from a flat soft scar area. The grafts are used to cover the defect after scar excision. Any flat noncongested scar area without hypertrophic reaction may be utilized. The donor area, in spite of having remnant skin islands, still requires a small number of postage stamp-sized skin grafts for coverage. Sometimes such a donor area may offer the possibility of repeated harvesting of free skin grafts.

As compared with the normal skin of intermediate thickness, the cicatricial free skin graft lacks elastic fibers, and thus the skin excised is just like a piece of thin paper. Upon excising the skin graft with a dermatome, it is not easy to raise the apparatus smoothly. To cut a thick piece is easier than a thin one; hence an expert technique is required. The reparative procedure requires a large piece of cicatricial skin. The back and abdominal regions are the sites most frequently used. The donor area is covered with pieces of skin left after the reparative procedure or with small split-thickness grafts from the scalp.

11 Skin Lesions Following Radiation Burn

Prolonged exposure to radiation or repeated small doses of radiation over a long period will cause radiation burn of the skin.

11.1 Clinical Manifestations

In the acute stage, the clinical manifestations of radiation burn of the skin resemble those of thermal burn. Frequently blisters are formed several days to 2 weeks after the radiation. The fluid from the blisters is tenacious and turbid. The earlier the blisters appear, the more severe are the clinical manifestations. Once a chronic ulcer is formed, it is hard to heal for several years and sometimes has marked pigment deposit. The larger the radiation dose and the longer the exposure to the radiation, the more severe the local skin damage. Early reactions consist of local numbness, general debility, nausea, vomiting, etc. The regional skin shows loss of hair, erythema, blister formation, or ulceration and necrosis. In the chronic stage the main manifestations are atrophy, capillary dilatation, cornification, and dryness of the skin with easy exfoliation. Sometimes the skin is transparent, thin, and with slight luster. There may at times be local eczematous changes which are liable to extend to the surrounding skin. Sensation of the local skin is poor. Its temperature is reduced and frostbite is apt to occur.

We have admitted six patients with radiation burns; the longest course reached 13 years, the shortest, 4 years. There were three patients with local chronic ulcers, two with keratinization and exfoliation, and one with scar formation. None showed malignant change upon biopsy.

Case Illustration. Female, aged 45. Seven years ago the patient presented with a piece of broken needle inside the sole of the foot. An attempt to remove the foreign body was made under fluoroscopy for more than 4 h. The radiation caused burn of the skin at the external malleolar region. Local pain was quite severe. The wound failed to heal, and repeated ulcerations occurred for 6 years. After admission to our hospital the foreign body was removed. Radical excision of the ulcer was performed, and a full-thickness skin graft was applied to the wound. Complete healing resulted.

Case Illustration. Female, aged 26. Four years ago the patient was injured by a car, with resultant contusion and avulsion of soft tissue of the left thigh. After the wound was healed, deep X-ray radiation was used to treat hypertrophic scar. Radiation burn was caused. The wound refused to heal for years. Radiography did not reveal any pathologic changes of the femur. After admission the wound was debrided with radical excision of the scar and the ulcer. A double pedicle skin flap (8 cm × 24 cm) was taken from the posterior surface of the same thigh to repair the tissue defect. The donor area was covered with pieces of free skin graft, and good healing resulted.

11.2 Principles of Treatment

11.2.1 General Treatment

The patient's nutritional status should be improved to enhance his (or her) general resistance and to promote the reparative capacity of the tissue. General reactions may be coped with by symptomatic treatment.

11.2.2 Local Treatment

Before the appearance of blisters, the chief measure is to prevent the occurrence of inflammatory reaction or to hasten its subsidence. Once the blisters have appeared, priority is given to maintaining the wound in an aseptic and dry condition and to protecting the blisters from breaking. For those with ulcer formation, early operation is recommended.

11.2.3 Surgical Treatment

The pathologic tissues should be excised, the defect repaired, and functions and appearance restored.

1. For those burns with clear-cut demarcations, an early operation is recommended before the appearance of ulceration. The burned area is excised and directly sutured, or it is covered with free skin grafts.

2. For those ulcers which refuse to heal for a long time, excision should be performed at an early stage. Depending on the degree of vascularization of the ulcer base, either free skin grafts or adjacent skin flaps may be used to cover the wound surface.

3. Should the tendon, nerve, or bone substance be exposed, pedicle skin flaps must be used for the repair. If there is insufficient tissue at an adjacent site, a distant pedicle flap must be transplanted to repair the local defect.

12 Transplantation of Free Skin Flaps

Free skin flaps were introduced into clinical use by Harii and Ohmori in 1972. They successfully transplanted a free skin flap 15 cm long and 3 cm wide from one side of the head to the other by anastomosis of the superficial temporal artery and vein. In 1973, first Daniel and then Yang accomplished free transplantation of flaps from the groin. In recent years, transplantation of free skin flaps has been widely and successfully used in our country as well as abroad.

12.1 Advantages of the Free Skin Flap

1. Comparing the free skin flap with the pedicle skin flap, the advantages of the former are that they obviate the need for repeated transfer operations, thus decreasing the patients' sufferings and shortening the course of treatment, not to mention lessening the financial burden.

2. Free skin flaps include the full thickness of the skin as well as the subcutaneous fat. Sometimes they may even include part of the muscles, nerves, and skeletal tissues. They are in reality composite grafts. They have ample blood supply and may therefore be used to repair complicated wounds in one stage.

3. Free skin flaps have their own circulation system; therefore besides supplying their own tissue with necessary blood and nutrition, they may also supply the recipient area with blood and nutrition. Consequently they are especially suitable for the plastic repair of radiation ulcers and complications of osteomyelitis.

4. When soft tissues are traumatized, tears and loss of tissue may take place, resulting in the exposure of bones, tendons, nerves, and blood vessels. Free skin flaps may cover all of these important tissues in one operation.

5. Free skin flaps may be taken from the unexposed parts of the body, i.e., the groin, back, chest, subaxillary region, etc. As a rule, the wound of the donor area may often be closed by direct suturing and healing by first intention may be expected. In comparison with the scars arising from adjacent or distant pedicle flaps, this procedure may be more willingly accepted by the patients.

6. By the use of this kind of procedure, fixation of the body and limbs during transfer of the flaps can be avoided.

7. Since free skin flaps include subcutaneous fatty tissues, they have a certain amount of pliability. The color of the skin is also more natural.

12.2 Requirements of the Donor Area

1. The donor area should have one or more pairs of artery and vein forming a closed circuit circulation of its own. The donor vessels for anastomosis ought to have a caliber of about 1 mm, and the vascular pedicle ought to be 2 cm–3 cm in length.

2. The vascular network of the donor flap should be rich enough to supply sufficient blood and nutrition after its transplantation.

3. The donor skin should be pliable and of normal color. There should be no scar or pigmentation. Hairy skin areas are not suitable as donor sites.

4. After the free flap is excised, the function of the donor site should not be disturbed. No ugly looking scars should be left.

12.3 Requirements of the Recipient Area

1. The walls of the blood vessels of the recipient area should be healthy. The vessels should carry sufficient blood supply to the transplanted free skin flap. The artery and vein should be comparatively close to each other and preferably there should be two reserve veins for emergency.

2. The diameter of the vessels of the recipient area should be similar to that of the vessels of the donor flaps, so that after the vessels are anastomosed the nourishment of the donor flap will not be influenced.

The tension of the anastomosed vessels should be maintained at a minimum. There should be no twisting or plication, otherwise the free flow of the blood may be interfered with or thrombosis of the vessels may occur. Anastomosis of the blood vessels may only be carried out in the surroundings of normal tissues; any traumatized tissue should be thoroughly removed until healthy tissues are reached. The frequently used free skin flaps include the groin flap (also called lower abdominal flap), the dorsalis pedis flap, the deltoid–pectoral flap, and the thoracodorsal axillary flap. Of these, we have found the thoracodorsal axillary flap to be the best.

12.4 Free Transplantation of the Thoracodorsal Axillary Flap for the Repair of Postburn Cicatricial Contraction

The thoracodorsal axillary flap was first used clinically by BOCKX, DECONINCK, and VANDERLINDER in 1976, followed by BAUDET, LEMAIRE, and DANIEL et al. We have used this type of free flap for the correction of postburn cicatricial contraction to achieve functional recovery, for the repair of deep tissue defects in acute electric injuries, and for the repair of intractable ulcers of the extremities with satisfactory results.

12.4.1 Advantages of Thoracodorsal Axillary Flaps

1. This type of flap can provide a comparatively large area of tissue. The largest flap may involve 200 cm^2–300 cm^2 of skin, which is equivalent to the size of one and half dermatome drums, that is, 24 cm in length and 11 cm in width.

2. Thoracodorsal axillary flaps have one or more pairs of blood vessels, the calibers of which are large (the diameter of the artery and vein may reach 1.7 mm–2.0 mm). The free ends of the vascular pedicles may be as long as 5 cm–7 cm. Owing to the large caliber of the vessels, operative procedures may be carried out under the naked eye, and the rate of patency after the anastomosis is high. We have transplanted 28 such flaps, and the patency rate of the anastomosed vessels was 100%.

3. The subaxillary donor area may be sutured directly. Neither postoperative sequelae nor disturbances of function have been observed. If the wound of the donor area is more than 10 cm in width, free skin grafts are needed for the repair.

4. In the case of thin patients, the subcutaneous fatty tissue of the thoracodorsal axillary flap is usually scanty. The flap is pliable and of good texture. Secondary trimming of subcutaneous fat is not necessary.

12.4.2 Regional Anatomy

The term "thoracodorsal axillary flap" refers to a flap of tissues of the lateral aspect of the chest below the axilla with the midaxillary line as its axis. The thoracodorsal artery and vein, being the continuation of the subscapular artery and vein, are its main nutrient vessels.

Subscapular Artery. The subscapular artery and vein arise from the third part of the axillary artery and vein. After the subscapular artery is divided, it runs along the lower border of the subscapular muscle to the inferior border of the scapula. The subscapular artery then continues to form the thoracodorsal artery. The latter runs downward to a triangular space (with the subscapular muscle at its back, the M. latissimus dorsi at its external border, and the M. serratus anterior at its internal border).

Thoracodorsal Artery. This artery is divided into two branches at about the level of the second intercostal space as follows:

1. The *cutaneous branch,* which follows the anterior border of the m. latissimus dorsi to the skin.

2. The *muscular branch,* which follows the nerve of the m. latissimus dorsi and perforates into the muscle near the scapula.

Venous Return: As a rule, one or two branches of the thoracodorsal vein ensure venous return in the flap.

1. The *muscular branch,* which receives the blood flow from the m. serratus anterior and m. latissimus dorsi.

2. The *cutaneous branch,* which takes up the blood return from the flap between the third and the seventh ribs. The diameter of this branch is usually greater than 1.2 mm. The diameter of the thoracodorsal vein is usually about 1.5 mm, and that of the subscapular vein, 1.7 mm–2.0 mm. In addition to these branches, the external mammary vein is also an important vessel for the venous return of the thoracodorsal axillary flap.

Nerves: The position of the nerve of m. latissimus dorsi, which is a motor nerve, is stationary. It runs from above obliquely downward laterally, accompanying the thoracodorsal vein. If the nerve cannot be preserved when the vascular pedicle of the free flap is constructed, it may be sectioned.

12.4.3 Surgical Procedure

1. *Posture:* For the operation, the patient is placed supine with the operative field of the lateral aspect of the chest slightly elevated to about 30°. The arm is abducted to 130° with the elbow moderately flexed.

2. *Designing the flap:* First one must palpate the axillary artery at the apex of the axilla and thus localized it. In designing the thoracodorsal axillary flap, the subscapular artery and vein as well as their continuation, the thoracodorsal artery and vein, must be included to serve as the axial vessels of the flap.

3. *Incision:* The skin is incised from the pulsating point at the apex of the axilla downward between the greater pectoral muscle and the m. serratus anterior to the distal end of the designed flap. The incision is then redirected to the flap's posterior border close to the free anterior edge of the m. latissimus dorsi. When the incision is made on the right axilla, its direction is clockwise; when it is made on the left axilla, it is counterclockwise.

4. *Landmarks:* At the point at which the subscapular vein arises from the axillary vein, there is usually a dilated venous bulb. The latter may serve as a landmark. Beginning from the venous bulb, dissection should be carried downward until the thoracodorsal artery and vein are completely exposed.

The key point of the dissection is at the crossing of the vascular pedicle and the nerve of the m. latissimus dorsi. At the level where the thoracodorsal artery itself is divided into two terminal branches, there are many small branches which should be meticulously separated and ligated individually. If there is a cutaneous branch, the musclar branch may be ligated. If the cutaneous branch is absent, the muscular branch should be preserved. It is necessary to elevate the free border of the m. latissimus dorsi together with an artery–vein pair and the skin flap in order that the flap will receive sufficient blood supply.

The cutaneous branches of the thoracodorsal axillary flaps are not constant in our cases. Thoracodorsal axillary flaps always have muscular branches. The thoracodorsal artery supplies principally the m. latissimus dorsi muscle; its main trunk runs along the anterior border of the m. latissimus dorsi and has abundant perforating branches to supply the thoracodorsal axillary flap with blood. If the muscular branches are well utilized and a small portion of the free border of the m. latissimus dorsi is transferred with the flap, the success of the operation can be assured.

Chapter XV Anesthetization of Burn Patients

HUANG ZONG-MING

Translated by WANG ZHI-ZENG

To anesthetize an extensively burned patient is a challenge to the courage and proficiency of anesthetists. But, since surgical removal of the burned tissue and immediate coverage of the wound surface remain the best method of treatment, accepting such a challenge is justifiable and rewarding.

The patient is usually febrile and weak and is undergoing adverse biochemical changes and metabolic disorders. It is often unbearable for such a patient to receive repeated anesthesia, to undergo protracted operations, and to suffer massive blood loss. Fortunately, however, operations can be staged, anesthesia does not need to be very deep, and muscular relaxation is usually unnecessary. These advantages offset or lessen the deleterious effects of anesthesia.

From 1966 to 1978 we performed anesthesia for burned patients 5,083 times, excluding local anesthesia. In 235 cases anesthesia was used more than five times, and in one case it was used 20 times. However, no anesthetic death has occurred. One patient who had severe burns of the respiratory tract accompanied by acute respiratory distress syndrome died immediately after surgery. As far as anesthesia itself was concerned, all the patients recovered uneventfully.

1 Preparation for Anesthesia

The role of the anesthetist is that of a consultant to the surgeon in respect of pharmacologic and physiologic problems. The anesthetist attends to the patient's physiologic changes during the operation, thereby permitting the surgeon to devote his whole attention and skill to the correction of burn lesions. Every patient who undergoes surgery must be visited by the anesthetist the day before the operation, but in a severe case operation is usually decided upon as an emergency. Even then preanesthetic evaluation is essential. There should be a complete assessment of the patient, with three distinct objectives in mind; namely, determination of the patient's physical condition, choice of anesthetic technique and agent, and estimation of operative risk.

Preanesthetic preparation includes correction of blood volume deficit, water and electrolyte disturbance, acid-base disorders, etc. Hypovolemia is common, due either to plasma deficit or to massive red cell destruction – and in many cases both may be present.

In extensively burned patients cardiovascular function may only be estimated by EKG, because measurement of blood pressure can hardly be carried out.

An EKG serves as a screening test. It is not a measure of functional capacity, but in such cases it gives a clue to many abnormalities, such as toxic myocarditis. It is of particular importance to estimate the respiratory function too. However, specific tests of pulmonary function, even if available, cannot be used in a debilitated burned patient to be submitted to surgery. Decreased ventilation is common, resulting both from obstruction of the respiratory tract and from interference of gas exchange in the alveoli. Pain may cause hyperpnea. Atelectasis, pulmonary edema, and pneumonitis should not be overlooked, as respiratory complications present real hazards and may increase the risks of surgery. Urinary output exceeding 25 ml per hour indicates that the renal function has remained normal and that the blood volume deficit is small.

In septicemia, the patient's physical condition is generally very poor, and complications are likely to ensue; consequently anesthetic management becomes more complicated. Furthermore, the mental attitude of a burn patient has a profound influence on the outcome of an operation. In concluding a visit, the patient should be reassured and the procedures of the forthcoming day should be explained so that the patient's confidence is increased and a rapport is achieved between the doctor and patient.

2 Premedication

Preanesthetic medication serves to prepare a patient for anesthesia by providing a state of acquiescence during the induction of anesthesia, and by obtunding the activity of the nervous system. It also serves to contribute to the anesthetic process or state itself and may reduce the anesthetic drug requirements. In extensively burned patients premedication is used in order to lessen apprehension, to reduce the amount of anesthetic required, to depress reflex excitability, and to lower basal metabolism. In the parenteral administration of drugs, intramuscular injection is satisfactory, except when the patient is in a state of vasoconstriction or there is impairment of peripheral perfusion; in such cases the intravenous route is recommended. Fifty milligrams meperidine and 50 mg promethazine are given intramuscularly as premedication 1 h before surgery, sometimes in combination with 0.1 g phenobarbital or 10 mg diazepam, which is administered intramuscularly. On the whole, selection of drugs should not be too restricted, as it largely depends upon the variety available, the anesthetist's preference, the personality of the patient, and his/her drug reaction.

3 Choice of Anesthesia

In extensively burned patients the variety of operations needed is numerous, but the principle of surgical technique, including anesthesia, is essentially similar. The majority of operations can be performed with the patient under light anesthesia because there is no need for muscular relaxation. However, the operations may be very time consuming. Patients with extensive burns and various complications may have to be submitted to the stress of repeated anesthesia and surgery at intervals of only a few days. Some of the patients may not be able to respond adequately; therefore, emphasis should be placed on the maintenance of a good milieu interne. At the same time anesthesia itself should be smooth in order to secure an uneventful recovery.

3.1 Regional Anesthesia

Regional anesthesia is particularly indicated in debilitated or even moribund patients, who tolerate anesthesia very badly. In selected cases brachial plexus nerve block as well as intravenous local anesthesia may be suitable for surgery on the extremities. The use of spinal or epidural analgesia is extremely limited in burn patients, because their wounds are often extensive and infected. If necessary, spinal or epidural anesthesia may be employed for plastic surgery in late stages and burn lesions limited to the lower part of the body.

3.2 General Anesthesia

For burn patients we are in favor of administering general anesthesia intravenously rather than by inhalation. In our experience, adequate ventilation with a patent airway can usually be maintained without tracheal intubation. Mechanical ventilation was seldom needed, but could be readily used if hypoventilation supervened or was suspected. As yet, intravenous anesthesia has been used in three-quarters of our cases. It has been the main choice in our burn unit for more than 10 years. There are three kinds of intravenous anesthetics, namely lytic cocktail, sodium γ-hydroxybutyrate, and thiopental sodium. When a combination of these anesthetics is used we refer to "combined intravenous anesthesia."

3.2.1 Lytic Cocktail

The lytic cocktail was first recommended by the French authors, Laborit and Huguenard, in 1950. They introduced a new concept based on selective blocking, not only of the cerebral cortex but also of certain cellular, autonomic, and endocrine mechanisms which are normally activated as a response to stress. A lytic cocktail is a mixture of a variety of neuroleptic drugs which are capable of causing multifocal inhibition to produce a state of rest in such structures as the cerebral cortex, the diencephalon, certain hormonal relays, and various ganglionic and terminal synapses. Laborit and Huguenard believed that the use of a lytic cocktail combined with mild hypothermia by physical cooling can produce a state of "artificial hibernation." M_4 is one of the commonest mixtures used. It is composed of 100 mg meperidine, 50 mg promethazine, and 2 mg acepromazine, dissolved in 250 ml–500 ml of 5% glucose or physiologic saline solution. After intravenous infusion of one unit of M_4, the effects of analgesia, hypnosis, and reduction of metabolism are obtained. The dosage of M_4 may be adjusted according to the body weight, age, and physical condition of the patient. Tachycardia and hypotension are frequently encountered, especially in the presence of hypovolemia and rapid infusion. We often use an "ether test" to confirm that artificial hibernation is underway, A negative ether test means that the patient has no response to cold; it indicates that the dosage is sufficient. If it is not negative, an additional dose should be supplemented. Apparently, artificial hibernation drug alone is not strong enough to fulfil the demands of an operation.

3.2.2 Sodium γ-Hydroxybutyrate (γ-OH)

The chemical formula of γ-OH is $OH-(CH_2)_3-COONa$. This substance is the sodium salt of a saturated fatty acid and is a natural product of lipid metabolism. γ-OH can easily penetrate the blood-brain barrier into brain tissues and induces sleep, as revealed by EEG. γ-OH is a white crystal and is easily dissolved in water. Its pH is approximately 7.4. The dosage ranges from 60 mg to 80 mg/kg body weight. The preparation used for intravenous injection is an aqueous solution of 20%. Its toxicity is low. Sleep lasts for approximately 1 h and can be prolonged by supplementary doses of 2 g each hour. The maximum total dosage is difficult to determine. In our cases, the largest total dosage was as high as 25 g. After intravenous injection of γ-OH, eyelid reflex is lost within 10 min–15 min, but corneal reflex and pharyngeal reflex are still present. The amplitude of respiration is shown to be increased. Relaxation of the jaw is moderate and permits intubation while the patient retains his spontaneous breathing. Sometimes it may induce bradycardia resulting from a transient parasympathomimetic effect. Its cardiotonic action may increase the cardiac output, thus resulting in a normal or even raised blood pressure. By potentiating narcotic and hypnotic durg, γ-OH can be considered to have a "sparing effect" as it reduces the amount of other agents required. When the drug is administered too rapidly, extrapyramidal gross muscular movements may occur, which can usually be prevented by the use of sodium pentothal prior to γ-OH.

3.2.3 Thiopental Sodium

Thiopental sodium is a short-acting barbiturate which was introduced into clinical practice by LUNDY and TOVELL in 1933. The pharmacologic properties of thiopental sodium are well known. The agent is directly administered into the bloodstream and consequently reaches the central nervous system quite rapidly. The solution currently in use is 2.5% for adults and 1%–1.5% for infants and children. We use thiopental sodium only as a supplement when anesthesia is insufficient. A small dose of 50 mg–100 mg is added in case surgical stimulus is intense. Total dosage is seldom higher than 1 g in adults and 0.5 g in children. Depression of respiration and hemodynamics will not take place if the drug is administered with strict caution.

3.3 Neuroleptanalgesia

A mixture, so-called Innovar or Thalamonal, is made by means of droperidol and fentanyl (50:1). The dosage of the fixed mixture is set at 0.1 mg/kg body weight, each milliliter containing 2.5 mg droperidol and 0.05 mg fentanyl. In high-risk or elderly patients the dose should be reduced by between one-third and one-half. With onset of sleep, N_2O-O_2 (1:1) mixture may be administered in a semiclosed system by mask or via an endotracheal tube, but we prefer γ-OH by the intravenous route in fractional amounts instead. When signs of lightening of the anesthesia are noted in response to surgical stress, additional doses of fentanyl (0.025–0.05 mg) are given intravenously to maintain the analgesic state. Prolonged surgical procedures can be carried out with a minimum of toxicity exerted by the neuroleptanalgesics. Also, analgesia is produced without serious cardiovascular impairment. The patient can be quickly awakened at the end of the operation. Nausea and vomiting in the postanesthetic recovery period are rarely seen. Although it is a relatively safe drug, fentanyl-induced respiratory depression may occur. In high-risk patients, hypotension may still take place during induction. Reducing the dosage of fentanyl may lead to incomplete analgesia. Extrapyramidal muscular movement may develop, which readily responds to atropine or other antiparkinsonian agents. As a rule, we use Innovar instead of lytic cocktail in debilitated patients, for hypotension and tachycardia may be prevented or ameliorated to some extent, but the analgesic effect of Innovar is less than that of lytic cocktail.

3.4 Ketamine

Ketamine is of value in the anesthetic management of a patient undergoing any of a variety of surgical procedures which evoke superficial somatosensory responses; it is particularly suitable for infants and children. A peculiar state of unconsciousness is produced in which the patient appears to be neither asleep nor anesthetized, but rather "disconnected" from his surroundings. The drug affects the neocortical–thalamic system intensely, followed by obtundation of the reticular activating and limbic system. Ketamine produces dissociation anesthesia, in which some areas of the brain are stimulated, while others are depressed simultaneously. Increases in arterial blood pressure and heart rate occur. However, in high-risk patients, myocardial depression may be predominant and hypotension develops. Respiratory depression should be anticipated when using ordinary doses in infants. Rapid bolus-type administration may cause apnea. Intravenous dosage is 2 mg/kg body weight of 1% solution for adults and 0.5 mg–1 mg/kg body weight for infants and children. The effect lasts 10 min. Intramuscular dosage is 4 mg–8 mg/kg body weight of 5% solution. The effect lasts 20 min or longer. Supplementary doses (one-half of the original dose) are given as needed for longer duration of anesthesia. Psychic effects do occur; they are infrequent in infants and children, but adults with emotion problems are prone to psychomotor activity and to unpleasant dreams.

4 Anesthetic Management

4.1 Measurement of Blood Pressure

In extensively burned patients it is difficult to measure blood pressure by the commonly used means. Noninvasive Doppler sphygmomanometry may sometimes be useful. Hemodynamics can only be monitored by EKG, hourly urinary output, CVP, etc., although these methods are not precise.

4.2 Clearance of Secretions from the Respiratory Tract

Tracheotomy is indicated prior to the administration of anesthesia when burns of the respiratory tract are suspected. It permits a much more thorough clearance of the tracheobronchial tree. Accumulation of secretions in the respiratory tract is harmful. It increases the chance of airway obstruction and may lead to interference with normal ventilation. If suction is used, it should never be prolonged for more than 15 s because it is dangerous for the very ill.

4.3 Maintenance of Ventilation

Hypoventilation can be corrected by assisted or controlled breathing either manually or mechanically. Administration of oxygen may help to offset the adverse effects of hypoxia and to increase arterial oxygen tension. However, respiratory acidosis cannot be corrected without hyperventilation. There is usually little doubt about the need for mechanical ventilation in patients with established respiratory failure. A pressure cycling ventilator is commonly used for such a case in which spontaneous respiration is still present, but the minute ventilatory volume is inadequate to meet the oxygen demands in the body. Positive end expiratory pressure of 5 cm–20 cm H_2O is an additional method to increase arterial oxygenation when the patient has been mechanically ventilated but severe hypoxemia continues to be present.

4.4 Restoration of Blood Volume Deficit

The amount of blood loss is always massive during excision of eschar. Active bleeding can often attract the surgeon's attention, who can then effectively control it, but oozing in the operative field may sometimes be overlooked. In these cases the concentration of hemoglobin and the red blood cell count are acutely lowered in the postoperative period, especially during the first 24 h. Transfusion is mandatory. Occasionally, two or three infusion sets are used simultaneously in order that sufficient amounts of blood can be infused into the body in a short period.

4.5 Changes in Body Temperature

Owing to extensive exposure of the body, administration of anesthesia, massive transfusion of cool bank blood, and air conditioning in the operating room, the body temperature of the patient is gradually lowered to below 35 °C. Temperature changes are particularly noticeable in infants and children. Such changes are often accompanied by bradycardia and sometimes induce hypotension and delayed return to consciousness.

4.6 Postural Hypotension

Changing the patient's position from supine to prone, or vice versa, is usually necessary during the operation for changing of dressings or for skin grafting. In spite of meticulous care, postural hypotension may still appear, partly owing to the action of neurolytic drugs. Ephedrine may be useful to combat hypotension induced by postural change. If the patient does not respond, strong vasoconstrictors should be administered without delay. It is likely that postural hypotension is more prone to occur in hypovolemia.

4.7 Use of Muscle Relaxants

As mentioned above, muscle relaxants are rarely used in surgery on burn patients. If intubation is indicated, muscle relaxants are helpful, but should be used with caution. Reports have demonstrated that succinylcholine may cause cardiac arrest in burned children, as hyperkalemia is present.

5 Anesthesia for Plastic and Reconstructive Surgery

Plastic and reconstructive surgery is usually undertaken in the late stage of burn injury. The patients are in convalescence; most of them are normal but still retain extensive scar formations. Unfortunately, some scar formations show contraction at sites such as face and neck. These patients are unable to open their mouths or extend their necks. Consequently intubation is difficult to carry out. Hence difficult intubation and prolonged anesthesia are two characteristics of plastic and reconstructive surgery in burned patients. Tracheal tubes may be introduced with the patient in the conscious state. Sometimes it is necessary to intubate by means of incising the contractured scar of both corners of the mouth and the anterior surface of the neck under local anesthesia, so that the mouth may open wider and extension of neck can be increased. "Combined intravenous anesthesia" is also employed for these patients with satisfactory effect. Light anesthesia may be maintained as there is no need for muscular relaxation. Surgery on the trunk and extremities may be undertaken under regional anesthesia such as nerve block and spinal or epidural analgesia.

Appendix I The Subeschar Bacterial Count

CHANG DE-ZHEN

Translated by YANG CHIH-CHUN

The following procedure must be carried out under sterile conditions:

1. Homogenization of the Specimen. a) A small block of eschar together with its subcutaneous fat is procured using a knife or a 0.3-cm trephine. A sharp knife is used to separate the eschar portion, which is then discarded. A piece of the subeschar portion weighing 0.1 g–0.2 g or 0.01 g–0.02 g (for microquantitation) is minced and put into a glass homogenizer.

b) Two milliliters of sterile physiologic saline is added, and the specimen is homogenized. This is called original homogenized specimen hereafter.

2. Gradient Dilution of the Homogenized Specimen. A series of tenfold dilution of the original homogenized specimen is made from 10^{-1} to 10^{-3} dilution. Before the diluted specimens are transferred, they must first be thoroughly homogenized. A fresh pipette should be used for each dilution.

In early cases, the expected subeschar bacterial count will be less than 1×10^{-6}/g if the wound infection is mild. The original specimen is used without dilution.

3. Inoculation and Incubation. Using a 0.001-ml calibrated loop, a separate loopful of inoculum is taken from the original homogenized specimen and from the 10^{-1} to 10^{-3} dilutions and is inoculated into the corresponding fan-shaped sectors of a blood agar plate (Fig. App. I.1). Sabouraud's agar is used for fungi.

Incubation at 37 °C is carried out for 18 h–24 h.

4. Calculation. Calculations are made according to the following equation:

$$B/g = N \times D \times L \times \frac{W+2}{W}$$

B/g: The bacterial count obtained from 1 g subeschar tissue by quantitation dilution
N: Number of colonies found
D: Fold of dilution of the homogenized specimen
L: Constant of calibrated loop = 0.001 or 10^{-3}
W: Weight of the specimen

Example: If eight colonies are found in the 10^{-2} sector, and the weight of the original specimen is 0.138 g, the subeschar bacterial count will be:

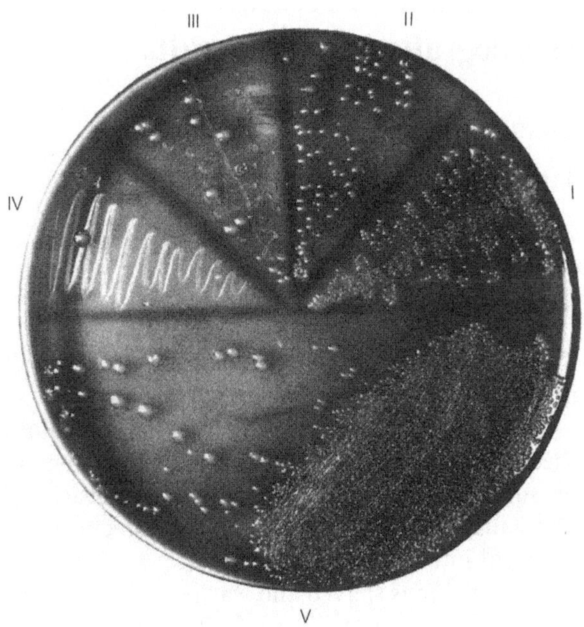

Fig. App. I.1. Quantitative determination plate. I, sector for original homogenized specimen; II, sector for 10^{-1} dilution; III, sector for 10^{-2} dilution; IV, sector for 10^{-3} dilution; V, sector for the identification of microorganisms. (Two colonies are found in the 10^{-3} sector of this agar plate; the weight of the specimen is 0.138 g, and the B/g will be 3.1×10^7)

$$B/g = 8 \times 10^2 \times 10^3 \times \frac{0.138+2}{0.138} = 1.2 \times 10^7$$

If no growth is revealed in the inoculum of a loopful of original homogenized specimen, the bacterial count should be less than 1×10^3/g. If a microspecimen of 0.01 g–0.02 g is used, a negative result implies that the bacterial count is less than 1×10^4. When using a microspecimen a quantitative pour plate of 1 ml original homogenized specimen should be made and incubated at 37 °C for 18 h–24 h. The quantitation of bacteria per gram of subeschar tissue is calculated according to:

$$B/g = N \times \frac{W+2}{W}$$

A negative report can only be made when no growth is revealed on the pour plate.

5. *Bacterial Swarming.* If there is swarming of *Proteus* on the blood agar plate, 10 ml of 10% chloral hydrate is added to each liter of media to inhibit the swarming.

Appendix II Preparation and Deep-freeze Storage of Allografts and Xenografts

YANG CHIH-CHUN and XIAO YU-RUI

Translated by YANG CHIH-CHUN

1. Preparation of Large Sheets of Allograft. The following method was introduced in 1960 and has been popularized since then.

a) Skin, together with part of the subcutaneous fat, is removed in large sheets from cadavers within 6 h postmortem (in winter the time limit may be suitably prolonged). The lines of incisions are shown in Fig. App. II.1. The cause of death should not be infectious disease, malignancies, jaundice, chemical intoxication, or cachexia.

b) The skin is shaved and washed with soap and tap water and then immersed into 1:1,000 chlorhexidine (Hibitane) for 20 min. After that, it is rinsed several times with sterile physiologic saline and stored at 4 °C (maximum time limit for preservation, 7 days).

c) On the day of operation, the stored skin is taken out and placed upside-down on a Padgett dermatome, with the epidermis facing the drum. The skin is cut to 0.2 mm–0.4 mm in thickness (0.2 mm for covering the granulation wound and 0.4 mm for a fresh wound after excision). A large sheet of partial-thickness graft is prepared by moving the whole skin all around (Fig. App. II.2).

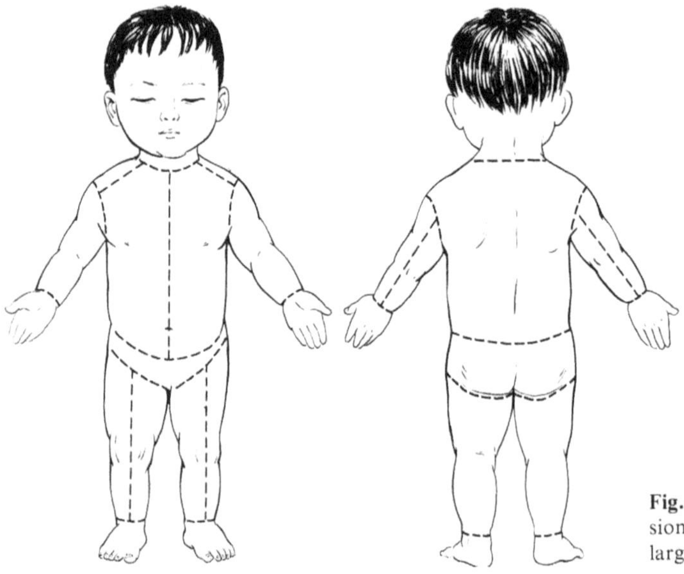

Fig. App. II.1. Lines of incision for the procurement of large sheets of allograft

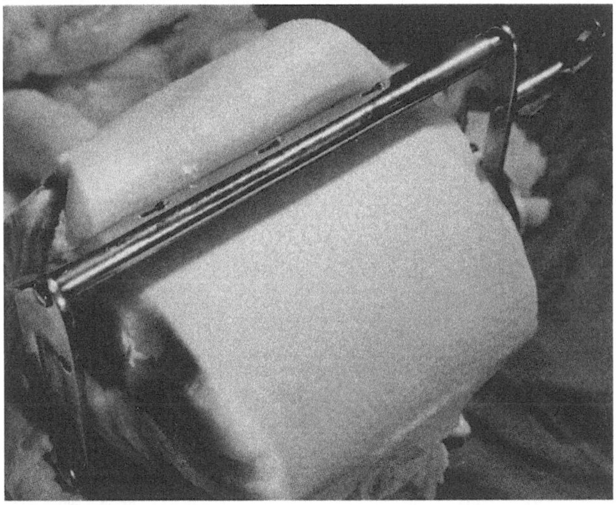

Fig. App. II.2. Method of preparing a large sheet of partial-thickness graft. For details, see text

The method of preparation of xenograft is the same as that of allograft.

2. Deep-freeze Storage. By the use of a slow-freezing and quick-thawing procedure, human skin stored in liquid nitrogen will give very satisfactory results provided that the skin is thin (0.2 mm thick) and is in small sheets (ca. 200 cm^2). If large sheets of thick partial-thickness skin (0.4 mm) are used, the result will be poor. Most of the epidermal cells of a thick, large preserved skin are dead, but after transplantation the dead epidermal layer will be "stuck" on the underlying dermis for some days.

After intermingled transplantation of the deep-freeze stored skin with autografts, the adjacent autoepidermis can creep on and "sandwich" the preserved allodermis as well. Therefore the preserved skin can also be used as a transplant after excision of the eschar. In order to achieve good results, the distance between the inserted autografts should be as small as possible (< 1 cm) and the size of the inlaid autografts should be as large as possible, ca. > 0.25 cm^2.

The procedure of deep-freeze storage is as follows:

a) Immerse prepared partial-thickness skin in 10%–15% DMSO–sodium bicarbonate–physiologic saline solution (v/v, e.g., 10 ml DMSO + 90 ml of sodium bicarbonate–physiologic saline solution). Balance at 4 °C for 10 min–15 min (if 10%–15% glycerine is employed as a cryoprotectant, 2 h is needed).

b) Seal the treated skin in a plastic bag. Before sealing, all the air should be driven out of the plastic bag.

c) Place the sealed plastic bags in metallic racks (Fig. App. II.3).

d) Place the racks in dry ice (−79 °C) or in a deep freezer (−60 °C–−80 °C); balance for 12 h.

e) Dip and preserve the plastic bags in a liquid nitrogen container (Fig. App. II.4).

f) For thawing, remove the plastic bag and immerse it in a 40 °C water bath. Immediately open the plastic bag and thaw the skin in a constant thermic

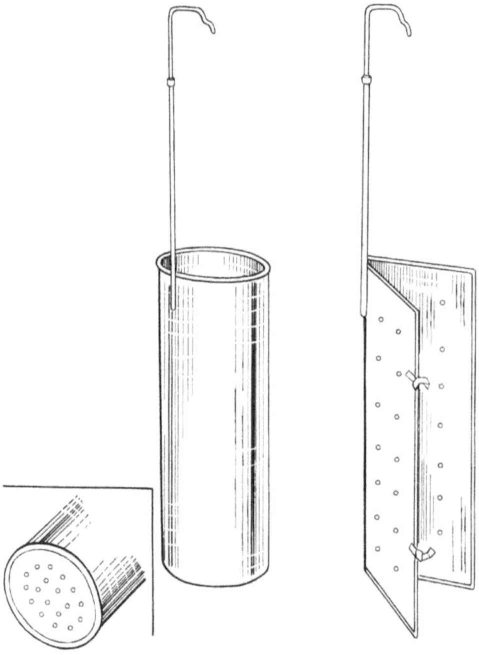

Fig. App. II.3. Metallic racks with insulated handles

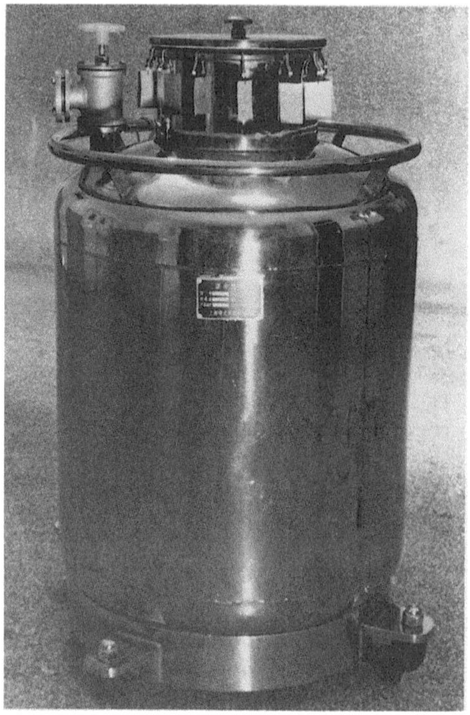

Fig. App. II.4. Liquid nitrogen container for the preservation of skin

water bath. Rinse repeatedly with physiologic saline. In the case of preserved thick split-thickness skin, in order to secure better "take" a thin layer of dermis is cut off before it is transplanted.

3. *Epidermal Cell Viability Test.* The percentage of living and dead epidermal cells is calculated before preservation and after thawing.

a) Triple wash 4 cm^2–8 cm^2 of partial-thickness skin with Hanks' solution, dry it with filter paper, and cut it into 0.25 cm^2 pieces.

b) Put the dermis side of the pieces of skin against a sterile Petri dish, and slowly pour a sufficient amount of 0.25% trypsin (pH 6.8–7) to float them. Incubate at 37 °C for 1 h–2 h.

c) Transfer the pieces of skin to another Petri dish containing a small amount of Hanks' solution.

d) Tear down the epidermal layer with pointed forceps and gently scrape down the remaining epidermal cells.

e) Add another few milliliters of Hanks' solution and stir by repeated pipetting for 10 min–15 min to disintegrate the epidermal layer. Filter with double layer gauze to remove the hornified debris.

f) Let the filtrates stand for 20 min.

g) Use the precipitate to make a smear; add 1 drop of trypan blue.

h) Observe under a light microscope; count 100 epidermal cells; find out how many cells are stained blue by the dye. (Dead cells are stained.)

Bibliography

Introductory Remarks

Barnes BA (1957) Mortality of burns at the Massachusetts General Hospital 1939–1954. Ann Surg 145:210–222

Baxter CR (1974) The current status of burn research. J Trauma 14:1–8

Bull JP, Fisher AJ (1954) A study of mortality in a burn unit: a revised estimate. Ann Surg 139:269–274

Bull JP, Squire JR (1949) A study of mortality in a burn unit: standards for the evaluation of alternative methods of treatment. Ann Surg 130:160–173

Pruitt BA Jr, Tumbusch WT, Mason AD Jr, Pearson E (1964) Mortality in 1,100 consecutive burns treated at a burn unit. Ann Surg 159:396–401

Chapter I. Early Management of Burn Patients

Artz CP, Reiss E (1957) General immediate care. In: Artz CP, Reiss E (eds) The treatment of burns. Saunders, Philadelphia London, pp 8–23

Berkow SG (1924) A method for estimating the extensiveness of lesions (burns and scalds), based on surface area proportions. Arch Surg 8:138–148

Burn Unit, Kwang-tze Hospital, Shanghai 2nd Medical College (1959) Treatment of severe burns. Shanghai Science and Technology Publisher, Shanghai, pp 24–36

Lund CC, Browder NC (1944) The estimation of areas of burns. Surg Gynecol Obstet 79:352–358

McManus WF (1979) Immediate emergency department care. In: Artz CP, Moncrief JA, Pruitt BA Jr (eds) Burns – a team approach. Saunders, Philadelphia London Toronto, pp 159–164

Moglan JA (1979) First aid and transportation of burned patients. In: Artz CP, Moncrief JA, Pruitt BA Jr (eds) Burns – a team approach. Saunders, Philadelphia London Toronto, pp 151–158

Chapter II. Burn Shock

Arturson G (1961) Capillary permeability in burned and nonburned areas in dogs. Acta Chir Scand [suppl] 274:55–103

Baxter CR (1974) Fluid volume and electrolyte changes of the early postburn period. Clin Plast Surg 1:693–703

Baxter CR (1978) Problems and complications of burn shock resuscitation. Surg Clin North Am 58:1313–1422

Burn Unit, Kwang-tze Hospital, Shanghai 2nd Medical College (1959) Management of severe burns. Chin Med J (Engl) 78:4–11, 134–143

Evans EI, Purnell OJ, Robinett PW, Batchelor A, Martin M (1952) Fluid and electrolyte requirements in severe burns. Ann Surg 135:804–815

Huang MK (1964) Early fluid replacement for extensive burns in adults (in Chinese). Chin J Surg 12:252

Li CL, Zhang XB, Wang L (1962) The preventive and therapeutic effect of dextran in burn shock (in Chinese). Chin J Surg 10:143–146

Li ZD (1964) Analysis of the blister contents of second degree burns (in Chinese). Chin J Surg 12:873

Monafo WW (1970) The treatment of burn shock by the intravenous and oral administration of hypertonic lactated saline solution. J Trauma 10:575–586

Moylan JA, Reckler JM, Mason AD (1973) Resuscitation with hypertonic lactate saline in thermal injury. Am J Surg 125:580–584

Moyer CA, Margraf HW, Monafo WW (1965) Burn shock and extravascular sodium deficiency – treatment with Ringer's solution with lactate. Arch Surg 90:799–811

National Burn Conference (1958) A Symposium (in Chinese). Chin J Surg 6:1314–1321

Pruitt BA Jr, Mason AD Jr, Moncrief JA (1971) Hemodynamic changes in the early postburn patient: the influence of fluid administration and of a vasodilator (hydralazine). J Trauma 11:36–46

Pruitt BA Jr (1978) Fluid and electrolyte replacement in the burn patient. Surg Clin North Am 58:1291–1312

Qu JH (1961) Experiences in fluid therapy in burns (in Chinese). Chin J Surg 9:766

Reiss E, Stirman JA, Artz CP, Davis JH, Amspacher WH (1953) Fluid and electrolyte balance in burns. JAMA 152:1309–1313

Shih TS (1960) Water and electrolyte balance in extensive burns under artificial hibernation. In: Collective papers (Medicine), vol VI (in Chinese). Shanghai Scientific and Technical Publisher, Shanghai, p 61

Chapter III. Management of Burn Wound

Artz CP, Reiss E, Davis JH, Amspacher WH (1953) The exposure treatment of burns. Ann Surg 137:456–464

Artz CP, Becker JM, Sako Y, Bronwell AW (1955) Postmortem skin homografts in the treatment of extensive burns. Arch Surg 71:682–687

Atulk K, Bhan AK, Reinisch CL, Devey RH, McCluskey RT, Schlossman SF (1975) T-cell migration into allografts. J Exp Med 141:1210–1215

Baker CF, Billingham RE (1973) Extension of skin homograft survival by prevention of graft-host skin contact. Transplant Proc 5:153–155

Bromberg BE, Song IC (1966) Homografts and heterografts as skin substitutes. Am J Surg 112:28–33

Bromberg BE, Song IC, Mohn MP (1965) The use of pig skin as a temporary biological dressing. Plast Reconstr Surg 36:80–90

Brown JB, Fryer MP, Landell P, Lu M (1963) Postmortem homografts as 'Biological dressings' for extensive burns and denuded areas – Immediate and preserved homografts as life-saving procedures. Ann Surg 138:618–630

Brown JB, McDowell F (1942) Massive repairs of burn with thick split-skin grafts: emergency "dressings" with homografts. Ann Surg 115:658–674

Burke JF, Bondoc CC, Quinby WC (1974) Primary burn excision and immediate grafting, a method shortening illness. J Trauma 14:389–395

Burke JF, Quinby WC, Bondoc CC, Cosimi AB, Russell PS, Szyfelbein SK (1975) Immunosuppression and temporary skin transplantation in the treatment of massive third degree burns. Ann Surg 182:183–197

Burn Unit, Rui Jin Hospital, Shanghai 2nd Medical College (1973) Treatment of extensive third degree burns (in Chinese). Chin Med J 4:195–199

Burn Unit, Rui Jin Hospital, Shanghai 2nd Medical College (1975) Burn treatment. Shanghai People's Publisher, Shanghai, pp 33–47

Burn Unit, Rui Jin Hospital, Shanghai 2nd Medical College (1978) Successful management of an extensive third degree burn patient (in Chinese). Shanghai Med J 3:3–6

Burn Unit, Rui Jin Hospital, Shanghai 2nd Medical College and Shanghai 3rd Traditional Chinese Pharmaceutical Factory (1973) Clinical observations on action of "wound healing ointment no 10" in separation of eschars (in Chinese). Chin Med J 4:226–228

Burn Unit, The Third Army Medical College (1977) Burns. People's Publisher, Beijing pp 137–138

Canizaro PC, Sawyer RB, Switzer WE (1964) Blood loss during excision of third degree burns. Arch Surg 88:800–802

Chambler K, Batchelor JR (1969) Influence of defined incompatibilities and area of burn on skin-homograft survival in burn-subjects. Lancet I:16–18

Colson P, Prunieras M, Leclercq P, Merigot P, Gangolphe M, Houot R (1960) Traitment de grand brûlés – comportement des greffes de peau (auto- et homogreffes) dans le procédé de Mowlem-Jackson. Lyon Chir 56:182–198

Colson P, Leclercq P, Gangolphe M, Houot R, Prunieras M (1962) Du rôle de l'homogreffe dans le procédé de Mowlem-Jackson. Acta Chir Belg 54:751–755
Davidson EC (1925) Tannic acid in treatment of burns. Surg Gynecol Obstet 41:202
DiVincenti FC, Curreri PW, Pruitt BA (1969) Use of mesh skin autografts in the burned patient. Plast Reconstr Surg 44:464–467
Fidler JP, Law E, MacMillan BG (1976) Comparison of carbon dioxide laser excision of burns with other thermal knives. Ann NY Acad Sci 267:254–262
Fidler JP, Law E, Rockwell RJ, MacMillan BG (1974) Carbon dioxide laser excision of acute burns with immediate autografting. J Surg Res 17:1–11
Girdner J (1958) Cited in Brown JB McDowell F Skin grafting. Pitman, London New York Toronto, p 262
Groves AR, Lawrence JC (1971) The tangential excision of burns: an experimental study using an animal model. Injury 3:30–39
Hagstrom WJ, Nassos TP, Boswick JA, Stuteville OH (1966) The importance of occlusive dressings in the treatment of mesh skin grafts. Plast Reconstr Surg 38:137–141
Hakim AA (1977) An immunosuppressive factor from serum of thermally traumatized patients. J Trauma 17:908–919
Hunt JL (1979) Early tangential excision and immediate mesh autografting of deep dermal hand burns. Ann Surg 189:147–151
Jackson D (1954) A clinical study of the use of skin homografts for burns. Br J Plast Surg 7:26–43
Jackson DM, Stone PA (1972) Tangential excision and grafting of burns – the method, and report of 50 consecutive cases. Br J Plast Surg 25:416–426
Janzekovic Z (1970) A new concept in the early excision and immediate skin grafting of burn. J Trauma 10:1103–1108
Janzekovic Z (1975) The burn wound from the surgical point of view. J Trauma 15:42–62
Levine N, Ger R, Stellar S, Levenson SM (1974) Use of a carbon dioxide laser for debridement of third degree burns. Ann Surg 179:246–252
Levine NS, Salisbury RE, Peterson HD, Pruitt BA (1975) Clinical evaluation of the carbon dioxide laser for burn wound excisions: a comparison of the laser, scalpel and electrocautery. J Trauma 15:800–807
Lawrence JC (1974) The healing of tangentially excised and grafted burns. Burns 1:75–81
Lawrence JC, Carney SA (1973) Tangential excision of burns: studies on the metabolic activity of the recipient areas for skin grafts. Br J Plast Surg 26:93–100
Lawrence JC, Stone PA (1973) The protection of damaged tissue by skin cover. Br J Plast Surg 26:101–105
MacMillan BG (1967) Early excision. J Trauma 7:75–79
MacMillan BG, Artz CP (1957) A planned evaluation of early excision of more than 25 per cent of the body surface in burn. Surg Forum 7:88
McClure RD, Lam CR, Romence H (1944) Tannic acid and the treatment of burns: an obsequy. Ann Surg 120:387–405
Monafo WW, Aulenbacher CE, Pappalardo C (1972) Early tangential excision of the eschars of major burns. Arch Surg 104:503–508
Moncrief JA, Switzer WE, Rose LR (1964) Primary excision and grafting in the treatment of third degree burns of the dorsum of the hand. Plast Reconstr Surg 33:305–316
Munster AW, Eurenius K, Katz RM, Canales L, Foley FD, Mortensen RF (1973) Cell-mediated immunity after thermal injury. Ann Surg 177:139–143
Neale HW (1974) Use of the nonexpanded mesh graft. J Trauma 14:247–251
Ninnemann JL, Fisher JC, Frank HA (1978) Prolonged survival of human skin allografts following thermal injury. Transplantation 25:69–72
Order SE, Moncrief JA (1965) The burn wound. Thomas, Springfield Illinois
Rapaport FT, Converse JM, Horn L, Ballantyne DL, Mulholland JH (1964) Altered reactivity of skin homografts in severe thermal injury. Ann Surg 159:390–395
Shuck JM (1979) Biologic dressing. In: Artz CP, Moncrief JA, Pruitt BA Jr (eds) Burns – a team approach. Saunders, Philadelphia, pp 211–223
Shuck JM, Pruitt BA Jr, Moncrief JA (1969) Homograft skin for wound coverage. A study in versatility. Arch Surg 98:472–479

Silvers WK (1974) The influence of removing lymphoid tissue in the persistence of tolerance of skin allograft in mice. J Immunol 113:804–809
Stellar S, Levine N, Ger R, Levenson SM (1973) Laser excision of acute third-degree burns followed by immediate autograft replacement: an experimental study in pig. J Trauma 13:45–53
Stone PA, Lawrence JC (1973) Healing of tangentially excised and grafted burns in man. Br J Plast Surg 26:20–31
Switzer WE, Moncrief JA, Mills W, Order SE, Lindbery RB (1966) The use of canine heterografts in the therapy of thermal injury. J Trauma 6:391–398
Taylor PH, Moncrief JA, Pugsley LQ, Rose LR, Switzer WE (1962) The management of extensively burned patients by staged excision. Surg Gynecol Obstet 115:347–352
Tanner JC, Vandeput J, Olley JF (1964) The mesh skin graft. Plast Reconstr Surg 34:287–292
Tavis MJ, Thornton J, Danet R, Bartlett RH (1978) Current status of skin substitutes. Surg Clin North Am 58:1233–1248
Wilmore DW, Mason AD Jr, Johnson DW, Pruitt BA Jr (1975) Effect of ambient temperature on heat production and heat loss in burn patients. Appl Physiol 38:593
Yang CC, Shih TS, Hsu WS, Kuo SY, Chao YF (1980) Emploi combiné d'hemogreffes et d'autogreffes cutanées dans le traitment des brulures étendues – Phénomène de Mowlem – Jackson. J Chir (Paris) 117:443–446
Yang CC, Shih TS, Hsu WS, Chu TA, Kao SY, Chao YF (1980) The intermingled transplantation of auto- and homografts in severe burns. Burns 6:141–145

Chapter IV. Infection in Burns

Abernathy RS (1973) Treatment of systemic mycoses. Medicine 52:385–394
Alexander JW, Fisher MW, MacMillan BG, Altemeier WA (1969) Prevention of invasive *Pseudomonas* infection in burns with a new vaccine. Arch Surg 99:249–256
Bjornson AB, Altemeier WA, Bjornson HS (1977) Changes in humoral components or host defense following burn trauma. Ann Surg 186:88–96
Bruck NM, Nash G, Foley FD, Pruitt BA Jr (1971) Opportunistic fungal infection of the burn wound with phycomycetes and aspergillus: a clinical-pathologic review. Arch Surg 102:476–482
Bruck HM, Nash G, Stein JM, Lindberg RB (1972) Studies on the occurrence and significance of yeast and fungi in burn wound. Ann Surg 176:108–110
Burn Unit and Burn Research Laboratory, Shanghai 2nd Medical College (1976) Pathological significance and treatment of postburn erythema gangrenosa (in Chinese). Med Exchange 3:26–27
Burn Unit, Rui Jin Hospital, Shanghai 2nd Medical College (1976) Treatment of infected wounds by "burn and scald ointment" in extensive burns – report of 39 cases (in Chinese). New Med Pharm J 8:25–27
Chu TA (1962) Postburn septicemia – report of 138 cases (Abstr) In: Symposium of the 8th national conference of surgery (in Chinese). Shanghai Science and Technology Publisher, Shanghai, p 103
Codish SD, Sheridan ID, Monaco AP (1979) Mycotic wound infections. Arch Surg 114:831–835
Codish SD, Tobias JS (1976) Managing systemic mycoses in the compromised host. JAMA 235:2132–2134
Codish SD, Tobias JS, Monaco AP (1979) Recent advances in the treatment of systemic mycotic infections. Surg Gynecol Obst 148:435–447
Feller I, Pierson C (1968) *Pseudomonas* vaccine and hyperimmune plasma for burned patients. Arch Surg 97:225–230
Fox CL Jr (1968) Silver sulfadiazine. A new topical therapy for *Pseudomonas* in burns. Arch Surg 96:184–188
Fox CL Jr, Rappole BW, Standford W (1969) Control of *Pseudomonas* infection in burns by silver sulfadiazine. Surg Gynecol Obstet 128:1021–1026
Foley FD, Shuck JM (1968) Burn-wound infection with phycomycetes requiring amputation of hand. JAMA 203:596
Law EJ, Kim OJ, Stricritz DD, MacMillan BG (1972) Experience with systemic candidiasis of the burned patient. J Trauma 12:543–552

Liu JX, Xu JY, Shu J (1964) Study on burn septicemia. II. Therapeutic results of anti-*Pseudomonas* sera in experimental *Pseudomonas* infection (in Chinese). Chin J Surg [Suppl] 12:178–180

Moncrief JA (1974) Topical antibacterial therapy of the burns wound. Clin Plast Surg 1:563–576

Moncrief JA, Lindberg RB, Switzer WE, Pruitt BA Jr (1966) The use of a topical sulfonamide in the control of burn wound sepsis. J Trauma 6:407–415

Moncrief JA, Teplitz C (1964) Changing concepts in burn sepsis. J Trauma 4:233–245

Majeski JA, MacMillan BG (1977) Fatal systemic mycotic infections in the burned child. J Trauma 17:320–322

Nash G, Foley D, Goodwin MN, Bruck HM, Greenwald KA, Pruitt BA Jr (1971) Fungal burn wound infection. JAMA 215:1664–1666

National Burn Conference (1958) A symposium (in Chinese). Chin J Surg 6:1314–1321

Neilan BA, Taddeini L, Strate RG (1977) T lymphocyte rosette formation after major burns. JAMA 238:493–496

Order SE, Mason AD, Walker HL, Lindberg RF, Switzer WE, Moncrief JA (1965) The pathogenesis of second and third degree burns and conversion to full-thickness injury. Surg Gynecol Obstet 120:983–991

Order SE, Mason AD, Walker HL, Lindberg RF, Switzer WE, Moncrief JA (1965) Vascular destructive effects of thermal injury and its relationship to burn wound sepsis. J Trauma 5:62–71

Order SE, Moncrief JA (1965) The burn wound. Thomas, Springfield, Illinois

Pruitt BA Jr, Foley FD (1973) The use of biopsies in burn patient care. Surgery 73:887–897

Rapaport FT, Milgrom F, Kano K, Gesner B, Solowey AC, Casson P, Silverman HI, Converse JM (1968) Immunologic sequelae of thermal injury. Ann NY Acad Sci 150:1004

Rose HD, Varkey B (1975) Deep mycotic infection in the hospitalized adult: a study of 123 patients. Medicine 54:499–507

Salisbury RE, Silverstein P, Goodwin MN (1974) Upper extremity fungal invasions secondary to large burns. Plast Reconstr Surg 54:654–659

Stone HH, Cuzzell JZ, Kolb LD, Moskowitz MS, McGowan JE (1979) *Aspergillus* infection of the burn wound. J Trauma 19:765–767

Stone HH, Kolb LD, Currie CA, Geheber CE, Cuzzell JZ (1974) *Candida* sepsis: pathogenesis and principles of treatment. Ann Surg 179:697–711

Stone HH, Martin JD, Huger WE, Kolb L (1965) Gentamicin sulfate in the treatment of *Pseudomonas* sepsis in burns. Surg Gynecol Obstet 120:351–352

Stone HH, Graber CD, Martin JD, Kolb L (1965) Evaluation of gamma globulin for prophylaxis against burn sepsis. Surgery 58:810–814

Shih TS (1961) Septicemia in severe burns. In: Symposium of annual meeting of Shanghai Medical Association, vol I (in Chinese). Shanghai Medical Association Publisher, Shanghai, p 248

Teplitz C (1965) Pathogenesis of *Pseudomonas* vasculitis and septic lesions. Arch Pathol 80:287–307

Teplitz C, Davis D, Mason AD (1964) *Pseudomonas* burn wound sepsis I. pathogenesis of experimental *Pseudomonas* burn wound sepsis. J Surg Res 4:200–216

Teplitz C, Davis D, Walker HL, Raulston GL, Mason AD, Moncrief JA (1964) *Pseudomonas* burn wound sepsis. II. Hematogenous infection at the junction of the burn wound and unburned hypodermis. J Surg Res 4:217–222

Volenec FJ (1977) Peripheral blood T and B lymphocytes in patients with burns. II. Sequential rosette analyses considering burn severity and *Pseudomonas* sepsis. Burns 4:7–13

Chapter V. The Traditional Chinese Medical Treatment of Burns

Burn Unit, Kwang-tze Hospital, Shanghai 2nd Medical College (1961) Treating extensive burns by discrimination of symptom and signs (in Chinese). Chin J Surg 9:126–129

Deng TT, Yang ZR, Cai R (1959) The theory and methods in treating scalds by Chinese traditional medicine (in Chinese). Chin Traditional Med J 11:39–42

Gu YS, Hsu WS (1959) Chinese traditional medicine in treatment of extensive burns. In: Burn Unit Kwan-tze Hospital, Shanghai 2nd Medical College (ed) Treatment of extensive burns (in Chinese). Shanghai Scientific Publisher, Shanghai, pp 10–14

Hsu WS (1965) Systemic treatment of burns and scalds by Chinese traditional medicine (in Chinese). Chin Traditional Med J Shanghai 4:37–40

Ren JH (1964) Discrimination of symptoms and signs in treatment of extensive burns by Chinese traditional medicine – analysis of 27 cases (in Chinese). Chin Traditional Med J Shanghai 7:15–20
Shanghai Traditional Medical College (1959) The theory and practice of Chinese traditional medicine in treatment of burns and scalds (in Chinese). Chin J Surg 7:7–10
Sun QY (1964) Experiences in burn treatment (in Chinese). Chin Traditional Med J Kiang-su 5:35–36

Chapter VI. Water-Electrolyte and Acid-Base Balance

Andersen OS, Engle K (1960) A new acid-base normogram. Scand J Clin Lab Invest 12:177–186
Andersen OS, Engel K, Jørgensen K, Astrup P (1960) A micro method for determination of pH, carbon dioxide tension, base excess and standard bicarbonate in capillary blood. Scand J Clin Lab Invest 12:172–176
Artz CP (1957) The treatment of burns. Saunders, Philadelphia, p 43
Baxter FC, Schwartz WB (1967) The syndrome of inappropriate secretion of antidiuretic hormone. Am J Med 42:790–806
Cope O, Moore FD (1947) The redistribution of body water and the fluid therapy of burned patient. Ann Surg 126:1010–1045
Curreri PW, Wilmore DW, Mason AD, Newsome TW, Asch MJ, Pruitt BA Jr (1971) Intracellular cation alterations following major trauma: effect of supranormal caloric intake. J Trauma 11:390–396
Hinton P, Allison SP, Littlejohn S. Lloyd J (1971) Insulin and glucose to reduce metabolic response to injury in burned patients. Lancet I:767
Hinton P, Allison SP, Littlejohn S, Lloyd J (1973) Electrolyte changes after burn injury and effect of treatment. Lancet II:218–221
Moore FD (1959) Metabolic care of the surgical patient. Saunders, Philadelphia, pp 868–920
Sevitt S (1957) Burn pathology and therapeutic application. Butterworth, London, p 237
Warden GD, Wilmore DW, Rogers PW, Mason AD, Pruitt BA Jr (1973) Hypernatremic state in hypermetabolic burn patients. Arch Surg 106:420–427
White MG, Asch MJ (1971) Acid-base effects of topical mafenide acetate in burned patient. N Engl J Med 284:1281–1286
Yang CC, Chu DA, Wang XY (1965) Acid and base disturbances in shock stage of extensively burned children (in Chinese). Chin J Surg 13:836–839

Chapter VII. Burns of Special Sites

Arch MJ, Moylan JM, Bruck HM, Pruitt BA Jr (1971) Ocular complications associated with burns: review of a 5 year experience including 104 patients. J Trauma 11:857–861
Arch MJ, Curreri PW, Pruitt BA Jr (1972) Thermal injury involving bone: report of 32 cases. J Trauma 12:135–139
Constable JD, Carroll JM (1970) The emergency treatment of the exposed cornea in thermal burns. Plast Reconstr Surg 46:309–312
DiVincenti FC, Pruitt BA Jr, Reckler JM (1971) Inhalation injuries. J Trauma 11:109–117
Dowling JA, Foley FD, Moncrief JA (1968) Chondritis in the burned ear. Plast Reconstr Surg 42:115–122
Gao XS, Chang TS, Fang ZY, Liu SK (1962) The early repairment of third degree burns of the hand (in Chinese). Chin J Surg 10:413–416
Harrison HN (1968) Respiratory tract injury, pathophysiology and response to therapy among burned patients. Ann NY Acad Sci 150:627–638
Hunt JL (1974) Early tangential excision and immediate mesh autografting of deep dermal hand burns. Ann Surg 189:147–151
Moncrief JA (1965) Burns of specific areas. J Trauma 5:278–291
Salisbury RE, Loveless S, Silverstein P, Wilmore DW, Moylan JA, Pruitt BA Jr (1973) Postburn edema of the upper extremity: evaluation of present treatment. J Trauma 13:857–862
Salisbury RE, Pruitt BA Jr (1975) Management of burns of the upper extremity. Saunders, Philadelphia
Silverstein P, Peterson HD (1973) Treatment of eyelid deformities due to burns. Plast Reconstr Surg 51:38–43

Wang SH, Chen XX, Yang KF (1963) Treatment of localized deep burns of the hand and forearm (in Chinese). Chin J Surg 12:564–567
Wexier MR, Yeshcua R, Neuman Z (1974) Early treatment of burn of the dorsum of the hand by tangential excision and skin grafting. Plast Reconstr Surg 54:268–273
Xu YH (1964) Respiratory burns (in Chinese). Chin J Surg 12:762–764

Chapter VIII. Electrical Injury

Artz CP (1967) Electrical injury simulates crush injury. Surg Gynecol Obstet 125:1316–1317
Baxter CR (1970) Present concepts in the management of major electrical injuries. Surg Clin North Am 50:1401–1418
Campbell JR, Campbell TS, Fletcher WS (1969) Severe electric burns. Am J Surg 35:780–788
DiVincenti GS, Moncrief JA, Pruitt BA Jr (1969) Electrical injuries: a review of 65 cases. J Trauma 9:497–507
Dossetor JB, Drummond JA, Allen AC, Celis TT, Baxter HA (1967) Prolonged oliguric renal failure after electric burns. Plast Reconstr Surg 40:67–71
Hartford CE, Ziffren SE (1971) Electrical injury. J Trauma 11:331–336
Hunt JL, Mason AD, Masterson TS, Pruitt BA Jr (1976) The pathophysiology of acute electrical injuries. J Trauma 16:335–340
Levine NS, Atkins A, McKeel DW Jr, Peck SD, Pruitt BA Jr (1975) Spinal cord injury following electrical accidents. J Trauma 15:459–463
Long JC (1963) Clinical and experimental study of electrical cataract. Am J Ophthalmol 56:108–131
Lynch JB, Wisner HK, Lewis SR (1971) Management of electrical injuries. South Med J 64:97–103
Peterson RA (1966) Electrical burns of the hand. J Bone Joint Surg 48 [Am]:407–423
Poate WJ, Macafee AL (1962) Gas gangrene following electrical burns: a report of two cases. Brit J Plast Surg 15:17–19
Robinson DW, Masters FW, Forrest WJ (1965) Electrical Burns: a review and analysis of 33 cases. Surgery 57:385–390
Rouse RG, Dimick AR (1978) The treatment of electrical injury compared to burn injury: a review of pathophysiology and comparison of patient management protocols. J Trauma 18:43–46
Skoog T (1970) Electrical injuries. J Trauma 10:816–830
Ugland OM (1966) Electrical injuries to peripheral nerves in animals: a preliminary report. Acta Chir Scand 131:432–437
Valdes RR, Torres VG, de Castro AB, Toribio JA (1974) Electric cataract. Burns 1:317

Chapter IX. Chemical Burns

Cason JS (1959) Report on three extensive industrial chemical burns. Br Med J 1:827–829
Dalderup LM (1973) Cyanide intoxication. Lancet II:625
Jelenko C (1974) Chemicals that "burn". J Trauma 14:65–72
Kwangtong Institute of Occupational Disease (1978) The prevention and treatment of industrial accidents. In: Industrial medicine and prevention of occupational diseases (in Chinese). People's Health Publisher, Beijing, pp 323–353
Lewis BK (1959) Chemical burns. Am J Surg 98:928–937
Naham BH (1972) Phosphorus burns. The antidote: a new approach. Br J Plast Surg 25:245–249
Naham BH, Applebaum J (1975) The phosphorus burns and its specific treatment. Burns 1:222–231
Zhou HD, Cheng CL, Gu JK, Ding XJ (1976) Intoxication by organic chemicals. In: Zhou HD (ed) Laboratory diagnosis of occupational diseases (in Chinese). People's Publisher, Beijing, pp 366–436

Chapter X. Burn Complicated with Trauma

Apley AG (1973) Principles of fracture. In: Apley AG (ed) A system of orthopaedics and fracture, 4th edn. Butterworths London Beccles Colchester, pp 350–386
Barr PO, Birke G, Liljedahl SO, Plantin LO (1967) Treatment of burn with warm dry air. Lancet I:1276
Barr PO, Birke G, Liljedahl SO, Plantin LO (1968) Oxygen consumption and water loss during treatment of burns with warm dry air. Lancet I:164–168

Barr PO, Birke G, Liljedahl SO, Plantin LO (1969) Studies on burns X changes in BMR and evaporative water loss in the treatment of severe burns with warm dry air. Scand J Plast Reconstr Surg 3:30

Birke G, Liljedhal SO (1971) Studies on burns XV treatment with warm dry air clinical results compared with those of earlier treatment series. Acta Chir Scand [Suppl] 422:5–16

Birke G, Garlson LA, Euler VS, Liljedhal SO, Plantin LO (1972) Studies on burns XII lipid metabolism catecholamine excretion basal metabolic rate and water loss during treatment of burn with warm dry air. Acta Chir Scand 138:321–333

Nealon TF (1969) Trauma to the chest. In: Gibbon JH, Sabiston DC, Spencer FC (eds) Surgery of the chest, 2nd edn. Saunders, Philadelphia London Toronto, pp 168–182

Zarem HA, Rattenborg CC, Harmel MH (1973) Carbon monoxide toxicity in human fire victims. Arch Surg 107:851–853

Chapter XI. Systemic Complications of Burns

Achauer BM, Allyn PA, Furnas DW, Bartlett RH (1973) Pulmonary complications of burns. Ann Surg 177:311–319

Artz CP (1969) Electrical injury simulates crush injury. Surg Gynecol Obstet 125:1316–1317

Back SM, Makabali GG, Bryan-Brown CW, Kusek J, Shoemaker WC (1975) The influence of parenteral nutrition on the course of acute renal failure. Surg Gynecol Obstet 141:405–408

Barry KG, Malloy JP (1962) Oliguric renal failure: evaluation and therapy by the intravenous infusion of mannitol. JAMA 179:510–513

Baskin TW, Rosenthal A, Pruitt BA Jr (1976) Acute bacterial endocarditis: a silent source of sepsis in the burn patient. Ann Surg 184:618–621

Biber TUL, Mylle M, Baines AD, Gottchalk CW (1968) A study by micropuncture and microdissection of acute renal damage in rats. Am J Med 44:664–705

Camerson JS, Miller-Jones CMH (1967) Renal function and renal failure in badly burned children. Br J Surg 54:132–141

Chernov M, Cook FB, Wool M, Hale HW (1972) Stress ulcer: a preventable disease. J Trauma 12:831–833

Chiu CJ, McArdle AH, Brown RA, Scott HJ, Gurd FN (1971) Gastric mucosal changes following burns in rats. Arch Surg 103:147–152

Choudhury M (1963) Two further cases of Curling's ulcer in major burns in children. Br Med J 5328:448–449

Coleman JB, Chang FC (1975) Pulmonary embolism: an unrecognized event in severely burned patients. Am J Surg 130:697–699

Conger JD (1975) A controlled evaluation of prophylactic dialysis in post-traumatic acute renal failure. J Trauma 15:1056–1063

Czaja AJ, McAlhany JC Jr, Pruitt BA Jr (1974) Acute gastroduodenal disease after thermal injury: an endoscopic evaluation of incidence and natural history. N Engl J Med 291:925–929

Czaja AJ, Rizzo TA, Smith WR, Pruitt BA Jr (1975) Acute liver disease after cutaneous thermal injury. J Trauma 15:887–894

Davies DM, Pusey CD, Rainford DJ, Brown JM, Bennett JP (1979) Acute renal failure in burns. Scand J Plast Reconstr Surg 13:189–192

Dossetor JB, Drummond JA, Allen AC, Celis TT, Baxter HA (1967) Prolonged oliguric renal failure after electric burns. Plast reconstr Surg 40:67–71

Drapanas T, Woolverton WC, Reeder JW, Read RL, Weichert R (1971) Experiences with surgical management of acute gastric mucosal hemorrhage: a unified concept in the pathophysiology. Ann Surg 173:628–639

Foley FD (1969) Fatal complication of burns. Am J Clin Pathol 52:1–13

He WS, Qian SC (1963) Postburn bone and joint changes. In: 8th national conference of surgery (symposium abstract) (in Chinese). Shanghai Science and Technology Publisher, Shanghai, p 103

Iaina A, Reisin E, Eliahou H (1975) Acute renal failure in combat injuries. J Trauma 15:281–284

Lordon RE, Burton JR (1972) Post-traumatic renal failure in military personnel in southeast Asia: experience at Clark USAF hospital, Republic of the Phillipines. Am J Med 53:137–147

Luo YG, Li L, Li CS (1964) Postburn complications of the circulatory system (in Chinese). Chin J Surg 12:870–872

McAlhany JC Jr, Czaja AJ, Pruitt BA Jr (1967) Antacid control of complications from acute gastroduodenal disease after burns. J Trauma 16:645–647
McElwee HP, Sirinek KR, Levine BA (1979) Cimetidine affords protection equal to antacids in prevention of stress ulceration following thermal injury. Surgery 86:620–624
McDowell RAW (1973) Pulmonary embolism and deep venous thrombosis in burned patients. Br J Plast Surg 26:176–177
Menguy R, Masters YF (1974) Mechanism of stress ulcer. III. Effects of hemorrhagic shock on energy metabolism in the mucosa of the antrum, corpus and fundus of the rabbit stomach. Gastroenterology 66:1168–1176
Muehrcke RC (1969) Management of the patients with acute oliguric renal failure. In: Muehrcke RC (ed) Acute renal failure: diagnosis and management. Mosby St Louis, pp 262–283
Mayers JK, Storrs D, Miller TB, Mueller CB (1966) The role of renal tubular flow in the pathogenesis of traumatic renal failure. Surg Gynecol Obstet 123:1241–1251
O'Neill JA, Pruitt BA Jr, Moncrief JA (1971) Studies of renal function during the early postburn period. In: Matter P, Barday TL, Konickova Z (eds): Research in burns. Huber, Bern Stuttgart Vienna, pp 95–99
Pruitt BA Jr, DiVincenti FC, Mason AD (1970) The occurrence and significance of pneumonia and other pulmonary complications in burned patients: comparisons of conventional and topical treatments. J Trauma 10:519–571
Pruitt BA Jr, Erickson DR, Morris A (1975) Progressive pulmonary insufficiency and other pulmonary complication of thermal injury. J Trauma 15:369–379
Pruitt BA Jr, Flemma RJ, DiVincenti FC, Foley FD, Mason AD (1970) Pulmonary complications of burn patients, a comparative study of 697 patients. J Thorac Cardiovasc Surg 59:7–20
Pruitt BA Jr, Foley FD, Moncrief JA (1970) Curling's ulcer. A clinical pathology study of 323 cases. Ann Surg 172:523–539
Rosenberg SA, Brief DK, Kinney JM, Herreca MG, Wilson RE, Moore FD (1965) Syndrome of dehydration, coma and severe hyperglycemia without ketosis in patients convalescing from burns. New Engl J Med 272:931–983
Sevitt S (1958) Hepatic jaundice after blood transfusion in injured and burned subjects. Br J Surg 46:68–74
Sevitt S (1965) Renal function after burning. J Clin Pathol 18:572–578
Sevitt S (1967) Duodenal and gastric ulceration after burning. Br J Surg 54:32–41
Skillman JJ, Gould SA, Chung RSK, Silen W (1970) The gastric mucosal barrier, clinical and experimental studies in critically ill and normal man and in the rabbit. Ann Surg 712:564–581
Vermillion SE, Gregg JA, Baggenstoss AH, Bartholomew LG (1969) Jaundice associated with bacteremia. Arch Intern Med 124:611–618
Wang QL (1959) Medical problems in burns (in Chinese). In: Burn Unit, Kwang-tze Hospital, Shanghai 2nd Medical College (ed) Treatment of extensive burns. Shanghai Science and Technology publisher, Shanghai, pp 74–85
Wilmore DW, Dudrick SJ (1969) Treatment of acute renal failure with intravenous essential L-amino acids. Arch Surg 99:669–673
Zimmerman LJE (1971) Respiratory failure complicating post-traumatic acute renal failure: etiology, clinical features and management. Ann Surg 174:12–18

Chapter XII. Nursing Care in Burns

Artz CP, Reiss E (1957) The treatment of burn. Saunders, Philadelphia London, pp 214–216
Burke JF, Quinby WC, Bondoc CC, Sheehy EM, Moreno HC (1977) The contribution of a bacterially isolated environment to the prevention of infection in seriously burned patients. Ann Surg 186:377–387
Curreri PW (1975) Metabolic nutritional aspects of thermal injury. Burns 2:16
Freeman JB, Egan MC, Millis BJ (1976) The elemental diet. Surg Gynecol Obst 142:925–932
Gump FE, Kinney JM (1971) Energy balance and weight loss in burned patients. Arch Surg 103:442–448
Hinton P, Littlejohn S (1971) Insulin and glucose to reduce catabolic response to injury in burned patients. Lancet I:767–769
Kinney JM (1975) Energy requirements of the surgical patient. In: Ballinger WF, Collins JA, Drucker WR, Dudrick SJ, Zeppa R (eds) Manual of surgical nutrition. Saunders, Philadelphia London Toronto, pp 236–266

Lennard ES, Alexander JW, Craycraft TK, MacMillan BG (1975) Association in burn patients of improved antibacterial defence with nutritional support by the oral route. Burns 1:98–107
Malcolm DE, Settle JAD (1978) Elemental feeding in severe burns: Monitoring a regime using vivonex. Burns 5:127–135
Newsome TW, Mason AD, Pruitt BA Jr (1973) Weight loss following thermal injury. Ann Surg 178:215–217
Pruitt BA Jr (1975) Postburn hypermetabolism and nutrition of the burn patient. In: Ballinger WF, Collins JA, Drucker WR, Dudrick SJ, Zeppa R (eds) Manual of surgical nutrition. Saunders, Philadelphia London Toronto, pp 396–412
Reckler JM, Bruck HM, Munster AM (1972) Superior mesenteric artery syndrome as a consequence of burn injury. J Trauma 12:979–985
Wretlind A (1978) Parenteral nutrition. Surg Clin North Am 58:1055–1070
Zaki MS, Burke JF, Trelstad RL (1978) Protective effects of adenosine triphosphate administration in burns. Arch Surg 113:605–610

Chapter XIII. Pathologic Anatomy of Burns

Boyd W (1970) Burns. In: Boyd Pathology, 8th edn. Kimpton, London, pp 73–75
Burn Unit, The Third Military Medical School (1977) Pathology of burns. In: Treatment of burns. People's Health Publisher, Beijing, pp 12–50
Cabanne F, Bonnefant BL (1980) Hyperthermie localisée brulure thermique. In: Anatomie pathologique. Maloine, Paris, pp 410–417
Cheng Z (1957) Pathology of burns – general considerations. Chin J Pathol 3:126–132
Foley FD (1970) Pathology of cutaneous burns. Surg Clin North Am 50:1201–1205

Chapter XIV. Plastic Surgery in Burns

Bakamjian VT (1965) A two-stage method for pharyngoesophageal reconstruction with a primary pectoral skin flap. Plast Reconstr Surg 36:173–184
Baudet J, Guemberteau JC, Nascimento E (1976) Successful clinical transfer of two free thoracodorsal axillary flaps. Plast Reconstr Surg 58:680–688
Baudet J, Lemaire JM (1978) Etude anatomique du lambeau axillaire et de son transfert par micro-chirurgie vascularie. Chirurgie 104:44–57
Carter PD (1962) Suture and non-suture methods of small vein anastomosis. Arch Surg 84:350–354
Daniel RK, Taylor I (1973) Distant transfer of an island flap by microvascular anastomoses. Plast Reconstr Surg 52:111–115
Daniel RK, Terzis J, Schwartz G (1975) Neurovascular free flap: preliminary report. Plast Reconstr Surg 56:13–20
Harii K, Ohmori K (1976) Free skin flap transfer. Clin Plast Surg 13:111–117
Harii K, Ohmori K, Ohmori S (1974) Successful clinical transfer of ten free flaps by microvascular anastomoses. Plast Reconstr Surg 53:259–270
Harii K, Ohmori K, Ohmori S (1974) Free deltopectoral skin flap. Br J Plast Surg 27:231–239
Ikuta Y, Watari S, Kawamura K, Shima R, Matsueshi Y, Miyoshi K, Tsuge K (1975) Free flaps transfer by end-to-side arterial anastomoses. Br J Plast Surg 28:1–3
McCraw JB, Furlow LT (1975) The dorsalis pedis arterialized flap. Plast Reconstr Surg 55:177–185
McGregor IA, Jackson IT (1972) The groin flap. Br J Plast Surg 25:1–3
Kernahan DA, Littlewood AHM (1961) Experience in the use of arterial flaps about the face. Plast Reconstr Surg 28:207–213
O'Brien BM, Macleod AM, HayHorst JW, Morrison WA (1973) Successful transfer of large island flaps from the groin to the foot by microvascular anastomoses. Plast Reconstr Surg 52:271–278
Taylor GI, Daniel RK (1975) Anatomy of several free donor sites. Plast Reconstr Surg 56:243–253

Chapter XV. Anesthesia for the Burn Patients

Belin RP, Karleen CI (1965) Cardiac arrest in the burned patients following succinylcholine administration. Anesthesiology 27:516–518
Blumenfeld M, Suntey RG, Harmel MH (1962) Sodium gamma-hydroxybutyric acid: a new anesthetic adjunct. Anesth Analg [Cleve] 41:721–726

Crossen G, Domino EF, Sweet RB (1964) Neuroleptanalgesia and Anesthesia. Anesth Analg [Cleve] 43:748–763
Finer BL, Nylen BO (1961) Cardiac arrest in the treatment of burns, and report on hypnosis as a substitute for anesthesia. Plast Reconstr Surg 27:49–55
Huang ZM (1978) Anesthesia for the burned patient. In: Wu C (ed) The practical anesthesiology (in Chinese). Shanghai Science and Technology Publisher, Shanghai, p 599
Kern ER (1965) Role of the anesthesiologist in the treatment of severe burns. Int Anesthesiol Clin 3:829–841
Knox JWD, Bovill JG, Clarke RSJ, Dundee JW (1970) Clinical studies of induction agents – ketamine. Br J Anaesth 42:875–885
Laborit H, Huguenard P (1951) Hibernation artificielle par moyens pharcodynamiques and physiques en chirugie. Presse Med 59:1329
Li XF, Wang ZZ, Shih TS (1960) Anesthetic management for severe burn – shock stage (in Chinese). Chin J Surg 8:331–333
Lowenstein E (1966) Succinylcholine administration in the burned patient. Anesthesiology 27:494–496
McCaughey TS (1962) Hazards of anaesthesia for the burned child. Can Anesth Soc J 9:220–233
Moncrief JA (1958) Complications of burns. Ann Surg 147:443–475
Wang ZZ (1959) Anesthetic management for severe burn. In: Burn Unit, Kwang-tze Hospital, Shangahi second Mediccal College (ed) Treatment of severe burn (in Chinese). Shanghai Science and Technology Publisher, Shanghai, p 101

Appendix I. The Subeschar Bacterial Count

Georgiade NG, Lucas MC, Osterhout S (1970) A comparison of methods for the quantitation of bacteria in burn wounds. Am J Clin Pathol 53:40–42
Moncrief JA, Teplitz C (1964) Changing concepts in burn sepsis. J Trauma 4:233–245
Robson MC, Heggers JP (1960) Bacterial quantification of open wounds. Milit Med 134:19–24
Teplitz C, Davis D, Mason AD, Moncrief JA (1964) *Pseudomonas* burn wound sepsis. I. Pathogenesis of experimental pseudomonas burn wound sepsis. J Surg Res 4:200–216

Appendix II. Preparation of Allo and Xenoskins and Their Deep-freezing Storage

Berggren RB, Lehr HB (1965) Clinical use of viable frozen human skin. JAMA 194:149–151
Billingham RE (1961) Free skin grafting in mammals. In: Billingham RE, Silver WK (eds) Transplantation of tissue and cells. Wistar Institute Press, Philadelphia, pp 1–24
Bondoc CC, Burke JF (1971) Clinical experience with viable frozen human skin and a frozen skin bank. Ann Surg 174:371–382
Lawrence JC (1972) Storage and skin metabolism. Br J Plast Surg 25:440–453
Lehr HB, Berggren RS, Letke PA, Coriell LL (1964) Permanent survival of preserved skin autografts. Surgery 56:742–746
Santoni-Rugiu P (1962) Compared studies on the viability of skin stored by different methods. Plast Reconstr Surg 30:586–594
Sherman JK (1965) Pretreatment with protective substances as a factor in freeze-thaw survival. Cryobiology 1:298

Subject Index

Figures are indicated by (f) and tables by (t).

Basic Problems in Burns

Proceedings of the Symposium for Treatment of Burns held in Prague, September 13–15, 1973
Editors: R. Vrabec, Z. Koníčková, J. Moserová
1975. 62 figures, 56 tables. XI, 224 pages
ISBN 3-540-07112-1

Contents: Surgery of the Burn Wound. – Anaesthesiology, Resuscitation and Intensive Care. – Septicaemia. – Complications of the Burn Illness.

D. L. Ballantyne, J. M. Converse

Experimental Skin Grafts and Transplantation Immunity

A Recapitulation
1979. 60 figures. XIX, 192 pages
ISBN 3-540-90425-5

Contents: Vacularization of Skin Grafts: Autografts and Allografts. – Acute Rejection of First-Set Allografts. – Chronic Reaction Patterns of First-Set Skin Allografts. – Reaction Patterns of Skin Xenografts. – Role of the Dosage Phenomenon in Allograft and Xenograft Reactions. – Behavior of Preserved Skin Grafts in Their Hosts. – Survival and Rejection of Second-Set Skin Allografts. – References. – Index.

E. Biemer, W. Duspiva

Reconstructive Microvascular Surgery

With Forewords by U. Schmidt-Tintemann, D. Buck-Gramcko
1982. 127 figures in 315 separate illustrations, some in color. Approx. 165 pages
ISBN 3-540-11320-7

Contents: Technicque of Microvascular Surgery and Preliminary Experimental Studies. – Clinical Microvascular Surgery: Replantation with Microvascular Anastomosis (Microreplantation). Tissue Transplantation with Microvascular Anastomosis. – Bibliography. – Index.

Springer-Verlag
Berlin
Heidelberg
New York

W.S. McDougal, C.L. Slade, B.A. Pruitt, Jr.

Manual of Burns

Medical Illustrators: M. Williams, C.H. Boyter, D.P. Russell

1978. 214 coloured figures, 4 tables. X, 165 pages
(Comprehensive Manuals of Surgical Specialties
ISBN 3-540-90319-4

Contents: Initial Treatment. - Wound Care. - Nutrition and Metabolism. - Special Types of Burn-Related Injury. - Systemic Complications of Burn Injury. - Complications Requiring Surgical Correction.

Microsurgery

By Chen Zhong-wei, Yang Dong-yue, Chang Di-sheng, Chao Yu-lin

1982. 366 figures. Approx. 500 pages
ISBN 3-540-11281-2

Contents: A General Review of Microsurgery. - The Operating Microscope and Magnifying Loupes. - The Instruments and Sutures of Microsurgery. - Basic Microsurgical Technique. - Microsurgical Suturing Technique. - Microsurgery and Pathology. - Replantation of Severed Limbs and Digits. - Free Toe Transfer. - Free Thumb Transfer. - Free Skin Flap Transfer. - Free Muscle Transfer. - Free Bone Grafting. - Transplantation of Intestinal Segment and Great Omentum. - Application of Microsurgical Technique in Tumor Surgery. - Microsurgical Techniques in Neurosurgery. - Application of Microsurgical Techniques in Otolaryngology. - Microsurgery in Ophthalmology. - Application of Microsurgical Techniques in Urological Surgery.

I. Pitanguy

Aesthetic Plastic Surgery of Head and Body

Water-colours: L.H. Schnellbächer

1981. 749 figures in 1494 separate illustrations, some in colour.
XVI, 412 pages
ISBN 3-540-08706-0

Contents: Body Contouring Surgery: Breast. Abdomen. Upper and Lower Extremities. - Aesthetic Plastic Surgery of the Head and Neck: General Introduction. Face. Rhinoplasty. Congenital and Acquired Deformities of the Ear. - Common Aesthetic Problems: Combined Aesthetic Procedures. Heamangioma. Giant Hairy Pigmented Naevi. Management of Soft Tissue Injuries and the Treatment of Scars. - List of Previously Published Illustrations. - Subject Index.

MIX
Papier aus verantwortungsvollen Quellen
Paper from responsible sources
FSC® C105338

If you have any concerns about our products,
you can contact us on
ProductSafety@springernature.com

In case Publisher is established outside the EU,
the EU authorized representative is:
Springer Nature Customer Service Center GmbH
Europaplatz 3, 69115 Heidelberg, Germany

Printed by Libri Plureos GmbH
in Hamburg, Germany